van g[o]
n[o]
In partnership with Audible Ed

DATE DUE

n the go
ngoNotes.

chapter reviews from
listen to them on any
ow wherever you are--
re doing--you can
ening to the following
ter of your textbook:

S: Your "need to
h chapter

Test: A gut
Big Ideas--
you need to keep

S: Audio "flashcards"
eview key concepts and

iew: A quick drill
e it right before your

VangoNotes.com

Pearson Nursing Reviews & Rationales

Mental Health Nursing

Third Edition

SERIES EDITOR

MaryAnn Hogan, MSN, RN

Clinical Assistant Professor
University of Massachusetts–Amherst
Amherst, Massachusetts

CONSULTING EDITORS

Theresa Przybylowicz, MS, RN, CNE

Professor
Springfield Technical Community College
Springfield, Massachusetts

Jenny Vacek, MSN, RN

Lecturer I, College of Nursing
The University of New Mexico
Albuquerque, New Mexico

PEARSON

Boston   Columbus   Indianapolis   New York   San Francisco   Upper Saddle River
Amsterdam   Cape Town   Dubai   London   Madrid   Milan   Munich   Paris   Montréal   Toronto
Delhi   Mexico City   São Paulo   Sydney   Hong Kong   Seoul   Singapore   Taipei   Tokyo

Cataloging-in-Publication Data on File with the Library of Congress

Director of Readypoint™: Maura Connor
Executive Editor: Jennifer Farthing
Developmental Editor: Elisa Rogers
Editorial Assistant: Deirdre MacKnight
Director, Digital Product Development: Alex Marciante
Media Product Manager: Travis Moses-Westphal
Vice President, Director Sales & Marketing: David Gesell
Senior Marketing Manager: Phoenix Harvey
Marketing Coordinator: Michael Sirinides

Director of Media Production: Allyson Graesser
Media Project Manager: Rachel Collett
Managing Editor, Production: Patrick Walsh
Production Editor: GEX Publishing Services
Manufacturing Manager: Ilene Sanford
Art Director/Cover Designer: Mary Siener
Composition: GEX Publishing Services
Printer/Binder: Edwards Brothers
Cover Printer: Lehigh/Phoenix Color Hagerstown

Notice: Care has been taken to confirm the accuracy of the information presented in this book. The authors, editors, and the publisher, however, cannot accept any responsibility for errors or omissions or for the consequences for application of the information in this book and make no warranty, express or implied, with respect to its contents.

The authors and the publisher have exerted every effort to ensure that drug selections and dosages set forth in this text are in accord with current recommendations and practice at time of publication. However, in view of ongoing research, changes in government regulations, and the constant flow of information relating to drug therapy and drug reactions, the reader is urged to check the package inserts of all drugs for any change in indications of dosage and for added warnings and precautions. This is particularly important when the recommended agent is a new and/or infrequently employed drug.

The authors and publisher disclaim all responsibility for any liability, loss, injury, or damage incurred as a consequence, directly or indirectly, of the use and application of any of the contents of this volume.

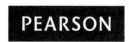

10 9 8 7 6 5 4 3 2 1

ISBN 13: 978-0-13-295687-1
ISBN 10: 0-13-295687-X

Contents

Welcome to the Pearson Nursing Reviews & Rationales Series!

This series has been specifically designed to provide a clear and concentrated review of important nursing knowledge in the following content areas:

- Anatomy & Physiology
- Fundamentals & Skills
- Nutrition & Diet Therapy
- Fluids, Electrolytes, & Acid–Base Balance
- Medical-Surgical Nursing
- Pathophysiology
- Pharmacology
- Maternal-Newborn Nursing
- Child Health Nursing
- Mental Health Nursing
- Health & Physical Assessment
- Community Health Nursing
- Leadership & Management

The books in this series are designed for use either by current nursing students as a study aid for nursing course work, for NCLEX-RN® exam preparation, or by practicing nurses seeking a comprehensive yet concise review of a nursing specialty or subject area.

This series is truly unique. One of its most special features is that it has been developed and reviewed by a large team of nurse educators from across the United States and Canada to ensure that each chapter is edited by a nurse expert in the content area under study. The series editor, MaryAnn Hogan, designed the overall series in collaboration with a core Pearson team to take full advantage of Pearson's cutting edge technology. The consulting editors for each book, also experts in that specialty area, then reviewed all chapters and test questions submitted for comprehensiveness and accuracy. Finally, MaryAnn Hogan reviewed the chapters in each book for consistency, accuracy, and applicability to the NCLEX-RN® Test Plan.

All books in the series are identical in their overall design for your convenience. As an added value, each book comes with a comprehensive support package, including access to additional questions online, complete eText, and a tear-out *NursingNotes* card for clinical reference and quick review.

Study Tips

Use of this book should help simplify your review. To make the most of your valuable study time, follow these simple but important suggestions:

1. Use a weekly calendar to schedule study sessions.
   - Outline the timeframes for all of your activities (home, school, appointments, etc.) on a weekly calendar.
   - Find the "holes" in your calendar, which are the times in which you can plan to study. Add study sessions to the calendar at times when you can expect to be mentally alert and follow your plan!
2. Create the optimal study environment.
   - Eliminate external sources of distraction, such as television, telephone, etc.
   - Eliminate internal sources of distraction, such as hunger, thirst, or dwelling on items or problems that cannot be worked on at the moment.
   - Take a break for 10 minutes or so after each hour of concentrated study both as a reward and an incentive to keep studying.
3. Use pre-reading strategies to increase comprehension of chapter material.
   - Skim read the headings in the chapter (because they identify chapter content).
   - Read the definitions of key terms, which will help you learn new words to comprehend chapter information.
   - Review all graphic aids (figures, tables, boxes) because they are often used to explain important points in the chapter.

4. Read the chapter thoroughly but at a reasonable speed.
   - Comprehension and retention are actually enhanced by not reading too slowly.
   - Do take the time to reread any section that is unclear to you.
5. Summarize what you have learned.
   - Use the accompanying online resource, NursingReviewsandRationales.com, to test yourself with hundreds of NCLEX-RN®-style practice questions.
   - Review again any sections that correspond to questions you answered incorrectly or incompletely.

Test-Taking Strategies

Test-taking strategies accompany the rationales for every question in the series. These strategies will assist you to select the correct answer by breaking down the question, even if you don't know the correct response. Use the following strategies to increase your success on nursing tests or examinations:

- Get sufficient sleep and have something to eat before taking a test. Avoid eating concentrated sweets, though, to prevent rapid upward and then downward surges in your blood glucose. Avoid also high-fat foods that will make you sleepy.
- Take deep breaths during the test as needed. Remember, the brain requires both oxygen and glucose as fuel.
- Read the question carefully, identifying the stem, the four options, and any key words or phrases in either the stem or options.
  - Key words in the stem such as "most important" indicate the need to set priorities, since more than one option is likely to contain a statement that is technically correct.
  - Remember that the presence of absolute words such as "never" or "only" in an answer option is more likely to make that option incorrect.
- Determine who is the client in the question; often this is the person with the health problem, but it may also be a significant other, relative, friend, or another nurse.
- Decide whether the stem is a true response stem or a false response stem. With a true response stem, the correct answer will be a true statement, and vice-versa.
- Determine what the question is really asking, sometimes referred to as the issue of the question. Evaluate all answer options in relation to this issue, and not strictly to the "correctness" of the statement in each individual option.
- Eliminate options that are obviously incorrect, then go back and reread the stem. Evaluate the remaining options against the stem once more to make a final selection.
- If two answers seem similar and correct, try to decide whether one of them is more global or comprehensive. If the global option includes the alternative option within it, it is likely that the more global response is the correct answer.

The NCLEX-RN® Licensing Examination

Upon graduation from a nursing program, successful completion of the NCLEX-RN® licensing examination is required to begin professional nursing practice. The NCLEX-RN® examination is a Computer Adaptive Test (CAT) that ranges in length from 75 to 265 individual (stand-alone) test items, depending on your performance during the examination. The blueprint for the exam is reviewed and revised every three years by the National Council of State Boards of Nursing using the results of a job analysis study of new graduate nurses practicing within the first six months after graduation. Each question on the exam is coded to a *Client Need Category* and an *Integrated Process*.

Client Need Categories   There are four categories of client needs, and each exam will contain a minimum and maximum percent of questions from each category. Each major category has subcategories within it. The *Client Needs* categories according to the NCLEX-RN® Test Plan effective April 2010 are as follows:

- Safe Effective Care Environment
  - Management of Care (16–22%)
  - Safety and Infection Control (8–14%)
- Health Promotion and Maintenance (6–12%)
- Psychosocial Integrity (6–12%)
- Physiological Integrity
  - Basic Care and Comfort (6–12%)
  - Pharmacological and Parenteral Therapies (13–19%)
  - Reduction of Risk Potential (10–16%)
  - Physiological Adaptation (11–17%)

Integrated Processes The integrated processes identified on the NCLEX-RN® Test Plan effective April 2010, with condensed definitions, are as follows:

- Nursing Process: a scientific problem-solving approach used in nursing practice; consisting of assessment, analysis, planning, implementation, and evaluation.
- Caring: client–nurse interaction(s) characterized by mutual respect and trust and that are directed toward achieving desired client outcomes.
- Communication and Documentation: verbal and/or nonverbal interactions between nurse and others (client, family, health care team); a written or electronic recording of activities or events that occur during client care.
- Teaching and Learning: facilitating client's acquisition of knowledge, skills, and attitudes that lead to behavior change.

More detailed information about this examination may be obtained by visiting the National Council of State Boards of Nursing website at http://www.ncsbn.org and viewing the *2010 NCLEX-RN® Detailed Test Plan.*[1]

[1]Reference: National Council of State Boards of Nursing, Inc. *2010 NCLEX Test Plan.* Effective April, 2010. Retrieved from http://www.ncsbn.org/2010_NCLEX_RN_TestPlan.pdf.

HOW TO GET THE MOST OUT OF THIS BOOK

Each chapter has the following elements to guide you during review and study:

- **Chapter Objectives** describe what you will be able to know or do after learning the material covered in the chapter.

Objectives

➤ Discuss at least three etiological theories of mood disorders.
➤ Differentiate between the primary behavioral characteristics of depressive disorders and manic disorders.
➤ Identify four specific treatment modalities used in the treatment of mood disorders.
➤ State examples of at least five nursing diagnoses frequently used in the management of clients experiencing mood disorders.

NCLEX-RN® Test Prep

Use the accompanying online resource, NursingReviewsandRationales, to test yourself with hundreds of NCLEX®-style practice questions.

Review at a Glance contains a glossary of key terms used in the chapter, with definitions provided up-front and available at your fingertips, to help you stay focused and make the best use of your study time.

Review at a Glance

anorexia nervosa an eating disorder in which a person attempts to lose weight by dramatically decreasing food intake and increasing physical exercise
autistic disorder a focus inward, excluding the external environment

binge eating episodes of continuous eating even when not hungry
bulimia nervosa an eating disorder in which a person attempts to manage weight through dieting, binge eating, and purging

encopresis fecal incontinence
enuresis incontinence of urine, especially nocturnal bedwetting
purging the act of self-induced vomiting to empty the stomach after eating
tic a sudden, repetitive movement, gesture, or utterance

Pretest provides a 10-question quiz as a sample overview of the material covered in the chapter and helps you decide in what areas you need the most—or the least—review.

PRETEST

1 The nurse is responsible for providing care to a group of clients with various personality disorders. The nurse should anticipate that a characteristic common to each client will be which of the following?

1. An ability to charm and manipulate people
2. A desire for interpersonal relationships
3. A diminished need for approval
4. A disruption in some aspect of his or her life

Practice to Pass questions are open-ended, stimulate critical thinking, and reinforce mastery of the chapter information.

Practice to Pass

How would knowledge about a genetic predisposition to schizophrenia be helpful?

NCLEX® Alert identifies concepts that are likely to be tested on the NCLEX-RN® examination. Be sure to learn the information highlighted wherever you see this icon.

Case Study, found at the end of the chapter, provides an opportunity for you to use your critical thinking and clinical reasoning skills to "put it all together." It describes a true-to-life client case situation and asks you open-ended questions about how you would provide care for that client and/or family.

Case Study

A seven-year-old male client is expected to die from leukemia. You are the nurse working in the home where the child has gone to prepare for death.

1. Based on the child's age, how would you expect him to view his impending death?

2. What assessment information would you expect to obtain from the child and family?

3. What would be the important nursing diagnoses for this child and family?

4. How would you determine the child and family have obtained goals?

5. Once the child has died, describe the bereavement, grief, and mourning by the family.

For suggested responses, see pages 301–302.

Posttest provides an additional 10-question quiz at the end of the chapter. It provides you with feedback about mastery of the chapter material following review and study. All pretest and posttest questions contain comprehensive rationales for the correct and incorrect answers, and are coded according to cognitive level of difficulty, NCLEX-RN® Test Plan category of client need, and integrated process.

POSTTEST

1 Which of the following is the most appropriate nursing diagnosis for a client with pain disorder who is homebound and unable to work in his previous profession for the past two years?

1. Impaired Role Performance
2. Anxiety
3. High Risk for Injury
4. Disturbed Sensory Perception

NCLEX-RN® Test Prep: NursingReviewsandRationales.com

For those who want to prepare for the NCLEX-RN®, practicing online will help you become more familiar with the computer-based testing experience, especially for the new alternate item formats such as audio, media-enhanced, hot spot, and exhibit questions. With this new edition, use the code printed inside the front cover of the book to access Nursing Reviews & Rationales, which offers 700 practice questions using all NCLEX®-style formats. This includes the practice questions found in all chapters of the book as well as 30 additional questions per chapter. Nursing Reviews & Rationales allows you to choose the two ways to prepare for the NCLEX-RN®. Both approaches personalize your practice experience according to what stage you are at in your NCLEX® preparation.

Nursing Reviews & Rationales includes the eText version of Pearson Nursing Mental Health Nursing, third edition. This eText is fully searchable and includes features like note-taking, highlighting, and more. The eText allows you to take your review with you anywhere you have an internet connection to NursingReviewsandRationales.com.

Pearson NursingNotes Card

This tear-out card provides a reference for frequently used facts and information related to the subject matter of the book. This is designed to be useful in the clinical setting, when quick and easy access to information is so important!

About the Mental Health Nursing Book

Chapters in this book cover "need-to-know" information about mental health nursing, including major diagnostic categories. Additional chapters focus on special topics such as crisis intervention and suicide, family violence and sexual assault, loss and grief, and the psychological adaptation to medical illness. Since mental health questions are unique and cause many students distress, Chapter 1 discusses effective test-taking techniques and strategies that will be specifically helpful when answering mental health questions. Mastery of the information in this book and effective use of the test-taking strategies described will help the student be confident and successful when answering psychosocial integrity questions on the NCLEX-RN®.

Acknowledgments

This book is a monumental effort of collaboration. Without the contributions of many individuals, this edition of *Mental Health Nursing: Reviews and Rationales* would not have been possible. Thank you to all the contributors and reviewers who devoted their time and talents to the third edition. The contributors for this edition are Theresa Przybylowicz, RN, MS, CNE, Springfield Technical Community College, Springfield, Massachusetts and Jenny Vacek, MSN, RN, University of New Mexico, Albuquerque, New Mexico. The reviewers for this edition are Ginette G. Ferszt, PhD, RN, PMHCNS BC, University of Rhode Island School of Nursing, Kingston, Rhode Island and Alexandra W. Winter, RN, MSN, Metropolitan Community College, Omaha, Nebraska.

Thanks also to the contributors and reviewers who assisted with the previous editions of this book: George Byron Smith, ARNP, MSN, PhD(c), Hillsborough Community College, Tampa, Florida; Susan Bobek, RN, PhD, University of North Alabama, Florence, Alabama; Jane E. Bostick, Doctoral Candidate, MSN, RN, University of Missouri–Columbia, Columbia, Missouri; Sara L. Campbell, DNS, RN, Illinois State

University, Normal, Illinois; Karma Castleberry, PhD, RN, APRN, BC, Radford University, Radford, Virginia; Pamela Gaurkee, RN, BSN, Alterra Wynwood, Bayside, Wisconsin; David S. Hodson, RN, MS, ARNP, St. Petersburg Junior College, St. Petersburg, Florida; Ann Koranda, RN, CNS, LADC, CGP, Mayo Foundation, Rochester, Minnesota; Linda Manfrin-Ledet, APRN, MN, CS, Nicholls State University, Thibodaux, Louisiana; Lee Murray, MSN, RN, CS, CADAC, Holyoke Community College, Holyoke, Massachusetts; Marybeth O'Neil, RN, MSN, CS, Mayo Foundation, Rochester, Minnesota; Mark D. Soucy, MS, RN, CS, The University of Texas, Health Science Center at San Antonio School of Nursing, San Antonio, Texas; Carol Stubblefield, RN, PhD, Jewish Hospital College of Nursing and Allied Health, St. Louis, Missouri; M. Crowell, PhD, RN, CS, CNAA, University of New Hampshire, Durham, New Hampshire; Susan B. Del Bene, Pace University, Pleasantville, New York; Marilyn S. Fetter, PhD, RN, CS, Villanova University, Villanova, Pennsylvania; Carol Holdcraft, DNS, RN, Wright State University–Miami Valley, Dayton, Ohio; Jaya Jambunathan, University of Wisconsin–Oshkosh, Oshkosh, Wisconsin; Michael Landry, RN, BS, BSN, MN, DNS, University of Louisiana–Lafayette, Lafayette, Louisiana; Melissa Lickteig, RN, MSN, Georgia Southern University, Statesboro, Georgia; Ruby J. Martinez, RN, PhD, CS, University of Colorado, Denver, Colorado; Jean Rubino, EdD, PN, APN, C, Seton Hall University, South Orange, New Jersey; Judi Sateren, RN, MSN, St. Olaf College, Northfield, Minnesota; Beatrice Crofts Yorker, JD, RN, MS, CS, FAAN, San Francisco State University, San Francisco, California. Their work will surely assist both students and practicing nurses alike to extend their knowledge in the area of mental health nursing.

I owe a special debt of gratitude to the wonderful team at Pearson Nursing for their enthusiasm for this project, as well as their good humor, expertise, and encouragement as the series developed. Maura Connor, Director of Readypoint™ was unending in her creativity, support, encouragement, and belief in the need for this series. Jennifer Farthing, Executive Editor, Readypoint™ coordinated this revision with insight, talent, and zeal, and fostered a culture of true collaboration and teamwork. Elisa Rogers, Developmental Editor, devoted many long hours to coordinating different facets of this project. Her high standards and attention to detail contributed greatly to the final "look" of the book. Editorial Assistant, Deirdre MacKnight, helped to keep the project moving forward on a day-to-day basis, and I am grateful for her efforts as well. A very special thank you goes to the designers of the book and the production team, led by Patrick Walsh, Managing Editor, who brought the ideas and manuscript into final form.

Thank you to the team at GEX Publishing Services, led by Michelle Durgerian, for the detail-oriented work of creating this book. I greatly appreciate their hard work, attention to detail, and spirit of collaboration.

Finally, I would like to acknowledge and gratefully thank my children, Michael Jr., Kathryn, Kristen, and William, who sacrificed precious hours of family time so this book could be revised. I would also like to thank my students, past and present, for continuing to inspire me with their quest for knowledge and passion for nursing. You are the future!

—*MaryAnn Hogan*

Overview of Psychiatric–Mental Health Nursing

1

Chapter Outline

Objectives

➤ Describe mental health and mental illness.
➤ Describe psychiatric–mental health nursing from a historical perspective.
➤ Identify basic theoretical assumptions of at least two theoretical approaches to mental illness.
➤ Explain the use of the nursing process as applied to psychiatric–mental health nursing.
➤ Identify the roles of neuroanatomy and neurophysiology in brain dysfunction.
➤ Describe effective communication techniques.
➤ Differentiate between normal age-related changes and mental health disorders in older populations.
➤ Explain the importance of understanding cultural diversity in mental illness.
➤ Describe key elements of legal/ethical issues in mental health nursing.

NCLEX-RN® Test Prep

Use the accompanying online resource, NursingReviewsandRationales, to test yourself with hundreds of NCLEX®-style practice questions.

Review at a Glance

aging the physiological changes occurring with age (diminished neurotransmitters, circulatory capacity, sensory acuity, and perception) that affect the brain

ageism a process of systematic stereotyping and discrimination against older people simply on the basis of their age

competency a legal determination that a client can make reasonable judgments and decisions about treatment and other significant areas of personal life

countertransference the emotional reaction by a member of the mental health team to clients based on feelings for significant people in the past

culture a pattern of learned behavior based on values, beliefs, and perceptions of the world taught and shared by members of a group or society

Diagnostic and Statistical Manual of Mental Disorders (DSM-IV-TR) a text that provides a classification of diagnoses of mental illness

discrimination prejudice that is expressed behaviorally

ethnicity ethnic affiliation and a sense of belonging to a particular cultural group

ethnocentrism the belief that one's own culture is more important than, and preferable to, any other

mental health an ability to see oneself as others do and to fit into the culture and society where one lives

mental illness an inability to see oneself as others do and not having the ability to conform to the norms of the culture and society

negative bias a refusal to recognize that there are other points of view

neurotransmitters chemical messengers of the nervous system; manufactured in one neuron, released from the axon into the synapse, and received by the dendrite of the next neuron

prejudice a negative feeling about people who are different from oneself

stereotypes a way of organizing information; arising out of negative biases, they are images frozen in time that cause us to see what we expect to see, even when the facts differ from our expectations

subculture a smaller group within a large cultural group that shares values, beliefs, behaviors, and language

therapeutic communication a process of influencing the behavior of others by sending, receiving, and interpreting messages

therapeutic relationship a nurse–client interaction that focuses on client needs and is goal specific, theory based, and open to supervision

transference an unconscious process of displaying feelings for significant people in the past onto the mental health team member in the present relationship

values a set of personal beliefs about what is meaningful and significant in life

PRETEST

1 The client states, "Who is confused? He said I should go, but I didn't. Is that weird?" Which response by the nurse would be best to clarify the client's statement?

1. "How did you feel before you talked with him?"
2. "When did you first notice yourself feeling confused?"
3. "Did he indicate to you exactly what he meant?"
4. "I don't understand. Can you explain in another way?"

2 During the initial interview with a client, the nurse begins to feel uncomfortable and realizes the client's behaviors and mannerisms remind the nurse of the nurse's abusive parent. The nurse concludes that the current situation represents which phenomenon?

1. Transference
2. Countertransference
3. Denial
4. Reaction formation

3 A client asks the nurse what to do about leaving the spouse. The nurse replies, "Why are you having trouble making a decision? It's easy to see that you should file for a divorce." The nurse manager overhearing the conversation would counsel this nurse because of which inappropriate element of the nurse's response? Select all that apply.

1. It restricts the client's opportunity for self-exploration and problem solving.
2. It belittles the client and the client's indecisiveness.
3. It challenges the client's belief system.
4. It assumes that the client is incapable of reaching an independent decision.
5. It positively reinforces the client's indecision.

4 While communicating with a client, the nurse decides to provide the client with feedback. What is the primary reason for the nurse to give appropriate feedback?

1. Present advice.
2. Explore feelings.
3. Provide information.
4. Explain behavior.

5 The nurse assesses a client as being on the mental health end of the mental health/mental illness continuum. Which statement by the client best supports this assessment? Select all that apply.

1. "I am satisfied with my life and life choices."
2. "My family thinks that I am a good person."
3. "Perhaps I would have been better off if I had remained single."
4. "I'm an average person leading a normal average life."
5. "I've always thought I should have been more successful."

6 A newly admitted adult client says, "No, I don't want that medicine. I won't take it." The nurse says, "Take it. It's good medicine." The nurse then places the cup in front of the client's mouth and forcefully presses it against the client's lips. In counseling this nurse, what important legal principle(s) can be applied to the nurse's action? Select all that apply.

1. If a client does not object a second time, a nurse can administer the medication.
2. If treatment is given without consent, legal charges of battery can be filed.
3. Clients have the right to be treated in the least restrictive manner possible.
4. Clients, unless declared legally incompetent, have the right to refuse medication.
5. Clients who wish to do so may establish psychiatric advance directives.

7 A client presents at a crisis clinic with reports of having crying spells and overwhelming feelings of loss. The client further relates that this extreme distress began one week ago when the client's parent developed an acute physical illness and died. The client speaks clearly and descriptively about the illness and death and verbalizes feelings readily. The nurse interprets that the client's behaviors suggest which of the following about the client?

1. Has suffered irreversible psychological damage
2. Is a candidate for long-term psychotherapy
3. Is highly anxious and depressed
4. Is a good candidate for short-term, focused psychotherapy

8 A client has purposefully attempted to embarrass a nurse by making a sexually explicit comment. What is the best response by the nurse?

1. Clarify the intention of the client.
2. Leave the situation altogether.
3. Refuse to talk with the client any further.
4. Continue to interact as if the comments did not cause embarrassment.

9 An emergency psychiatric client presents with amnesia, hyperthermia, and unexplained loss of appetite. Accompanying family members state that the client suffered a head injury while falling from a ladder several days ago. The nurse concludes that the client's symptoms are consistent with trauma to which area of the brain?

1. Thalamus
2. Hypothalamus
3. Cerebrum
4. Cerebellum

10 The nurse has explained to a client the biologic theories of depression. The nurse concludes that the teaching has been effective if the client says that depression may be caused from which of the following? Select all that apply.

1. Excessive serotonin activity in the central nervous system (CNS)
2. Insufficient serotonin activity in the CNS
3. Excessive acetylcholine in the CNS
4. Insufficient acetylcholine activity in the CNS
5. A genetic mutation on chromosome 6

➤ *See pages 23–25 for Answers and Rationales.*

I. OVERVIEW OF PSYCHIATRIC–MENTAL HEALTH NURSING

   A. *Mental health*: an ability to see oneself as others do and fit into the culture and society where one lives; indicators of mental health include positive attitudes toward self, growth, development, self-actualization, integration, autonomy, reality perception, and environmental mastery

   B. *Mental illness*: an inability to see oneself as others do and not having the ability to conform to the norms of the culture and society

   1. Medical diagnoses of mental illness are classified according to the ***Diagnostic and Statistical Manual of Mental Disorders***, 4th edition text revision (***DSM-IV-TR***), of the American Psychiatric Association

Box 1-1

DSM-IV Axes

Axis I: Adult and child clinical disorders; conditions not attributable to a mental disorder that are a focus of clinical attention
Axis II: Personality disorders; mental retardation
Axis III: General medical conditions
Axis IV: Psychosocial and environmental problems
Axis V: Global assessment of functioning (0–100)

2. The *DSM-IV-TR* uses a multiaxial system that addresses various mental disorders, general medical conditions, aspects of the environment, and areas of functioning that might be overlooked if the focus were exclusively on assessing a single mental illness problem (see Box 1-1)

C. **Mental health and mental illness** can be viewed as end points on a continuum, with movement back and forth throughout life

D. **The mental health–mental illness continuum** cuts across physical, personal, interpersonal, and societal levels
   1. Physical level: in the structure and function of the brain
   2. Personal level: in caring for and about the self
   3. Interpersonal level: in interactions with others
   4. Societal level: in social conditions and the cultural context

E. **On the mental health–mental illness continuum**, each level is so intertwined with the others that it is often difficult to pinpoint the original source of distress; review Figure 1–1 to see how personal, interpersonal, and cultural factors interact in ways that produce movement toward mental health or mental illness

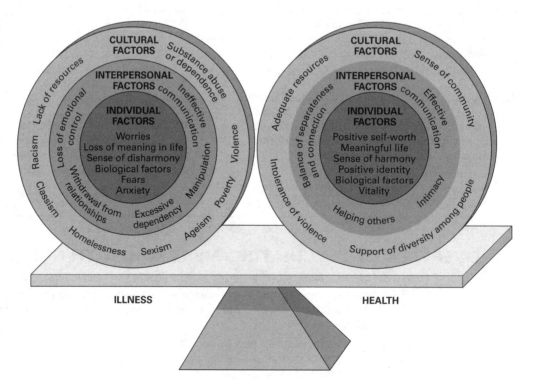

Figure 1-1

Factors contributing to the mental health–mental illness continuum

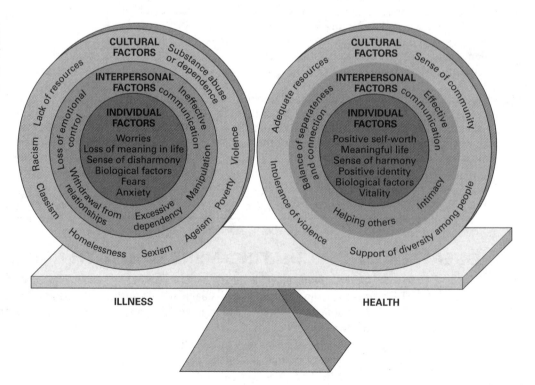

F. Mental health is not a concrete goal to be achieved; instead, it is a lifelong process and includes a sense of harmony and balance for the individual, family, friends, and community; it is more than the mere absence of a mental disorder; rather, it also entails a continuous process of growing toward one's potential

G. Mental health statistics

1. In the United States, approximately one in four Americans will suffer a serious mental disorder during his or her lifetime (25% lifetime chance)
2. Approximately one in five adults 18 years and older have a diagnosable mental disorder in a given year
3. Nearly one-third of the homeless population has a psychiatric disability
4. The majority of the 29,000 Americans who commit suicide each year have a mental disorder
5. Mental illness accounts for more than 15% of the burden of disease in established market economies, such as the United States

Practice to Pass

You are conducting a class on mental health and mental illness with a group of well adults in the community. How would you use the mental health–mental illness continuum?

II. HISTORICAL PERSPECTIVE

A. Mental illness

1. Historically the care of the mentally ill in Western society has been characterized by a lack of understanding of mental illness; this led to clients being treated in inhumane ways (see Table 1-1 for historical timeline)
2. Prior to enactment of the Community Mental Health Act (1963), mental health treatment was provided in state or private hospitals for the mentally ill that were usually isolated and located away from well-populated areas
3. The Community Mental Health Act (1963) shifted the focus of funding and treatment away from these large hospitals to newly established community mental health centers, which provided emergency services, inpatient hospitalization, outpatient services, community support, and education
4. Currently, treatment for mental illness is focused on managing care of clients with mental disorders across the continuum of care and services

   a. Managed behavioral health care utilizes case management, utilization management, and interdisciplinary treatment planning to ensure the coordination and resource management of services

   b. The least restrictive care setting is the goal for placement of clients; the aim of treatment is to manage the severity of mental illness and assist the client to live at the highest, most independent level of functioning within the community

   c. The Americans with Disabilities Act (ADA) of 1990 was enacted to ensure that people with disabilities, including mental illnesses, were able to fully participate in the economic and social mainstream of society; the ADA has been able to ensure these rights for the medical disabled but has had less success with ensuring the rights of the mentally ill

   d. Consumer organizations have worked to remove the stigma of mental illness in U.S. society and have promoted a legislative agenda to protect rights of the mentally ill and to ensure parity for mental illness coverage

   e. The decade of the 1990s was titled the "Decade of the Brain," and produced great promise in the treatment and recovery of mental disorders; more medications and treatments have been discovered, which have offered individuals with mental illness more options and opportunities for treatment and recovery

Table 1-1	Mental Health Illness and Psychiatric–Mental Health Nursing Historical Developments		
Time Period	**Significant Change in Thinking**	**Mental Health/Mental Illness**	**Psychiatric–Mental Health Nursing**
1800s	• The mentally ill were no longer treated as less than human. • Human dignity was upheld. • Scientific studies held promise for treating and curing mental health problems.	• Treatment of the mentally ill was provided in asylums. • The study of the mind and the effectiveness of treatment approaches to psychiatric conditions flourished.	• Linda Richards, the first psychiatric nurse, directed a school of psychiatric nursing at the McLean Psychiatric Asylum (1880).
1950–1960	• Least restrictive environment of care evolved. • Patient rights for the mentally ill began to be discussed and evolve.	• Significant psychotropic medications, including lithium, chlorpromazine, monoamine oxidase inhibitors (MAOIs), haloperidol, tricyclic antidepressants (TCAs), and benzodiazepines, were discovered.	• Hildegarde Peplau developed a framework for psychiatric nursing with an emphasis on the nurse–client relationship and theoretical constructs to explain client problems and provided the foundation for psychiatric nursing practice. • ANA established the Conference Group on Psychiatric Nursing, which defined the practice of psychiatric–mental health nursing.
1960–1980	• The Deinstitutionalization Movement began. • People with mental illness had a right to be treated in their own communities.	• Community Mental Health Centers Act was passed (1963). • Treatment shifted from long-term hospital care to shorter inpatient stays, followed by community-based treatment after discharge.	• The American Psychiatric Nurses Association was founded. • ANA first published standards of mental health and psychiatric nursing practice (1973).
1980–Present	• Significant changes in mental health treatment and delivery across the continuum occurred. • Population-based community care focused on mental illness prevention and mental health promotion.	• Behavioral managed health care evolved, leading to reduction in number of days of inpatient hospitalization. • Delivery of care focused on case management and critical pathways or interdisciplinary planning. • "Decade of the Brain" (1990) focused on mental illness as a brain disease.	• Coalition of Psychiatric Nursing Organizations and the ANA jointly published a description of two levels of practice, the generalist and the specialist (1994).

B. Psychiatric–mental health nursing (refer again to Table 1-1 for historical timeline)
   1. Psychiatric–mental health nursing can be traced as far back as the late seventeenth century
   2. Linda Richards (1880) was credited with being the first U.S. psychiatric nurse; she spent much of her professional career developing nursing care in psychiatric hospitals and directed one of the first schools of psychiatric nursing at the McLean Psychiatric Asylum in Massachusetts

3. Harriet Bailey (1920) wrote the first psychiatric nursing textbook, *Nursing Mental Diseases*
4. Hildegarde Peplau (1952) wrote *Interpersonal Relations in Nursing*, the first nursing framework for psychiatric nursing practice, in which she defined nursing as "a significant, therapeutic, interpersonal process…an educative instrument, a maturing force, that aims to promote forward movement of personality in the direction of creative, constructive, productive, personal, and community living"

III. PSYCHIATRIC–MENTAL HEALTH NURSING PRACTICE

A. **Generalist**: requires a baccalaureate degree in nursing with validation of clinical competencies
   1. Works with individuals, families, groups, and the community to assess mental health needs; develop diagnoses; and plan, implement, and evaluate nursing care
   2. The psychiatric–mental health generalist uses interventions that include the following:
      a. Health promotion and maintenance
      b. Assessment and evaluation
      c. Case management
      d. Provision of a therapeutic milieu
      e. Education of clients about factors that influence mental health and mental illness
      f. Promotion of self-care and independence
      g. Administration and monitoring of psychobiological treatment regimens
      h. Crisis intervention and counseling
      i. Engaging in social and community mental health efforts
   3. Practice settings include the following:
      a. Psychiatric hospitals
      b. Community mental health centers
      c. General hospitals
      d. Community health agencies (i.e., home health, primary-care centers, homeless clinics, etc.)
      e. Outpatient services
      f. Senior centers and daycare centers
      g. Schools
      h. Prisons
      i. Health maintenance organizations (HMOs)
      j. Emergency and crisis centers
B. **Specialist**: requires a master's degree in psychiatric–mental health nursing with validation of clinical competencies
   1. Psychiatric nurse practitioners (APN or APRN) provide primary care including both medical and mental health services
   2. Clinical nurse specialists (CNS) provide direct care as therapists or indirect care as consultants, educators, or researchers
C. **Standards of care and practice**: ANA (2000) devised standards of clinical practice for psychiatric–mental health nursing
   1. Standards of care
      a. Identify the function of the psychiatric–mental health nurse
      b. Outline the activities and accountability for both the psychiatric–mental health generalist and specialist nurses

   2. Standards of professional performance
   a. Identify the role of the psychiatric–mental health nurse
   b. Include such things as quality of care, performance appraisals, education, collegiality, ethics, research, and resource utilization

IV. THEORETICAL CONTRIBUTIONS SIGNIFICANT TO PSYCHIATRIC–MENTAL HEALTH NURSING

A. Intrapersonal theory

Practice to Pass

A client who was hospitalized after a narcotic overdose states, "I really wasn't trying to kill myself, I had just had a very stressful day and drank a few too many beers." You suspect the client is using which defense mechanism?

   1. Intrapersonal theory focuses on the behaviors, feelings, thoughts, and experiences of each individual
   2. Sigmund Freud divided all aspects of consciousness into three categories: conscious, preconscious, and unconscious; he theorized that there were three components of the personality: the id, ego, and superego
   a. Freud defined anxiety as a feeling of tension, distress, and discomfort produced by a perceived or threatened loss of inner control
   b. He identified processes called defense mechanisms, which protect the ego from anxiety by denying, misinterpreting, or distorting reality; for the most part, defense mechanisms operate at an unconscious level
   c. See Table 1-2 for definitions and examples of defense mechanisms
   3. Erik Erikson saw personality as developing throughout the entire lifespan rather than stopping at adolescence; he felt personality was shaped by conflict between needs and culture; Erikson identified eight development stages: sensory, muscular, locomotor, latency, adolescence, young adult, adulthood, and maturity; see Table 1-3 for Erikson's stages of growth and development
   4. Intrapersonal models provide a way of looking at how individuals develop, how they are still trying to achieve developmental tasks, and how they have learned to cope with anxiety

B. Social-interpersonal theory

   1. The focus of social-interpersonal theory is on relationships and events in the social context
   2. Harry Stack Sullivan believed that personality could not be observed apart from interpersonal relationships; he identified three principal components of the interpersonal sphere: dynamisms, personifications, and cognitive processes
   3. Abraham Maslow identified basic physiological needs and growth-related meta-needs; his humanistic theory emphasized health rather than illness

Practice to Pass

A 72-year-old retired and recently widowed man is hospitalized on a geropsychiatric unit for major depression. He says, "My life is meaningless now that my wife is gone. What do I have to live for? There is no hope for the future now." Using Erikson's stages of growth and development, which stage is this client in and how would you assist him?

   a. Maslow conceptualized these needs on a hierarchy, often symbolized by a pyramid
   b. There are five levels of needs in the hierarchy; these are identified (from bottom to top of the pyramid) as physiological needs, safety needs, love and belonging needs, esteem and recognition needs, and self-actualization needs
   1. Physiological needs include the needs for oxygen, food, water, sleep, shelter, and sexual expression
   2. Safety needs include physical safety, avoiding harm, and attaining security and order
   3. Love and belonging needs include companionship, the giving and receiving of affection, and identification with a group
   4. Esteem and recognition needs include self-esteem, the respect of others, prestige, and success at work
   5. Self-actualization is the fulfillment of one's unique potential

4. Hildegarde Peplau saw nursing as an interpersonal process, with the therapeutic nurse–client relationship at its core; the major components of her theory are growth, development, communication, and roles

Table 1-2 **Defense Mechanisms**

Defense Mechanism	Example
Compensation. Covering up weaknesses by emphasizing a more desirable trait or by overachievement in a more comfortable area	A high school student who is too small to play football becomes the star long-distance runner for the track team.
Denial. An attempt to screen or ignore unacceptable realities by refusing to acknowledge them	A woman, though told her father has metastatic cancer, continues to plan a family reunion 18 months in advance.
Displacement. The transferring or discharging of emotional reactions from one object or person to another object or person	A husband and wife are fighting, and the husband becomes so angry he hits a wall instead of his wife.
Identification. An attempt to manage anxiety by imitating the behavior of someone feared or respected	A student nurse imitates the nurturing behavior she observes one of her instructors using with clients.
Intellectualization. A mechanism by which an emotional response that normally would accompany an uncomfortable or painful incident is evaded by the use of rational explanations that remove from the incident any personal significance and feelings	The pain over a parent's sudden death is reduced by saying, "He wouldn't have wanted to live disabled."
Introjection. A form of identification that allows for the acceptance of others' norms and values into oneself, even when contrary to one's previous assumptions	A seven-year-old boy tells his sister, "Don't talk to strangers." He has introjected this value from the instructions of parents and teachers.
Minimization. Not acknowledging the significance of one's behavior	A person says, "Don't believe everything my wife tells you. I wasn't so drunk I couldn't drive."
Projection. A process in which blame is attached to others or the environment for unacceptable desires, thoughts, shortcomings, and mistakes	A mother is told her child must repeat a grade in school, and she blames this on the teacher's poor instruction.
Rationalization. Justification of certain behaviors by faulty logic and ascription or motives that are socially acceptable but did not in fact inspire the behavior	A mother spanks her toddler too hard and says it was all right because he could not feel it through the diaper anyway.
Reaction Formation. A mechanism that causes people to act exactly opposite to the way they feel	An executive resents his bosses for calling in a consulting firm to make recommendations for change in his department but verbalizes complete support for the idea and is exceedingly polite and cooperative.
Regression. Resorting to an earlier, more comfortable level of functioning that is characteristically less demanding and responsible	An adult throws a temper tantrum when he does not get his own way.
Repression. An unconscious mechanism by which threatening thoughts, feelings, and desires are kept from becoming conscious; the repressed material is denied entry into consciousness	A teenager, seeing his best friend killed in a car accident, becomes amnesic about the circumstances surrounding the accident.
Sublimation. Displacement of energy associated with more primitive sexual or aggressive drives into socially acceptable activities	A person with excessive, primitive sexual drives invests psychic energy into a well-defined religious value system.
Substitution. The replacement of a highly valued, unacceptable, or unavailable object by a less valuable, acceptable, or available object	A woman wants to marry a man exactly like her dead father and settles for someone who looks a little bit like him.
Undoing. An action or words designed to cancel some disapproved thoughts, impulses, or acts in which the person relieves guilt by making reparation	A father spanks his child and the next evening brings home a present for the child.

Source: Adapted from Fontaine, K. L. (2009). *Mental health nursing* (6th ed.). Upper Saddle River, NJ: Pearson Education, Inc., pp. 12–13.

Table 1-3 **Erik Erikson's Stages of Social Growth and Development**

Stage of Development	Period	Developmental Task	Defining Characteristics
Sensory	Birth–1 year	Trust vs. mistrust	Child learns to develop trusting relationships
Muscular	1–2 years	Autonomy vs. shame and doubt	Child starts the process of separation; starts learning to live autonomously
Locomotor	3–5 years	Initiative vs. guilt	Child learns about environmental influences; becomes more aware of own identity
Latency	6–11 years	Industry vs. inferiority	Energy is directed at accomplishments, creative activities, and learning
Adolescent	12–19 years	Identity vs. role confusion	Transitional period; movement toward adulthood; adolescent starts incorporating beliefs and value systems that have been acquired previously
Young Adult	20s, 30s	Intimacy vs. isolation	Person learns the ability to have intimate relationships
Adulthood	40s, 50s	Generativity vs. stagnation	Emphasis on maintaining intimate relationships; movement toward developing a family
Maturity	60 years and older	Integrity vs. despair	Acceptance of life as it has been; acceptance of both good and bad aspects of past life; maintaining a positive self-concept

Source: Adapted from Fontaine, K. L. (2009). *Mental health nursing* (6th ed.). Upper Saddle River, NJ: Pearson Education, Inc., pp. 12–13.

5. Feminist theory is an androgynous model of mental health; theorists examine how gender roles limit the psychological development of all people and inhibit the development of mutually satisfying and noncoercive intimacy
6. Social-interpersonal models enable the nurse to assess the influences of culture, social interaction, gender stereotypes, and support systems on the behavior of clients

C. **Behavioral theory**
1. The focus of behavioral theory is on a person's actions, not on thoughts and feelings
2. The major emphasis of B. F. Skinner's theory is the functional analysis of behavior
   a. Positive reinforcements are stimuli that lead to an increase in a behavior; negative reinforcements are stimuli that lead to a decrease in the behavior
   b. The principle of reinforcement states that a response is strengthened when reinforcement is given
3. Behavioral models are helpful in planning client education and designing programs for a variety of mental health clients and families

D. **Cognitive theory**
1. Cognitive theory explains how we interpret our daily lives, adapt and make changes in our thinking, and develop the insights to make those changes
2. Jean Piaget thought that children learn by the changing stimuli that challenge their experiences and perceptions; he identified four major stages of cognitive development: sensorimotor, preoperational, concrete operational, and formal operational
3. Aaron Beck's cognitive theory focuses on how people view themselves and their world; he identified cognitive schemas as personal controlling beliefs that influence the way people process data about themselves and others; cognitive distortions result from the cognitive triad of an inadequate view of self, a negative misinterpretation of the present, and a negative view of the future

4. Albert Ellis's work with cognitive restructuring is often used as part of treatment today

5. Cognitive models help the nurse assess clients' learning capabilities; they also help the nurse analyze cognitive distortions that are symptoms of a number of mental disorders

E. Biogenic theory

1. In studying genetic factors in mental disorders, researchers must first establish that there is a higher-than-expected rate of incidence within the family and then must identify what parts are caused by genetic factors and what parts are caused by environmental factors

2. Biogenic theory looks at how genetic factors, neuroanatomy, neurophysiology, and biological rhythms relate to the cause, course, and prognosis of mental disorders

   a. The cerebrum compromises the majority (60%) of the brain and is composed of two cerebral hemispheres with each hemisphere being divided into four lobes

      1) Frontal lobe: primary functions—higher-order thinking, abstract reasoning, decision making, speech, and voluntary muscle movement

      2) Parietal lobe: primary functions—sensory function and proprioception (body position information)

      3) Occipital lobe: primary function—visual function

      4) Temporal lobe: primary functions—judgment, memory, smell, sensory interpretation, and understanding sound

   b. Diencephalon: extends from the cerebrum and sits above the brainstem; the diencephalon has three primary structures

      1) Thalamus: receives and relays sensory information and plays a role in memory and in regulating mood

      2) Hypothalamus: controls the body homeostasis; it regulates the autonomic nervous system, body temperature, appetite, water balance, biologic rhythms and drives, and hormonal output of the anterior pituitary gland

      3) Limbic system: comprised of the limbic lobe and the numerous structures functioning with it, including the frontal cortex, hypothalamus, amygdala, hippocampus, brainstem, and autonomic nervous system; the limbic system is primarily responsible for regulating emotional responses

3. Mental disorders are often related to dysfunctional neuronal receptors or a deficiency, excess, or imbalance of **neurotransmitters** (chemical messengers of the nervous system, manufactured in each neuron and released from the axon into the synapse and received by the dendrite of the next neuron); a synapse is the gap between one membrane of one neuron and the membrane of another and is the point at which nerve impulse transmission occurs

   a. Serotonin (5-HT) is involved primarily in depressive and anxiety disorders, and possibly eating disorders and psychotic disorders; many antidepressants target the synapses to increase serotonin levels; newer antipsychotic agents known as atypical antipsychotic agents block serotonin receptors

   b. Norepinephrine (NE) is a catecholamine neurotransmitter of the sympathetic nervous system, which mediates fight-or-flight response; depressive disorders, including bipolar disorder, are involved with changes in norepinephrine levels

   c. Dopamine (DA) is involved with schizophrenic disorders and attention-deficit hyperactivity disorder (ADHD); many antipsychotic medications block dopamine from binding to its receptors; stimulant medications enhance dopamine transmission

   d. Acetylcholine (ACH) is a major neurotransmitter of the parasympathetic nervous system, which controls muscles, memory, and coordination; changes in acetylcholine levels are involved with Alzheimer's disease

   e. Gamma-aminobutyric acid (GABA) is an inhibitory neurotransmitter; antianxiety medications increase the effects of GABA

Practice to Pass

You are conducting a medication education group for a group of clients who are experiencing major depression. How would you explain this disease as a chemical imbalance in the brain?

      f. Glutamate is an excitatory neurotransmitter; excessive glutamate leads to neuron toxicity

    4. Biological rhythms: circadian rhythms are regular fluctuations of a variety of physiological factors over a period of 24 hours

      a. Temperature, energy, sleep, arousal, motor activity, appetite, hormones, and mood all demonstrate circadian rhythms

      b. The "biological clock" is located in the hypothalamus and may be desynchronized by external or internal factors

      c. Some mental disorders demonstrate alterations in adrenal rhythm, temperature patterns, and sleep patterns

V. THE NURSING PROCESS

    A. Provides the boundaries for psychiatric–mental health nursing and a scientific method for the delivery of nursing care

    B. The steps of the nursing process

      1. Assessment: establishing a database about a client, family, or community

        a. Observation is extremely important in assessing clients with mental illness; clients are observed in terms of their behavior, affect, cognition, interpersonal relationships, and physiology

        b. The psychosocial assessment includes the client's and family's definition of the problem(s), history of the present problem(s), family and social history, spiritual considerations, cultural assessment, physical assessment, and strengths and competencies

        c. The mental status assessment provides more specific information about the client's appearance, activity, speech, emotional state, cognitive functioning, and perception

      2. Diagnosis: identifying the client's health care needs and selecting goals of care; psychiatric–mental health nursing diagnoses are applicable to individuals, families, groups, and communities; they include the etiologies and standard nursing interventions

      3. Outcome identification: establishing criteria for measuring achievement of desired outcomes; client outcomes are specific behavioral measures by which the nurse, clients, and significant others determine progress toward a goal

      4. Planning: designing a strategy to achieve the goals established for client care

        a. In psychiatric–mental health nursing, safety needs often are more of a priority than physiological needs; clients must be assessed for exhaustion, poor judgment, self-mutilation, and violence and suicide potential

        b. Goals are planned with client input, although some clients may be too ill to participate in this process; they must be included as soon as they are physically and mentally able to participate

      5. Implementation: initiating and completing actions necessary to accomplish the defined goals; nurses assume several roles in assisting clients to grow and adapt, such as socializing agent, teacher, role model, advocate, counselor, role player, and milieu manager

      6. Evaluation: determining the extent to which the goals of care have been achieved

        a. Formative evaluation is an ongoing process for maintaining, modifying, or expanding the nursing care plan

        b. Summative evaluation is a terminal process; summative evaluations are written in the form of discharge summaries

     c. All steps in the nursing process pertinent to the client must be documented in the client's record; some of the most critical documentation involves falls, seclusion, restraints (both physical and chemical), and suicidal or violent behaviors

VI. THERAPEUTIC RELATIONSHIP

  A. A *therapeutic relationship*: is a nurse–client interaction that focuses on client needs and is goal specific, theory based, and open to supervision

  B. **The therapeutic relationship has three phases**: introduction, working, and termination

    1. The introduction phase of the therapeutic relationship includes establishing a contract, discussing confidentiality, assessing thoroughly, and developing the preliminary nursing care plan

    2. During the working phase, the care plan is implemented through the process of therapeutic alliance

      a. Client **transference** is the unconscious process of displacing feelings for significant people in the past onto the clinician (nurse, psychologist, psychiatrist, recreational therapist, etc.) in the present relationship

      b. **Countertransference** is the clinician's emotional reaction to clients based on feelings for significant people in the past

    3. The primary goal of the termination phase of the therapeutic relationship is to review the client's progress and plans for the immediate future

    4. The physical component of the relationship includes all procedures and technical skills that nurses do for clients

    5. The psychosocial component involves qualities such as positive regard, nonjudgmental attitude, acceptance, warmth, empathy, and authenticity

    6. The spiritual component is the feeling of connectiveness with clients and the respect for the diversity of spiritual needs among clients

    7. The power component includes beliefs about external and internal locus of control

VII. THERAPEUTIC COMMUNICATION

  A. *Therapeutic communication* is the process of influencing the behavior of others by sending, receiving, and interpreting messages; feedback and consideration of the context complete the cycle; see Figure 1-2 for a diagram of the therapeutic communication process

  B. **Therapeutic communication** is the foundation of interpersonal relationships and is a key process needed to use the nursing process

    1. Communication includes spoken words, paralanguage, the thinking process, emotions, non-verbal behavior, and the culture of the individuals sending and receiving the message

    2. Non-verbal communication includes body language, eye contact, personal space, and the use of touch

    3. Listening means paying attention to what the person is saying, acknowledging feelings, holding back on what the nurse has to say, avoiding interruption, and controlling the urge to give advice

    4. Characteristics of effective helpers include a nonjudgmental approach, acceptance, warmth, empathy, authenticity, congruency, patience, trustworthiness, self-disclosure, and humor

    5. Techniques that facilitate effective communication include broad openings, giving recognition, minimal encouragement, offering self, accepting, making observations, validating perceptions, exploring, clarifying, placing the event in time or sequence, focusing, encouraging the formulation of a plan of action, suggesting collaboration,

Figure 1-2

The communication process

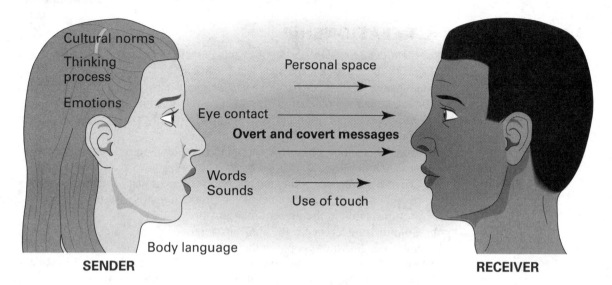

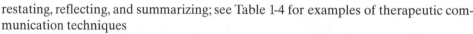

SENDER   **RECEIVER**

restating, reflecting, and summarizing; see Table 1-4 for examples of therapeutic communication techniques

6. Techniques that contribute to ineffective communication include stereotypical comments, parroting, changing the topic, disagreeing, challenging, requesting an explanation, false reassurance, belittling expressed feelings, probing, advising, imposing values, and double/multiple questions; see Table 1-5 (p. 16) for examples of ineffective communication techniques

VIII. OLDER ADULTS

A. Etiology

1. Between 15 and 25% of older adults living in the community have symptoms of mental disorders
2. Almost 20% of the population over 65 years of age experience significant anxiety that may be related to anxiety disorders or to medical illness
3. Although depression is common, it may not be recognized in older adults and may be confused with dementia
4. Older adults with Parkinson's disease and cerebrovascular accidents are at risk for a concurrent depression
5. Alcohol abuse is a problem for 10 to 15% of older adults, and it is often underdiagnosed
6. As the aging population grows, there will be an inevitable increase in age-related mental disorders such as dementia
7. **Aging** is a process of physiological changes occuring with age (diminished neurotransmitters, circulatory capacity, sensory acuity, and perception) that affect the brain
8. Aging causes a decrease in a number of neurotransmitters, which may be a factor in mood disorders among older adults
9. **Ageism** is a process of systematic stereotyping and discrimination against older people simply on the basis of their age; it contributes to the incidence of depression among older adults

Practice to Pass

You are working with an 82-year-old client who is experiencing dementia. She is oriented to self only. She wanders the halls and is often found in other clients' rooms both lying in their beds and going through their clothes. Many of the clients have become angry with her and have threatened to hurt her if she does not stop stealing from them. Based on this data, what are the top three nursing diagnoses for this client?

Table 1-4	Effective Communication Techniques
Technique	**Examples**
Broad opening	"What would you like to work on today?" "What is one of the best things that happened to you this week?"
Giving recognition	"I notice you're wearing a new dress. You look very nice." "What a marvelous afghan that is going to be when you finish."
Minimal encouragement	"Go on." "Ummm." "Uh-huh."
Offering self	"I'll sit with you until it's time for your family session." "I have at least 30 minutes I can spend with you right now."
Accepting	"I can imagine how that might feel." "I'm with you on that [nodding]."
Making observations	"Mr. Robinson, you seem on edge. You are clenching your fist and grinding your teeth." "I'm puzzled. You're smiling, but you sound so resentful."
Validating perceptions	"This is what I heard you say. . . . Is that correct?" "It sounds like you are talking about sad feelings. Is that correct?"
Exploring	"How does your girlfriend feel about your being in the hospital?" "Tell me about what was happening at home just before you came to the hospital."
Clarifying	"Could you explain more about that to me?" "I'm having some difficulty. Could you help me understand?"
Placing the event in time or sequence	"Which came first . . . ?" "When did you first notice . . . ?"
Focusing	"Could we continue talking about you and your dad right now?" "Rather than talking about what your husband thinks, I would like to hear how you're feeling right now."
Encouraging the formulation of a plan of action	"What do you think you can do the next time you feel that way?" "How might you handle your anger in a nonthreatening way?"
Suggesting collaboration	"Perhaps together we can figure out . . ." "Let's try using the problem-solving process that was presented in group yesterday."
Restatement	*Client*: Do you think going home will be difficult? *Nurse*: How difficult do you think going home will be?
Reflection	*Client*: I keep thinking about what all my friends are doing right now. *Nurse*: You're worried that they aren't missing you? *Client*: He laughed at me. My boss just sat there and laughed at me. I felt like such a fool. *Nurse*: You felt humiliated?
Summarizing	"So far we have talked about . . ." "Our time is up. Let's see, we have discussed your family problems, their effect on your schoolwork, and your need to find a way to decrease family conflict."

Source: Fontaine, K. L. (2009). *Mental health nursing* (6th ed.). Upper Saddle River, NJ: Pearson Education, Inc., p. 133.

Table 1-5 **Ineffective Communication Techniques**

Technique	Examples
Stereotypical comments	"What's the matter, cat got your tongue?"
	"Still waters run deep."
Parroting	*Client*: I'm so sad.
	Nurse: You're so sad.
Changing the topic	*Client*: I was so afraid I was going to have another panic attack.
	Nurse: What does your husband think about your panic attacks?
Disagreeing	"I don't see any reason for you to think that way."
	"No, I think that is a silly response to your mother."
Challenging	"Is that a valid reason to become angry?"
	"You weren't really serious, were you?"
Requesting an explanation	"Why did you react that way?"
	"Why can't you just leave home?"
False reassurance	"Don't worry anymore."
	"I doubt that your mother will be angry about your failing math."
Belittling expressed feelings	"That was four years ago. It shouldn't bother you now."
	"You shouldn't feel that all men are bad."
	"It's wrong to even think of your mother like that."
Probing	"I'm here to listen. I can't help you if you won't tell me everything."
	"Tell me what secrets you keep from your wife."
Advising	"You sound worried. I think you'd better talk to your doctor or your rabbi."
	"I think you should divorce your husband."
Imposing values	*Client*: [With head down and low tone of voice.] I was going to go on the cruise, but my mother is coming to stay with me.
	Nurse: You must be looking forward to her arrival.
Double/multiple questions	"What makes you feel that you should stay? How would you get along if you left?
	"Would you rent an apartment or move in with a friend?"

Source: Fontaine, K. L. (2009). *Mental health nursing* (6th ed.). Upper Saddle River, NJ: Pearson Education, Inc., p. 136.

B. Assessment
1. It is imperative to carefully assess older adults to differentiate between dementia, delirium, and depression
2. Older adults may have loss of hearing that may lead to incorrect or bizarre responses when they are unable to hear questions clearly
3. Assess the older adults' ability to accomplish physical and instrumental activities of daily living (e.g., shopping, cooking, financial management, etc.)

C. Nursing diagnoses: related to the behavioral, affective, cognitive, sociocultural, and physiological changes that occur with aging and life events; see Box 1-2 for nursing diagnoses for older adults with mental health problems

Box 1-2	
Psychosocial Nursing Diagnoses for Older Adults	• Chronic Confusion related to changes in brain function; being in an unfamiliar environment • Chronic Low Self-Esteem related to lack of acceptance of the retirement role; continuous feelings of despair • Chronic Sorrow related to loss of life partner and possessions; isolation from social support • Disturbed Body Image related to multiple physiological losses; changes in body composition • Disturbed Sexuality Patterns related to poor body image; loss of life partner, ageism • Fear related to the inevitability of mortality • Hopelessness related to isolation from significant others; overwhelming stress • Impaired Adjustment related to retirement from active work responsibilities; non-supportive relationships with significant others • Impaired Memory related to disturbed mood; changes in brain function • Ineffective Coping related to unsuccessful attempts at forming a philosophy of life; multiple losses • Powerlessness related to inadequate finances and economic burdens; inadequate societal provisions for older adults • Relocation Stress Syndrome related to having to sell family home and move into an assisted living facility • Risk for Isolation related to loss of social support; multiple losses • Spiritual Distress related to the inability to find meaning in life; hopelessness and despair in the life review

D. Interventions

1. Older adults are more prone to the side effects and toxic effects of many medications
   a. Many times medications are given at half the normal adult doses
   b. The key to starting older adults on psychopharmacologic medication therapy is to reduce the dose and progress any increases in dosage slowly
2. Physical restraints increase agitation, confusion, incontinence, pressure ulcers, feelings of anger and fear, and even death from accidental strangulation
3. Electroconvulsive therapy (ECT) is highly successful for treating mood disorders among treatment-resistant older adults
4. Reminiscence therapy can raise self-esteem and increase social intimacy

IX. CULTURAL CONSIDERATIONS

A. *Culture* is a pattern of learned behavior based on values, beliefs, and perceptions of the world; culture is taught and shared by members of a group or society
   1. A **subculture** is a smaller group within a large cultural group that share values, beliefs, behaviors, and language

   2. **Ethnicity** is ethnic affiliation and a sense of belonging to a particular cultural group
   3. **Ethnocentrism** is the belief that one's own culture is more important than, and preferable to, any other

B. **Culture and mental health**
   1. Ideas about mental health, mental illness, psychiatric problems, and treatments are based on cultural values and understanding
   2. What is considered normal or abnormal depends on the specific cultural viewpoint

C. *Values*: a set of personal beliefs about what is meaningful and significant in life
   1. They provide general guidelines for behavior and are standards of conduct in which people or groups of people believe
   2. Every society has basic values about the relationship between humans and nature, sense of time, a sense of productivity, and interpersonal relationships

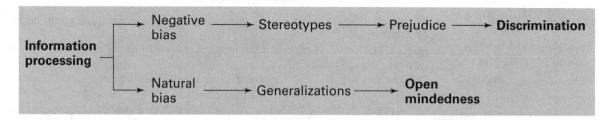

Figure 1-3

Pathways to open-mindedness and discrimination

   3. Predominant U.S. values have historically tended to represent European American, middle-class, Judeo-Christian, male values; nursing as a discipline tends to have the same values as middle-class U.S. or European American background

D. Attitudes and perceptions

   1. Natural biases refer to how nurses' points of view cause them to notice some things and not others

   2. Negative bias is a refusal to recognize that there are other points of view

   3. Generalizations are a way of organizing information; arising out of natural biases, they are changeable starting places for comparing typical behavioral patterns with what is actually observed

   4. Stereotypes are also a way of organizing information; arising out of negative biases, they are images frozen in time that cause us to see what we expect to see, even when the facts differ from our expectations; stereotypes can be favorable or unfavorable, and either kind is potentially harmful

   5. Prejudice is negative feelings about people who are different from oneself

   6. Discrimination is prejudice that is expressed behaviorally; examples are racism, ageism, homosexism, and sexism

   7. Open-mindedness is a positive outcome in an attempt by the nurse to be more sensitive to diverse cultural groups and being willing to support clients in their own cultural beliefs and practices; see Figure 1–3 for diagram of pathways to open-mindedness or discrimination

E. Caring for a culturally diverse population

   1. Effective advocacy for culturally diverse groups depends on a balance of knowledge, sensitivity, and skills

   2. Nurses must understand their own ethnocentrism and acquire knowledge about other cultural groups

   3. Sensitivity includes examining how our own attitudes, values, and prejudices affect our own nursing practice

   4. Communication is an important skill in caring for clients from diverse backgrounds; it includes learning clients' level of fluency in spoken and written English, and determining the most important style of communication

   5. Becoming culturally competent and confident in managing diversity requires practice and patience

X. LEGAL AND ETHICAL ISSUES

   A. Client autonomy and liberty must be ensured by treatment in the least restrictive setting by active client participation in treatment

   B. Voluntary admission occurs when a client consents to confinement in the hospital and signs a document indicating as much

C. **Commitment or emergency (involuntary) admission** may be implemented on the basis of dangerousness to self or others; some states also have the criterion of prevention of significant physical or mental deterioration for involuntary admission

D. **Competency**: a legal determination that a client can make reasonable judgments and decisions about treatment and other significant areas of personal life
   1. An adult is considered competent unless a *court* rules the client incompetent; in such cases, a guardian is appointed to make decisions on the person's behalf
   2. Clients who are committed are still capable of participating in health care decisions

E. **Informed consent**: a client's right to be given enough information to make a decision, to be able to understand the information, and to communicate his or her decision to others; in an emergency situation with no time to obtain consent without endangering health or safety, a client may be treated without legal liability

F. **Adherence to the principle of confidentiality** is extremely important in the practice of psychiatric nursing
   1. There are federal rules regarding chemical dependence confidentiality; staff members are not allowed to disclose any admission or discharge information
   2. Confidentiality is violated by telling others that a client has been admitted to a psychiatric facility
   3. Some states require written consent before human immunodeficiency virus (HIV) tests may be performed; states have laws regarding when HIV test results or the diagnosis of acquired immunodeficiency syndrome (AIDS) may be disclosed
   4. The duty to disclose is the health care professional's obligation to warn identified individuals if a client has made a credible threat to harm someone
   5. Ways in which client confidentiality may be compromised
      a. Speaking about client to others who are not members of the client's treatment team
      b. Leaving clinical documents where others may see them
      c. Careless handling of medical information after client signs release of information to other health care providers

G. **Nursing ethics**
   1. Nurses are required to make numerous ethical decisions every day; client differences in values, culture, and lifestyles often present nurses and other health care providers with an ethical dilemma
   2. Competent care involves knowing what and how to perform skills, being open to criticism, and a willingness to seek appropriate education when there are known knowledge deficits
   3. The perspective of principalism in ethics ignores the socioeconomic and cultural contexts and is too abstract to have practical application in clinical practice
   4. Nursing is based on ethics of care, including medical indications, client preferences, quality of life, and contextual factors

XI. NCLEX® TEST-TAKING TIPS FOR PSYCHIATRIC–MENTAL HEALTH NURSING QUESTIONS

A. **NCLEX® questions for psychiatric–mental health nursing**: primarily test on two levels— application and analysis
   1. Application: the process of using information to know why a phenomenon occurs; effective application relies on the use of understood memorized facts to verify intended action; application is the progression from facts to nursing action; Box 1-3 gives an example of an application question
   2. Analysis: the ability to use abstract or logical forms of thought to show relationships and to distinguish cause and effect between variables in a situation; Box 1-4 gives an example of an analysis question

Box 1-3 **Application Question**	A client who is hospitalized for panic disorder is experiencing increased anxiety. The client exhibits selective inattention and tells the nurse, "I'm anxious now." The nurse determines that the degree of the client's anxiety is **1.** mild. **2.** *moderate.** **3.** severe. **4.** panic. *The nurse must know the facts related to levels of anxiety. The nurse must be able to differentiate the correct level of anxiety the client is experiencing in order to implement appropriate nursing actions.

Box 1-4 **Analysis Question**	A hospitalized client with depression who has a weekend pass asked the nurse, "Do you think I should go home this weekend?" The nurse uses the technique of reflection when the he or she responds: **1.** *"Should you go home for the weekend?"** **2.** "Home means . . . ?" **3.** "It sounds as if you haven't decided whether or not to go home this weekend." **4.** "Do you think you are ready to go home this weekend?" *The nurse must know the relationship of reflection in order to distinguish the cause and effect between it and the other communication techniques used in the situation.

3. The components of a question include a background statement, a stem, and a list of four options; most psychiatric–mental health nursing NCLEX® test questions have two or more right answers; therefore, the question usually targets a BEST answer; the key to answering these questions is to understand the *what* or the *how* the question is attempting to elicit
   a. First read the background statement, noting key concepts or conditions, and then read the stem again, noting critical words
   b. Attempt to answer the question *before* reviewing the list of four options; if an option matches your hypothesized answer, that is the most likely correct response; if no option matches your hypothesized answer, then re-review the question, noting the critical concepts and words
   c. With physiological NCLEX®-type questions, when all answer choices are equal in importance, the *priority* or the correct answer often follows the rule of the "ABCs"—Airway, Breathing, Circulation; in psychological NCLEX®-type questions, when all answer choices are equal in importance, the *priority* or the correct answer often follows the rule of the "SEAs"—Safety, Expressing feelings, Assisting with problem solving
   d. Questions that elicit an effective response by the nurse (refer back to Section VII, Therapeutic Communication) follow these general rules:
      1) Do not solve the clients' problems; the nurse's role is to assist clients in solving their own problems
      2) Correct responses often encourage clients to examine their own thoughts or feelings
      3) Often the correct response is to restate the client's comments or to reflect back to the client the content and/or feelings behind the client's comments
      4) Do not change the subject or topic; if the client brings up an unsettling topic, then the client is ready to discuss or address the issue

5) The nurse's role is to support clients as they develop an understanding of their own feelings and thoughts as well as to assist clients in forming their own solutions to problems

6) Do not discount the client's feelings or thoughts; a client who verbalizes sadness is not going to become less sad or happy because the nurse simply states "Don't worry," or "Don't be sad," or "Cheer up, it could be worse."

7) Feelings are not good or bad, they just *are*; the behaviors that the client exhibits make the situation good or bad; for example, anger is not a "bad" feeling; anger can motivate a client to change a stressful situation or to get out of a dangerous circumstance; however, an angry client who threatens to harm others or does harm to others may be placed in jail

Case Study

A female nurse approaches a depressed female client on a psychiatric unit. The nurse introduces herself and asks if it is all right if she sits with the client. The nurse asks, "How are you doing today?" The client leans away, maintains a rigid posture, avoids eye contact, and shrugs her shoulders. The nurse leans back to give the client her space and crosses her arms over her chest to create a less threatening posture. After several minutes of silence, the nurse explains to the client that she has an hour that she can spend with her today. Following another long period of silence, the nurse says, "I guess you're not in the mood to talk today, so I'll see you tomorrow." The nurse leaves after spending 25 minutes with the client.

1. What actions by the nurse demonstrate respect for the client?

2. What actions by the nurse, if any, did not represent therapeutic communication skills and could decrease the client's confidence and trust in the nurse?

3. How would you interpret the client's body language and silence during this first session?

4. How could the nurse's interaction with the client have been improved?

5. Why do you think the nurse decided to leave after 25 minutes?

For suggested responses, see pages 295–296.

POSTTEST

1 A client was quite upset the entire time she was pregnant and made it clear that she did not want her unborn child. However, since the birth, she has become overly protective and refuses to let anyone else near the infant. Which ego defense mechanism does the nurse recognize in the client's behavior?

1. Denial
2. Projection
3. Reaction formation
4. Displacement

2 The client has had an elective abortion. The nurse wishes to assist the client to manage post-abortion emotional responses. Which nursing approach is most appropriate?

1. Reassure the client that having an abortion was the best possible decision.
2. Teach the client how to use effective methods of birth control.
3. Encourage the client to express feelings of loss and grief.
4. Suggest that the client rely on a higher power for spiritual support.

3 A 63-year-old male client expresses feelings of hopelessness and helplessness about his spouse's illness and anticipated death. On which issues should the nurse initially assist the client to focus?

1. The nature of the spouse's present illness
2. The client's responses to past losses
3. The dying spouse's feelings about impending loss and death
4. The client's relationship with the spouse

4 The mental health nurse is conducting an assessment with a client who has a history of anxiety. The nurse concludes that the client's use of defense mechanisms is adaptive when the client remains psychologically and physically safe and does which of the following?

1. Experiences fewer direct manifestations of anxiety
2. Seeks social isolation to avoid stress
3. Displaces anxiety onto other persons or situations
4. Identifies the personal level of anxiety

5 The client with body dysmorphic disorder says, "My ugly nose horrifies everyone." The nurse should conclude that the client is using which defense mechanisms? Select all that apply.

1. Conversion
2. Somatization
3. Symbolism
4. Projection
5. Sublimation

6 A mental health client who experienced a brief psychotic reaction was treated as an inpatient for one week and then discharged to an outpatient day hospital program for follow-up treatment. The nurse explains to the client's family that the outpatient treatment setting approach is based on the principle of providing which of the following?

1. Compliance with the Americans with Disabilities Act as it applies to mental health clients
2. Mental health care in the least restrictive setting possible
3. Community-based care for non-chronically ill mental health clients
4. Non-pharmacologic treatment modalities for mental health clients in outpatient settings

7 A nurse completing a cultural assessment of the client recognizes a personal tendency to engage in stereotyping and countertransference responses. The nurse should further recognize that these behaviors are likely to lead the nurse to do which of the following?

1. Anticipate the unmet needs of the individual client
2. Be open and honest while responding to the client's concerns
3. Fail to recognize unmet needs of the individual client
4. Facilitate the treatment process

8 In order to deal effectively with the spiritual needs of a client, what should be the nurse's initial strategy?

1. Refer the client to an appropriate clergy.
2. Clarify own spiritual beliefs and values.
3. Use a spiritual assessment tool.
4. Discuss own religiosity with the client.

9 During a team meeting, the nurse develops the outcomes of care for a depressed male client. Which of the following is the most appropriately stated outcome for the client within three days?

1. Feel less depressed.
2. Reduce self-rating on a depression scale by 10%.
3. State he has significantly more insight into his problems.
4. Feel supported as he deals with grief issues.

10 An older adult grieving the loss of a family member reports all of the following symptoms to the nurse. To plan appropriate nursing interventions, the nurse needs to determine which symptoms need to be addressed first. Put the following client symptoms in order from highest to lowest priority.

1. Occasional feelings of tightness in the chest
2. Expressed thoughts of being better off dead
3. Statements of guilt about a loved one's death
4. A morbid preoccupation with feelings of worthlessness

➤ *See pages 25–27 for Answers and Rationales.*

ANSWERS & RATIONALES

Pretest

1 **Answer: 4** **Rationale:** Asking the client to explain it another way is correct. It uses the clarifying technique, because the nurse is attempting to determine, or clarify, the exact meaning the client is attempting to convey. The client's original statement does not convey a clear meaning. Asking the client how he or she felt utilizes the technique of exploring. It is not useful in this situation because it diverts the focus of the conversation away from the present concern of the client. Asking the client when the feelings of confusion began employs the techniques of exploring and attempting to place an event in time and sequence. This response is inappropriate because the particular meaning of the client's statement is unclear. Rather than assuming that the client is referring to being in a confused state, the nurse should clarify and determine exactly what message the client is attempting to convey. Asking the client if the person indicated what he meant is incorrect because it changes the focus from the client to another person. The focus of the nurse should be on the client. **Cognitive Level:** Applying **Client Need:** Psychosocial Integrity **Integrated Process:** Caring **Content Area:** Mental Health **Strategy:** Does the client's statement leave you feeling confused about an intended message? Communicate that to the client clearly and simply. **Reference:** Fontaine, K. (2009). *Mental health nursing* (6th ed.). Upper Saddle River, NJ: Prentice Hall, pp. 131–134.

2 **Answer: 2** **Rationale:** Countertransference is correct. Countertransference is the phenomenon in which the helper in a therapeutic relationship (in this case, the nurse) responds emotionally to clients based on feelings for persons who have been (or are) significant in the helper's life. It is likely that this type of response to the client will interfere with the progress of the nurse–client relationship. Transference is the unconscious process of the client's displacing feelings for significant people in the past onto a person in a present relationship. In this instance, the client would displace feelings to the nurse. When transference occurs in a nurse–client relationship, it is likely to interfere with normal processes of the therapeutic relationship. Denial is a defense mechanism used by individuals in an attempt to screen or ignore unacceptable realities by refusing to acknowledge them. Reaction formation is a defense mechanism that causes people to act exactly opposite to the way they feel. **Cognitive Level:** Applying **Client Need:** Psychosocial Integrity **Integrated Process:** Caring **Content Area:** Mental Health **Strategy:** Recall basic concepts in psychoanalytic theory. Notice that the feeling originates in the nurse, not the client, to make the correct selection. **Reference:** Varcarolis, E., &

Halter, M. (2010). *Foundations of psychiatric mental health nursing: A clinical approach* (6th ed.). St. Louis, MO: Saunders Elsevier, pp. 26–27.

3 **Answer: 1, 2, 4** **Rationale:** Advising clients prevents them from taking responsibility and using the problem-solving process. The nurse should not offer personal opinions to clients, even if asked to do so. Instead, the nurse should use the technique of reflection to redirect the topic back to the client. Belittling the client and the client's indecisiveness shows that the nurse is responding nontherapeutically in a critical way. The tone of the nurse's response demonstrates neither appreciating the difficulty of the client's situation nor valuing the client as an individual. The nurse's response will have a negative impact on the client. Assuming that the client is incapable of reaching an independent decision transfers responsibility for decision making from the client to the nurse. Advising prevents clients from using the problem-solving process, reaching independent decisions, and taking responsibility. Regarding a challenge to the client's belief system, the nurse should accept a client's belief system without challenge. However, there is no indication in this situation that the client's behavior is related to a particular belief system. The nurse's response is inappropriate, but not because he or she is challenging the client's belief system. A positive reinforcer increases the likelihood that a behavior will be repeated. This comment, which is opinionated and critical, is not a positive reinforcer. **Cognitive Level:** Applying **Client Need:** Psychosocial Integrity **Integrated Process:** Nursing Process: Evaluation **Content Area:** Mental Health **Strategy:** Notice the critical word *inappropriate* in the stem of the question. **Reference:** Varcarolis, E., & Halter, M. (2010). *Foundations of psychiatric mental health nursing: A clinical approach* (6th ed.). St. Louis, MO: Saunders Elsevier, pp. 174–175, 179–184.

4 **Answer: 3** **Rationale:** Feedback provides the opportunity for the nurse to offer clients information about their verbal and non-verbal responses as they have been seen, heard, and understood by the nurse. When offered appropriately, feedback enhances the communication process. Regardless of whether feedback has been given, the nurse should avoid giving clients personal advice. Instead the nurse should assist clients to solve their own problems. Exploring feelings is definitely a part of therapeutic communication, but it is not the same as feedback. Appropriately offered feedback may set the stage for the exploration of feelings, but feelings are not explored during feedback. The purpose of feedback is to report observations made during the communication process. When providing feedback, the nurse will offer information about the verbal and non-verbal responses of the client as they have been seen, heard, and understood by the nurse. Appropriately offered feedback may facilitate the development of explanations for behavior, but it does not explain behavior. **Cognitive Level:** Applying **Client Need:** Psychosocial Integrity **Integrated Process:** Caring **Content Area:** Mental Health **Strategy:** Do not be misled by the words *explore feelings,* which are very often the correct response. Look back at what the question is asking for. Put this into your own words if necessary. **Reference:** Kneisl, C., Wilson, H., & Trigoboff, E. (2009). *Contemporary psychiatric-mental health nursing* (2nd ed.). Upper Saddle River, NJ: Prentice Hall, pp. 202–203.

5 **Answer: 1, 4** **Rationale:** Mental health is growing toward potential with an inner feeling of satisfaction. Mental health is accepting and feeling satisfaction with the self. Mental health is absent of regret, displeasure, or dissatisfaction, which are characteristics of placement toward the unhealthy end of the mental health continuum. Stating that the family thinks the client is a good person suggests that the individual may not hold the same opinion as the family. The client's statement does not indicate that the client feels personal satisfaction, which characterizes the more mentally healthy person. The statement about remaining single suggests regret and dissatisfaction, which are characteristics of a person whose position on the mental health continuum is more toward the unhealthy end. The statement expressing an expectation of being more successful is regretful and indicates dissatisfaction with the status of the individual's life, which is characteristic of poor mental health. **Cognitive Level:** Applying **Client Need:** Health Promotion and Maintenance **Integrated Process:** Caring **Content Area:** Mental Health **Strategy:** Look for behaviors that are optimal and keep your focus on the client. **Reference:** Kneisl, C., Wilson, H., & Trigoboff, E. (2009). *Contemporary psychiatric-mental health nursing* (2nd ed.). Upper Saddle River, NJ: Prentice Hall, pp. 187–188.

6 **Answer: 2, 4** **Rationale:** According to the law, pressing a cup against the client's mouth could be considered battery or offensive touching. Unless an emergency situation is present, psychiatric–mental health clients cannot be touched or treated without their consent. Psychiatric–mental health clients, when legally competent, have the right to refuse treatment, including medication. The lack of a client's objection upon a second request is not a legal principle. Therefore, it cannot be included among correct answers for this question. Forceful administration of medication to this client would meet the legal criteria for battery. The right to be treated in the least restrictive manner possible is an accurately stated legal principle; however, it does not apply in this situation, where no information is given about most restrictive or least restrictive options. The principle of least restrictive alternatives refers to providing sufficient care to the client with the least restrictive methods in the least restrictive treatment setting. It is true that clients who wish to establish psychiatric advance directives may do so, but it does not relate to the situation that is described in the

question. **Cognitive Level:** Analyzing **Client Need:** Management of Care **Integrated Process:** Nursing Process: Implementation **Content Area:** Mental Health **Strategy:** Notice that the nurse forcefully presses the cup to the client's mouth. Identify common legal principles that apply in the psychiatric–mental health area. **Reference:** Fontaine, K. (2009). *Mental health nursing* (6th ed.). Upper Saddle River, NJ: Prentice Hall, pp. 86–90.

7 **Answer: 4** **Rationale:** Short-term, focused psychotherapy is correct. This client's problems are not long-standing ones. Instead, they are newer ones that are clearly focused on the recent death of the parent. Subsequently, this client would be a good candidate for short-term, focused psychotherapy. Grief counseling and crisis intervention would be appropriate for this client, who would be expected to reestablish equilibrium in a reasonable period of time. There is nothing in the client's statement that suggests irreversible psychological trauma. Rather, it appears that the client is in an early stage of active grieving, which is considered a normal reaction to a recent loss. There is nothing in the client's statement that suggests a need for long-term psychotherapy. The client is experiencing a normal grief response to a recent sudden and unexpected loss. Extreme feelings of distress and being overwhelmed, accompanied by crying, are normal expected displays of grief. The fact that the client is able to verbally express his feelings is a positive indicator to a healthy adaptation. Although the client does show some probable signs of anxiety (crying spells and sleeplessness), this client shows no manifestations of depression. Instead, this client appears to be in the active stages of early grieving, which is a normal and time-limited response to loss. **Cognitive Level:** Analyzing **Client Need:** Health Promotion and Maintenance **Integrated Process:** Caring **Content Area:** Mental Health **Strategy:** Notice that the client's symptoms began very recently. Identify what preceded the onset of the symptoms to guide decision making. **Reference:** Varcarolis, E., & Halter, M. (2010). *Foundations of psychiatric mental health nursing: A clinical approach* (6th ed.). St. Louis, MO: Saunders Elsevier, pp. 715–721.

8 **Answer: 1** **Rationale:** Clarifying the client's intention communicates to the client that all behaviors have meaning and gives the nurse the opportunity to set boundaries. Three options are incorrect. Leaving the situation or continuing to interact with the client without acknowledging the comment may reinforce the behavior as being acceptable and inadvertently reinforce the dynamics between nurse and client. Refusing to interact with the client harms the nurse–client relationship and should only be an option after the nurse has clearly set boundaries with the client. **Cognitive Level:** Analyzing **Client Need:** Psychosocial Integrity **Integrated Process:** Caring **Content Area:** Mental Health **Strategy:** Consider that this is probably manipulative behavior on the part of the client and that the client is likely to have conscious awareness of underlying motivations. Recall that setting limits is necessary when manipulation is occurring. **Reference:** Fontaine, K. (2009). *Mental health nursing* (6th ed.). Upper Saddle River, NJ: Prentice Hall, pp. 503–504.

9 Answer: 2 Rationale: The hypothalamus is located in the diencephalon and is responsible for regulating temperature and appetite, as well as integrating the functions of the autonomic nervous system. The thalamus is located in the diencephalon, and its functions are primarily concerned with sensation and coordination. The cerebrum's primary functions include higher-order thinking, abstract reasoning, visual function, judgment, memory, and sensory function. The cerebellum is primarily responsible for balance and coordination. The nurse should not assume that the fall was caused by cerebellar dysfunction. Additionally, none of the presenting symptoms of the client suggest current cerebellar abnormalities. **Cognitive Level:** Applying **Client Need:** Physiological Adaptation **Integrated Process:** Nursing Process: Diagnosis **Content Area:** Mental Health **Strategy:** Identify the clinical presentation of the client. Recall particulars of brain structure and function from anatomy and physiology. **Reference:** Kneisl, C., Wilson, H., & Trigoboff, E. (2009). *Contemporary psychiatric–mental health nursing* (2nd ed.). Upper Saddle River, NJ: Prentice Hall, pp. 88.

10 Answer: 2, 3 Rationale: Insufficient serotonin activity in the CNS is associated with depression. Current research suggests that a variety of other neurotransmission abnormalities also exist when depression is present. These include dysregulation of catecholamines, dopamine, acetylcholine, and GABA. Excesses of acetylcholine in the CNS are associated with depression, excessive inhibition, and somatic complaints. Excessive serotonin in the CNS is not associated with depression. Reduced levels of acetylcholine in the CNS are not associated with depression, but rather with elevated mood. Depression is not associated with genetic mutation of chromosome 6. **Cognitive Level:** Analyzing **Client Need:** Psychosocial Integrity **Integrated Process:** Nursing Process: Evaluation **Content Area:** Mental Health **Strategy:** Recall basic functions of neurotransmitters. Do not assume that because the client is depressed, both answers should involve deficiency. **Reference:** Varcarolis, E., Carson, V., & Shoemaker, N. (2010). *Foundations of psychiatric mental health nursing: A clinical approach* (6th ed.). St. Louis, MO: Saunders Elsevier, pp. 250–252.

Posttest

1 Answer: 3 Rationale: Reaction formation is an ego defense mechanism that causes people to act exactly opposite to the way they originally felt. The behaviors of the person utilizing this defense mechanism are often excessively intense and appear somewhat unbelievable to others. Denial is an attempt to screen or ignore unacceptable realities by refusing to acknowledge them. The client is not denying the presence or reality of the baby. Projection is a process in which unacceptable personal desires, actions, thoughts, shortcomings, or mistakes are attributed

to others or the environment. There is no indication that this client is doing this. Displacement is the transferring or discharging of emotional reactions from one object or person to another. The recipient of the displaced emotion then assumes a symbolic significance to the individual who is displacing the emotion. There is no indication that the client is doing this. **Cognitive Level:** Applying **Client Need:** Psychosocial Integrity **Integrated Process:** Nursing Process: Diagnosis **Content Area:** Mental Health **Strategy:** Notice the vast contrast between the behaviors and attitudes of the mother during the pre- and post-delivery periods. Simply define each of the defense mechanisms and look for a fit between your definition and information you know about the mother. **Reference:** Fontaine, K. (2009). *Mental health nursing* (6th ed.). Upper Saddle River, NJ: Prentice Hall, p. 12.

2 Answer: 3 Rationale: Encouraging the client to express feelings of loss and grief will allow the client to manage any post-abortion emotional responses. The post-abortion client will normally be faced with a number of strong emotions, including loss and guilt. When and if the grieving process should occur, and the nurse can facilitate it by encouraging free expression of feelings. Telling the client that this was the best decision provides false reassurance and offers the nurse's probable personal opinion and approval. Although counseling the client about effective birth control methods is appropriate later, the timing is not right for this to occur now. The issues to be dealt with at this time are "here-and-now" emotional issues that could lead to a crisis state if left unexpressed and unaddressed. The client is in a situation where many people welcome spiritual support. However, the nurse should not assume that the client has a belief system involving a higher power, nor should the nurse impose personal spiritual beliefs on the client. The nurse should conduct a spiritual assessment, and if appropriate, arrange for a spiritual counselor who can assist the client within the client's own personal belief system. **Cognitive Level:** Applying **Client Need:** Psychosocial Integrity **Integrated Process:** Nursing Process: Implementation **Content Area:** Mental Health **Strategy:** Recognize that this client will experience loss and grief and use this knowledge as the basis for evaluating each option. **Reference:** Varcarolis, E., & Halter, M. (2010). *Foundations of psychiatric mental health nursing: A clinical approach* (6th ed.). St. Louis, MO: Saunders Elsevier, p. 715.

3 Answer: 2 Rationale: The nurse should help the client identify past experiences with loss, as well as coping strategies used at those times. This will allow the nurse and client to identify strengths, social supports, and effective coping strategies that could be used at this time. It will also help the client to look at the current situation rationally while drawing from experiences of the past. Focusing on the nature of the spouse's illness will neither facilitate expression of the client's feelings nor provide an opportunity for discussing healthy coping strategies. Medical and historical facts about the ill spouse would be gathered, but the feelings of "hopelessness and helplessness" verbalized by the client would not be acknowledged, validated, or relieved. While it is indeed important to support a dying client through the anticipatory grieving of impending death, the nurse should stay focused on the client in this case (the non-dying spouse). At another time, however, the dying spouse could become the client. While relationship issues might be a part of grief counseling, the most pressing need of the client at this time is to talk about the client's own feelings about the current situation. This will assist the client to identify familiar coping strategies, such as seeking social support, that have been effective in past situations of loss and grief. **Cognitive Level:** Analyzing **Client Need:** Psychosocial Integrity **Integrated Process:** Nursing Process: Planning **Content Area:** Mental Health **Strategy:** Keep your focus on who is the client in the question. In this case, it is the person whom the nurse is interacting with, not the dying spouse. Keep this in mind when evaluating options. **Reference:** Kneisl, C., Wilson, H., & Trigoboff, E. (2009). *Contemporary psychiatric-mental health nursing* (2nd ed.). Upper Saddle River, NJ: Prentice Hall, p. 421.

4 **Answer: 1** **Rationale:** The purpose of defense mechanisms is to reduce anxiety levels and allow the client to function adequately. Seeking social isolation to avoid stress is an unhealthy maladaptive strategy that can actually lead to increased anxiety. When anxiety is displaced onto other persons or situations, anxiety may be temporarily decreased. However, the reduction in anxiety frequently lasts only a short time, especially since displacement is often injurious to others. While identifying the level of anxiety will be generally beneficial to the client, unless the client can connect the anxiety to personal relief-seeking behaviors, this is not an adaptive technique. **Cognitive Level:** Applying **Client Need:** Psychosocial Integrity **Integrated Process:** Nursing Process: Diagnosis **Content Area:** Mental Health **Strategy:** Notice that you are looking for a positive behavioral change that would indicate adaptation. **Reference:** Fontaine, K. (2009). *Mental health nursing* (6th ed.). Upper Saddle River, NJ: Prentice Hall, p. 226.

5 **Answer: 3, 4** **Rationale:** Symbolization is the unconscious process by which one object or idea comes to represent another. In this case, the client's nose symbolizes everything distasteful and unacceptable to the client. Projection is the unconscious process by which an individual attributes one's own intolerable wishes, emotions, or motivations to another person. In this case, the client says that other people are horrified by the appearance of the client's nose, but it is actually the client who is horrified. Conversion, somatization, and sublimation are not shown in this situation. Conversion is an unconscious defense mechanism in which anxiety is expressed as a physical symptom, which results in an alteration of physical function and that has no organic cause.

Somatization is the expression of psychological stress through physical symptoms. Sublimation is the redirecting of unacceptable impulses (may be sexual or aggressive) into a constructive outlet in a socially acceptable fashion. **Cognitive Level:** Analyzing **Client Need:** Psychosocial Integrity **Integrated Process:** Nursing Process: Assessment **Content Area:** Mental Health **Strategy:** Recognize that when individuals have body dysmorphic disorder, they usually have a normal appearance. They are preoccupied with an imagined defective body part. **Reference:** Varcarolis, E., & Halter, M. (2010). *Foundations of psychiatric mental health nursing: A clinical approach* (6th ed.). St. Louis, MO: Saunders Elsevier, pp. 26–27.

6 **Answer: 2** **Rationale:** Mental health laws specify that mental health clients are to be treated in the least restrictive environment in which appropriate care measures can be delivered. This means that the client should be discharged from the inpatient setting as soon as stabilization has occurred and an appropriate outpatient treatment setting can be arranged. It is possible that active symptoms may still exist at this point. The Americans with Disabilities Act does not specify where mental health clients are to be treated. Instead, it is intended to ensure that all persons with disabilities, whether physical or mental, have adequate opportunities to participate in the economic and social mainstream of society. Federal and state laws stipulate that community-based care is made equally available to mental health clients who are acutely ill and to those who have chronic mental illnesses. No information in the stem of this question indicates that the client will or will not receive medication. **Cognitive Level:** Applying **Client Need:** Management of Care **Integrated Process:** Nursing Process: Planning **Content Area:** Mental Health **Strategy:** Note the progressive decrease in the level of intensity of treatment and correlate that with the less restrictive phrase in the correct option. **Reference:** Kneisl, C., Wilson, H., & Trigoboff, E. (2009). *Contemporary psychiatric-mental health nursing* (2nd ed.). Upper Saddle River, NJ: Prentice Hall, pp. 254–256.

7 **Answer: 3** **Rationale:** Stereotyping arises out of negative biases. Stereotypes are images frozen in time that cause us to see what we expect to see, even when the actual facts differ from our preconceived notions. Countertransference is the nurse's emotional reaction to a client based on feelings for significant people in the nurse's past. Both countertransference and stereotyping will decrease the nurse's sensitivity to the client's needs and the culture they represent. Hence, the client's need remains unmet. Both countertransference and stereotyping will decrease the nurse's sensitivity to the client. Instead of responding to the client needs, the nurse will make automatic responses based on preconceived ideas and expectations. The nurse is unable to be open and honest about client's concerns because responses will be governed by stereotyping or countertransference. Stereotyping and countertransference can be expected to interfere with the treatment process. Because the nurse will not be able to recognize characteristics of the individual that are readily identifiable to others and because the nurse is unable to address the client's unmet needs, the treatment process will be inevitably affected negatively. **Cognitive Level:** Applying **Client Need:** Psychosocial Integrity **Integrated Process:** Caring **Content Area:** Mental Health **Strategy:** Since stereotyping and countertransference are negative characteristics, expect the correct option to be one that has a negative tone. **Reference:** Fontaine, K. (2009). *Mental health nursing* (6th ed.). Upper Saddle River, NJ: Prentice Hall, p. 23.

8 **Answer: 2** **Rationale:** The first priority of nurses in assisting clients to manage any area of their lives is to understand themselves and clarify their own spiritual beliefs and values. This does not mean, however, that the nurse should attempt to impose his or her spiritual belief and value system on the client. Rather, the nurse must assist the client to best utilize the client's own belief and value system. The nurse should complete a spiritual assessment tool with the client before making the decision to refer the client to a member of the clergy. The nurse should not assume that the client will be comforted by contact with a clergy member. The spiritual assessment tool is useful for determining the client's spiritual needs and beliefs before working with the client to develop a plan for meeting spiritual needs of the client. However, this activity should be undertaken after the nurse has self-examined personal spiritual beliefs. The nurse's own religious and spiritual belief systems should not be imposed on the client. The nurse must carefully refrain from making any attempt to change the client's belief system. **Cognitive Level:** Analyzing **Client Need:** Psychosocial Integrity **Integrated Process:** Caring **Content Area:** Mental Health **Strategy:** Consider the importance of self-awareness in all nursing intervention situations. **Reference:** Varcarolis, E., & Halter, M. (2010). *Foundations of psychiatric mental health nursing: A clinical approach* (6th ed.). St. Louis, MO: Saunders Elsevier, pp. 774–775.

9 **Answer: 2** **Rationale:** Outcomes must be specific, measurable, and observable. This outcome is written in specific measurable terms. Using the self-rating scale would allow any nurse who is caring for the client to be able to compare recent and prior results on the same tool. This in turn would facilitate assessing client progress and determining if the outcome has been met. The nurse would not be required to have prior knowledge of the client, but rather of the client's prior depression scale score. Specific observable descriptors would be required for the nurse to know the client is less depressed. More insight is an immeasurable term, and there are few objective ways of validating the presence of more insight. As for feeling supported as he deals with grief issues, the outcome is immeasurable as written (feel supported), and the option also assumes that the depressed client is dealing with grief issues. Grief and depression are two separate phenomena, with grief being an expected and normal human response, and depression being a pathologic human response. **Cognitive Level:** Analyzing **Client Need:** Psychosocial Integrity **Integrated Process:** Nursing Process: Planning **Content Area:** Mental Health **Strategy:** Look for the option that would allow any nurse to recognize the client's attainment of the outcome. **Reference:** Kneisl, C., Wilson, H., & Trigoboff, E. (2009). *Contemporary psychiatric-mental health nursing* (2nd ed.). Upper Saddle River, NJ: Prentice Hall, pp. 711–712.

10 **Answer: 3, 1, 4, 2** **Rationale:** The correct ranking is as follows: Expressed thoughts of being better off dead is first priority. The nurse should recognize that any person who expresses thoughts of death or being better off dead should be viewed as being at risk for self-directed violence. Safety concerns for such persons take priority over all psychological and sociologic needs, as well as many physiologic needs. A morbid preoccupation with feelings of worthlessness is second priority. Grieving and depressed persons can be excessively preoccupied with feelings of worthlessness. This statement would be of concern once safety needs are met because of the word *morbid*. Occasional feelings of tightness in chest is third priority. Everyone experiences grief differently and older adults often experience grief somatically. However, physiologic dysfunction is a possibility to be concerned about as cardiac problems are more common in the older age group. If the client's discomfort continues, intensifies, or evidence of organic disease presents, then this option would become the number one priority. Statements of guilt about a loved one's death is fourth priority. Following the death of a significant person, the individual often feels guilty and fears having failed to do everything possible to prevent the death. These feelings are typically not pathological, but rather part of the normal grieving experience. With the passage of time, and the gradual acceptance of the loss, they usually diminish. **Cognitive Level:** Analyzing **Client Need:** Psychosocial Integrity **Integrated Process:** Nursing Process: Planning **Content Area:** Mental Health **Strategy:** Remember that you are looking to rank manifestations that are most dangerous to least dangerous. **Reference:** Varcarolis, E., & Halter, N. (2010). *Foundations of psychiatric mental health nursing: A clinical approach* (6th ed.). St. Louis, MO: Saunders Elsevier, pp. 711–712, 715.

ANSWERS & RATIONALES

References

American Psychiatric Association (2000). *Diagnostic and statistical manual of mental disorders* (4th ed. text revision). Washington, DC: American Psychiatric Association.

Beck, A. (1976). *Cognitive therapies and the emotional disorders.* New York, NY: International Universities Press.

Ellis, A. (1973). *Humanistic psychotherapy: The rational-emotive approach.* New York, NY: The Julian Press.

Erikson, E. (1963). *Childhood and society.* New York, NY: W. W. Norton.

Fontaine, K. (2009). *Mental health nursing* (6th ed.). Upper Saddle River, NJ: Pearson Education.

Freud, S. (1936). *The problem of anxiety.* New York, NY: W. W. Norton.

Kniesl, C., Wilson, H., & Trigoboff, E. (2009). *Contemporary psychiatric-mental health nursing* (2nd ed.). Upper Saddle River, NJ: Pearson Education.

Menninger, K. (1963). *The vital balance.* Newark, NJ: Viking Press.

Peplau, H. (1952). *Interpersonal relations in nursing.* New York, NY: G. P. Putnam's Sons.

Piaget, J. (1974). *The origins of intelligence in children.* New York, NY: International Universities Press.

Shives, L. (2012). *Basic concepts of psychiatric–mental health nursing* (8th ed.). Philadelphia, PA: Lippincott Williams & Wilkins.

Skinner, B. F. (1953). *Science and human behavior.* New York: Macmillan.

Stuart, G. (2009). *Principles and practice of psychiatric nursing* (9th ed.). St. Louis: Elsevier Science.

Sullivan, H. S. (1953). *Interpersonal theory of psychiatry.* New York, NY: W. W. Norton.

Townsend, M. (2011). *Essentials of psychiatric mental health nursing* (5th ed.). Philadelphia, PA: F. A. Davis.

Varcarolis, E. & Halter, M. (2010). *Foundations of psychiatric mental health nursing: A clinical approach* (6th ed.). Philadelphia: Saunders.

Venes, D. J. (2010). *Taber's Cyclopedic Medical Dictionary* (21st ed.). Philadelphia, PA: F. A. Davis.

Crisis Intervention and Suicide

2

Chapter Outline

Overview of Crisis

Nursing Process during Crisis

Psychopharmacology as
Treatment during Crisis

Overview of Suicide

Nursing Process for Persons
at Risk for Suicide

Psychopharmacology as
Treatment to Prevent
Suicide

Objectives

➤ List five characteristics of a crisis situation.

➤ State four goals for crisis intervention and crisis stabilization.

➤ Outline the steps involved in crisis intervention.

➤ Formulate six intervention strategies for clients experiencing
a crisis.

➤ Describe six common myths of suicide.

➤ Identify at least two populations at high risk for suicide.

➤ Describe the therapeutic milieu for a client on suicide precautions.

NCLEX-RN® Test Prep

Use the accompanying online resource,
NursingReviewsandRationales, to test
yourself with hundreds of NCLEX®-style
practice questions.

Review at a Glance

appraisal of stressor subjective
meaning of how an individual perceives
the stressful event

coping a conscious attempt to manage stress and anxiety; may be physical,
cognitive, or affective

completed suicide the taking of
one's own life

crisis an experience of being confronted
by a stressful event in which an individual
is unable to cope or solve problems

crisis intervention a therapeutic
framework for intervention that includes
short-term, action-oriented facilitation

equilibrium a state of psychological
and physiological balance; a condition in
which contending forces are equal

hardiness an individual's level of
commitment, control, and challenge
when confronted with stressful situations

fight or flight response aggressive action/behavior a person would take
or withdrawal that would occur if confronted with moderate to severe stress;
autonomic physiological responses occur
(i.e., increased blood pressure, increased
heart rate, dilated pupils)

helplessness a state that may arise
when a client has a condition in which he
or she is dependent on an outside source
for life support

hopelessness a subjective state in
which an individual sees limited or no
alternatives or personal choices available and is unable to mobilize energy on
own behalf

internal locus of control individual believes that his or her behaviors
are guided by his or her own choices
and efforts

locus of control individual believes
that destiny is controlled either by internal or external forces

resilience the ability to not only survive, but bounce back from traumatic
experiences, and also grow emotionally
and psychologically beyond the precrisis (stressor)

Seyle stress response three
phases can occur during stress and
include alarm (reaction to stress), resistance (organism does self-repair and
stores bodily energy), and exhaustion

suicidal ideation thoughts about,
plans, and/or actual attempts to take
one's life

suicidal threat a direct or indirect
warning that an individual is planning to
take one's life

PRETEST

1 A client presents in the mental health clinic saying, "I didn't expect it. They just told me this morning that I don't have a job any more. I can't think straight. I feel like I'm going crazy." The nurse documents that the client is experiencing which type of crisis?

1. Adventitious
2. Maturational
3. Situational
4. Cultural

2 The client is in a crisis state. At the beginning of the initial assessment interview, what should the nurse assist the client to identify? Select all that apply.

1. Current feelings
2. The realistic nature of the event
3. Others who might be affected by the event
4. An immediate action plan
5. Past emotional traumas

3 A client with suicidal ideation and a specific lethal plan for self-harm was admitted to the hospital. The client's spouse died recently after a very brief illness. The client states, "There's no reason to go on living. My best friend is gone, and I'm all alone now. We did everything together. Now I have no one to turn to or do things with." Which nursing diagnoses are appropriate? Select all that apply.

1. Helplessness related to suicidal attempt
2. Decisional Conflict related to loneliness
3. Risk for Suicide related to hopelessness
4. Social Isolation related to the loss of support system
5. Acute Grief caused from risk for suicide

4 A client seeks assistance at a crisis center. The client describes being intensely anxious and sleepless since assisting with cleanup activities at a school where a student fatally shot a classmate. To assist the client to cope more effectively, what should be the first intervention of the nurse?

1. Arrange for a member of the clergy to visit the client.
2. Advise the client to avoid going near the school for at least six weeks.
3. Send the client to the emergency department for further evaluation.
4. Allow ventilation of feelings.

5 When the nurse is working with a client in crisis, which nursing action is most important?

1. Obtaining complete assessment of the client's past history
2. Remaining focused on the client's immediate problem
3. Determining the relationship of early life experiences and the crisis state
4. Developing an action plan for the client

6 For the third time within a month, a client with borderline personality disorder took a handful of pills, called 911, and was admitted to the emergency department. The nurse overhears an unlicensed staff member say, "Here she comes again. If she was serious about committing suicide, she'd have done it by now." The nurse determines there is a need to teach the staff member which of the following?

1. Clients with personality disorders rarely kill themselves.
2. Each suicidal attempt should be taken seriously.
3. Exploration of suicidal ideas and intent should be avoided.
4. The nurse should prepare the client for direct inpatient admission.

7 A client has been treated in the surgical intensive care unit after sustaining a self-inflicted gunshot wound. The client is now admitted to a psychiatric unit. The nurse schedules time to meet with the client on a one-to-one basis to assist the client with which goals? Select all that apply.

1. Explore current life events that led to the suicide attempt.
2. Initiate contact with the nurse spontaneously.
3. Discuss past suicidal ideations and behavior.
4. Enter into a contract for safety with the nurse.
5. Identify post-discharge living arrangements.

8 A client who admits to having frequent suicidal ideations is admitted to the psychiatric inpatient unit. During the assessment interview, the client says, "I really don't need to be here. I'm very much at peace with myself now." The nurse should make which interpretation about this client?

1. Has resolved suicidal feelings and is no longer at risk for self-harm
2. Is ready to be discharged from the inpatient setting
3. Continues to be at significant risk for suicide
4. Has concluded that the risk for self-harm is no longer present

9 A female client presents to the crisis center as a victim of attempted rape earlier that day. She is initially distressed, but after venting her feelings with the nurse, she states she will be able to overcome the incident. She says she feels she has control over her emotions, and has had to deal with stressful events in the past. She states "I guess this is not as bad as what I've been through in the past. I left my abusive husband five years ago; it motivated me to get my master's degree." The nurse considers that which characteristics are potentially facilitating a healthy recovery for the client from this event? Select all that apply.

1. Resilience
2. External locus of control
3. Hardiness
4. Internal locus of control
5. Appraisal of stressor

10 A suicidal client is placed on one-to-one observation. When the nurse accompanies the client to the bathroom, the client loudly shouts, "I'm sick of being followed around and treated like a child who can't be trusted." What would be the best response by the nurse?

1. "I understand that you do not like this, but I must be able to see you at all times to make sure you are safe."
2. "You don't have to be so loud. I do trust you, but I can't change the rules for you."
3. "Since this is upsetting to you, leave the door open and I'll wait outside it for you."
4. "Being angry and uncooperative won't change anything. I can't leave a suicidal client alone."

➤ *See pages 42–45 for Answers and Rationales.*

I. OVERVIEW OF CRISIS

    A. Definition of *crisis*: an experience of being confronted by a stressful event in which the individual is unable to mobilize **coping** actions and problem solving

1. Crises are self-limiting, lasting from four to six weeks, during which time there is a potential for either increased psychological vulnerability, return to the precrisis state, or personal growth (i.e., strengthened sense of self and/or newfound problem-solving abilities)
2. Change or loss threatens the individual's **equilibrium**; all crises have some aspect of loss, whether perceived or actual; loss can include a person, object, hope, or a dream
3. Tension, mild to moderate anxiety, and/or panic accompany a crisis, making it challenging and difficult to cope and problem solve
4. Feelings of hopelessness and/or helplessness result from anxiety or panic and are accompanied by emotional and cognitive disorganization
5. Due to this disorganization, ineffective coping occurs; the individual is incapable of exploring alternatives and problem solving; loss of psychological and/or physiological equilibrium ensues, which further evokes physiological, cognitive, and/or affective responses
6. Examples of physiological responses during stress include the interaction of neuroendocrine axes, the **fight or flight response**, and/or the **Seyle stress response**
7. Examples of cognitive responses during stress include positive reactions (i.e., **resilience**, **hardiness**) and/or negative responses (i.e., disorganized thought, poor judgment)

8. Examples of affective responses during stress include (i.e., sadness, anger, hostility, avoidance)
9. During a crisis, communication with significant others is often interrupted, decreased, or completely terminated

B. Developmental phases of crisis
1. Initial increase in tension and/or anxiety as the stimulus continues, discomfort is experienced and endures
2. Failure to succeed in coping with the untoward stimulus contributes to an already distressful and anxious state
3. Additional tension and/or mild to moderate anxiety forces mobilization of internal and external resources, and physiological energy whereby emergency problem-solving efforts are attempted; the client outcome at this time will be either of the following:
   a. Redefining the problem
   b. Resigning oneself from attempts of achieving set goals, as they are now viewed as unattainable
4. If the problem cannot be suppressed, or resolved, or if the anxiety escalates too far, the client may reach a state of severe anxiety or may panic

C. Characteristics of a crisis
1. The stimulus or threat is beyond the person's usual experiences
2. The precipitating event (threat, stimuli) is usually identified
3. Previously developed coping mechanisms are ineffective and fail
4. Mild to moderate anxiety, tension, and panic
5. Client perceives a threat to own integrity (may seem as life threatening) and/or a threat to established goals
6. Crisis are classified as maturational, situational, or cultural
7. Maturational crises involve normal life transitions that evoke changes in an individual's self-perception in role, status, and/or integrity; crisis occurs when the person is unable to adapt to functioning at the new maturational level; examples of transitional periods in one's life include adolescence, parenthood, and marriage
8. Situational crises involve an external event that disturbs the person's equilibrium (i.e., loss, change) and threatens consistency between self-behaviors, values, and/or beliefs
9. Situational crises can be either accidental or unexpected events; examples of situational crises include loss of a job, loss of a loved one, or divorce; examples of unexpected events include natural and man-made disasters (crises resulting from unexpected environmental and other disasters are sometimes referred to also as *adventitious crises*)
10. Cultural crises may coexist with culture shock; this occurs when adapting to a new culture or returning to one's own culture after being assimilated into another culture; an example of a culture shock is when a soldier returns home to his or her family and country after being on active duty for two years

D. Balancing factors determining the client's response to crisis
1. The individual's **appraisal of stressor** (perception of the event)
2. The individual's past experiences with coping mechanisms
3. The individual's **locus of control**: research has shown that persons with an **internal locus of control** (when realistic) tend to have increased self-determination
4. The individual's preestablished coping mechanism
5. The individual's protective factors: history of resilience, hardiness, current support systems, and available resources and/or ability to access and accept help

E. Individual risk factors
1. Intensity and degree of impact of exposure
2. History of traumatic events/abuse

Practice to Pass

List and define two types of crises. Give an example of each.

3. History of or current psychiatric illness
4. History of violence to self or others
5. Poverty
6. Deficiency in or lack of resources
7. Weak (or lack of) support systems

F. **Goals for treatment**

1. The client will remain free of self-harm
2. The client will not harm others
3. The client will identify the specific problem(s) related to the event/problem
4. The client will verbalize thoughts and feelings related to the event

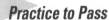

Practice to Pass

Identify balancing factors that determine the client's response to a crisis situation.

5. The client will analyze the event/problem and express own perceptions of the event
6. The client will identify and seek help from support systems
7. The client will explore alternative solutions for coping with the crisis
8. The client will participate in choosing an action plan to help get through the crisis
9. The client will implement an action plan
10. The client will experience decreased anxiety and tension
11. The client will begin to verbalize enhanced self-esteem
12. The client will return to the precrisis state

II. NURSING PROCESS DURING CRISIS

A. **Assessment**

1. Identify the history of the presenting problem
   a. Focus on the nature of the crisis—not on the past history
    b. Facilitate client to identify the immediate problem(s) at hand
   c. Determine the client's perception of problem (appraisal of stressor)—how threatened is he or she?
   d. Assess the client's communicative response for emerging past memories (experiences, trauma, loss) that may be magnifying the problem
   e. Assess the client's communicative response for emerging themes
   f. Assess the client's cognitive appraisal of event—identify any faulty thinking, delusions, or misinterpretations
2. Identify the client's current feelings, strengths, and resources
   a. Encourage client in a nonjudgmental manner to express current feelings
   b. Validate the client's current feelings as real and assist client to accept them
   c. Facilitate the client to express personal strengths
   d. Acknowledge the client's strengths
   e. Acknowledge that the client ultimately makes own decisions
   f. Assess client's resources (i.e., intellectual, educational, and financial)
3. Assess client's support systems (i.e., family members, friends, religious community)
   a. Identify client's living situation and relationships with persons whom he or she lives with
   b. Identify available resources
   c. Identify spiritual and religious belief systems
4. Assess for potential for violence to self
5. Ask the client if he or she has ever been treated for depression
6. Ask the client if he or she has any other psychiatric history or current illness
7. Ask the client if he or she has a problem with substance use, dependence, or abuse
   a. Ask the client in a matter-of-fact, direct manner if he or she has had suicidal thoughts

      b. Determine if the client has the means to harm/kill self (i.e., guns in house, access to medications with potential for overdose); determine lethality

      c. Determine if client can contract with nurse to maintain safety and identify an action plan if suicidal ideation increases or client feels he or she will act on ideas to harm self

  8. Refer client immediately for psychiatric evaluation if suicide risk; *do not leave client alone*

B. Nursing diagnoses useful during a crisis

  1. Nursing diagnoses related to safety/harm

      a. Risk for Self-Directed Violence

      b. Risk for Other-Directed Violence

      c. Risk for Self-Mutilation

  2. Nursing diagnoses related to coping

      a. Anxiety

      b. Ineffective Individual Coping

      c. Defensive Coping

      d. Coping, Compromised Family

      e. Hopelessness

      f. Powerlessness

         1) Stress Overload

         2) Risk for Post-trauma Syndrome

         3) Situational Low Self-Esteem

      g. Risk for Spiritual Stress

      h. Risk for Comprised Human Dignity

      i. Readiness for Enhanced Power

  3. Nursing diagnoses related to cognitive, perceptual, and communication problems

      a. Acute Confusion (i.e., disorientation)

      b. Decisional Conflict

      c. Sensory/Perceptual Alterations (i.e., visual or auditory hallucinations)

      d. Disturbed Thought Process (i.e., illusions, delusions, ideas of reference, inability to make decisions)

      e. Impaired Verbal Communication

      f. Readiness for Enhanced Self-Concept

  4. Nursing diagnoses related to behavioral responses

      a. Impaired Social Interaction

      b. Social Isolation

      c. Powerlessness

      d. Ineffective Role Performance

C. Planning and implementation for clients in crisis

  1. Crisis intervention may be useful in deterring the impact of short- and long-term trauma

      a. Examples of types of crisis interventions

         1) Psychological first aid (PFA): this preventive approach is for persons who survive disaster; principles of PFA are calmness, promoting safety, community effectualness, social connectedness, and optimism; psychological first aid may alleviate short- and long-term untoward psychological problems of trauma exposure

         2) Individual approach: this approach involves nurse addressing client's individual characteristics; interventions work to rehabilitate psychological integrity, provide education, restore effective coping mechanisms, and mobilize support systems

Practice to Pass

List five biological responses to stress or a crisis.

          3) Generic approach: this approach targets individuals and large groups as efficiently as possible; interventions include debriefing that works toward recalling the event, purging of feelings related to the event, crisis psychoeducation, and support groups

   2. General principles of planning and crisis intervention

      a. Mutual goal planning between nurse and client/family and/or significant other; often the nurse must use a directive approach

      b. Goals are set based on the specific assessment data and nursing diagnoses

      c. Overarching goals

         1) Establishing a relationship with the client

         2) Identifying the current problem(s) at hand

         3) Identifying and reducing any perceptual distortions the client may have

         4) Alleviating/reducing the level of anxiety

         5) Promoting engagement of support systems (i.e., family and friends)

         6) Reinforcing healthy coping behaviors, enhancing self-esteem

         7) Validating client's ability to problem solve

      d. Examine any client feelings that may interfere with or block the ability to cope adaptively

      e. Teach the client how to ask for help from others and utilize available resources

      f. Identify previously acquired adaptive coping strategies and assist the client to modify and expand these coping strategies

      g. Teach and encourage the use of expression of feelings, comfort strategies, and self-care activities

      h. Focus on problem resolution in a step-by-step, concrete way, first focusing on alternative solutions to problem solving, then selecting and acting on realistic potential solutions

      i. Consider involving the client in a crisis group, which helps clients feel less isolated and engages in group problem solving to identify alternatives

      j. Involve family in crisis intervention, as other members of the family often experience the crisis

D. Evaluation/outcomes for clients in crisis: measured by comparing actual outcomes to the goals of treatment and client response to nursing interventions

   1. The client will remain free of self-harm

   2. The client will not cause harm to others

   3. The client has clearly identified the current problem(s) at hand

   4. The client's perceptual distortions have been identified and resolved

   5. The client verbalizes a stable sense of self-esteem

   6. The client is able and willing, and perceives the ability to work on the problem

   7. The client's anxiety level has been reduced by use of effective coping strategies

   8. The client will identify, if willing and able, unhealthy coping mechanisms

   9. The client acknowledges his or her need for help, and asks others for help

  10. The client identifies and verbalizes any past and current feelings that may arise related to the crisis

  11. The client demonstrates self-care behaviors

  12. The client verbalizes or writes down a specific action plan

  13. The client begins to implement the action plan

E. Potential for growth

   1. The client identifies and practices new coping skills that may be useful in the future in dealing with stressful and potentially traumatic events

   2. The client verbalizes a renewed or enhanced sense of self-worth

III. PSYCHOPHARMACOLOGY AS TREATMENT DURING CRISIS

 A. Treatment with pharmacologic interventions should not interfere with crisis intervention strategies

  B. A crisis is not a psychiatric illness, nor a prolonged condition; therefore pharmacologic interventions are not the intervention of choice, but may be prescribed for symptom management, and if psychosocial intervention alone is not effective

 C. Pharmacologic agents may be used to treat target symptoms that interfere with the client's ability to function but should not be used as a substitute for crisis interventions

 D. Anxiolytics, specifically benzodiazepines, may be used for anxiety, panic, and anxiety disorders that are exacerbated during a crisis

  1. Common drugs include short-acting anxiolytics: alprazolam (Xanax) and lorazepam (Ativan), and the long-acting anxiolytic clonazepam (Klonopin)

  2. Potential untoward side effects include dizziness and sedation; they may be contraindicated with alcohol use

  3. Potential concern is decreased tolerance and abuse

  4. Dosing must be decreased to one-half in geriatric populations

 E. Hypnotics may be prescribed for short-term treatment of insomnia; examples include zolpidem (Ambien) or eszopiclone (Lunesta)

 F. Antipsychotics may be used during a crisis

  1. Psychosis is not typically caused by a crisis (may see some syptoms in acute stress states); psychotic features may be exacerbated during a crisis in clients who have a preexisting psychotic disorder

  2. Examples of atypical antipsychotics include aripiprazole (Abilify), clozapine (Clozaril), olanzapine (Zyprexa), olanzapine/fluoxetine (Symbyax), risperidone (Risperdal), ziprasidone (Geodon), and quetiapine (Seroquel)

  3. Examples of typical antipsychotics comprise Haldol, thioridazine hydrochloride (Mellaril), chlorpromazine hydrochloride (Thorazine), and fluphenazine (Prolixin)

IV. OVERVIEW OF SUICIDE

 A. *Completed suicide*: the intentional and voluntary taking of one's life

 B. Suicide statistics

  1. Suicide is the tenth leading cause of death in people of ages 1–85+ years in the United States, and is the fourth leading cause of death in the United States in people of ages 18–65 years

  2. Whites are more likely to die from suicide than non-whites

  3. Men are three to four times more likely to commit suicide than women, and the elderly are four times more likely to complete a suicide than those younger

  4. Gay teens are at increased risk of suicide

  5. Pediatric, adolescent, and young adult suicide is the fourth leading cause of death in people ages 10–14 years, and the third leading cause of death in people ages 15–24 years

 C. Characteristics of clients contemplating suicide

  1. Often perceive themselves as isolated; this isolation may be by maintaining physical distance from others and/or manifested by interpersonal discord

  2. There are often feelings of **helplessness**, loss of self-esteem, worthlessness, and **hopelessness**, the latter being most predictive of suicide

  3. Often a **suicidal threat**/plan is the result of a desire to be free from psychic pain

  D. Warning signs of suicide

  1. Personal warning signs that may indicate risk for suicidal ideations and self-injurious behavior include changes in personal habits such as appetite, sleep patterns, personal

appearance, personality, use of alcohol and other drugs, as well as bodily complaints, self-depreciating comments, formulating a will, and/or giving away personal/meaningful belongings.

2. Academic/occupational warning signs include truancy/absenteeism, decline in academic/occupational performance, boredom, apathy, disruptive classroom or work behavior, and anger/hostility toward authority figures

3. Family and social relationship warning signs include decreased interactions with peers and friends; a change in the people the individual is spending time with, and a lack of or absence of romantic relationship

E. **The single most predictive psychiatric disorder for suicide is the** presence of a mood disorder

F. **Anxiety is also a predictor of suicide** and is related to the impulsivity one often feels when anxious

G. **Common myths of suicide**

1. People who talk about suicide won't actually commit suicide
2. People who are serious about suicide will show warning signs or give clues
3. Children do not commit suicide
4. An improvement in mood indicates the risk for suicide is resolved
5. Only people who are depressed commit a completed suicide
6. A written or verbal safety contract is a guarantee that the client will *not* commit suicide

H. **Conscious and unconscious suicidal intention**

1. Conscious **suicidal ideation** includes the client's awareness of the following:
   a. The potential outcomes or results of the suicidal behavior
   b. The potential response of others to the suicidal threats or suicidal attempts
   c. The lethality index of the chosen method of suicidality
   d. The potential rescue possibilities

2. Unconscious suicidal ideation may be more difficult to assess than conscious suicidal ideation
   a. The client's desire to cause self-harm or self-destruction may be beyond conscious awareness
   b. The client may engage in high-risk behaviors that are a way of acting out the unconscious desire for self-harm (e.g., drinking and driving and engaging in potentially lethal activity)
   c. The nurse must pay careful attention to direct and/or indirect means in which the client communicates unconscious suicidal ideations

V. NURSING PROCESS FOR PERSONS AT RISK FOR SUICIDE

A. **Suicide assessment**

1. During initial assessment, question client about any thoughts or feelings related to self-harm; this will include inquiring past history of suicidal attempts, determining suicidal ideations, help the client has sought, and specifics regarding the type of plan the client has made, the client's mental status, available support systems, and lifestyle
   a. Ask questions like "Have you had any thoughts about life not being worth living?" (passive suicidal ideation)
   b. Move from general to specific questions like "Have you had any ideas about killing yourself?"
      1) It is a mistaken impression that the client will volunteer this information without being asked
      2) The nurse must be comfortable asking these questions directly and in a matter-of-fact way

     c. If the client answers yes, ask the client, "Have you thought of or made any plans on how you might harm or kill yourself?"

     d. Levels of lethality may be assessed based on answers to the above questions; ask the client "Do you have access to means to self-harm?" (i.e., do you have a gun in your home?)

     e. Evaluate the lethality of the means (i.e., access to pills, gun)

     f. Take a careful history of previous self-harming behaviors by asking the client such questions as "Have you ever tried to harm yourself or kill yourself in the past?"

     g. Assess perceptions/attitude about death

     h. Complete a mental status assessment to determine evidence of other psychological risk factors; include an assessment of mood, affect, perceptions, thought content, thought process, level of consciousness, memory, level of concentration, intelligence, judgment, and insight

2. Many people experience ambivalence about committing suicide; assessment of these ambivalent feelings is an important role of the nurse

3. Clients may lack emotional or psychic energy to act on suicidal ideations as a result of negative or neurovegetative symptoms they experience; thus the nurse must be aware that a sudden sense of peace or wellness reported by the client may indicate that the client has sufficient psychic energy to carry out a suicidal act

B. Nursing diagnosis related to suicidal ideation/threats

    1. Risk for Self-Directed Violence

    2. Ineffective Coping

    3. Hopelessness

    4. Powerlessness

    5. Chronic Low Self-Esteem

    6. Impaired Thought Process

    7. Social Isolation

    8. Defensive Coping

    9. Risk for Spiritual Distress

C. Goal setting for clients at risk for suicide

    1. The client will remain safe and free of self-harm

    2. The client will verbalize suicidal ideations and discuss these with nursing staff

    3. The client will develop a safety plan with the nursing staff and other members of the treatment team that identifies steps to keep him- or herself safe and ask for help before acting out suicidal/self-harm thoughts

    4. The client will verbalize a decrease or absence in suicidal ideations

    5. The client will verbalize a desire to live and state reasons for living

    6. The client will identify a plan following discharge that includes a commitment to follow up with psychotherapy and adherence to psychopharmacologic interventions

    7. The client will identify a support system

D. Nursing interventions to reduce risk of suicide

    1. Inpatient treatment is indicated if the client is assessed to be at high risk for self-directed violence; inpatient treatment may include voluntary or involuntary admission

    2. Inpatient interventions include providing a safe milieu in which the client's ability to act out on suicidal ideations is minimized

     a. The unit is locked, self-contained, and supervised by trained staff

     b. The unit is kept free of any objects that could be used to cause harm

     c. Prior to, or on admission to the unit, the client is assessed for any items that could cause self-harm; these will be removed, kept in a safe place, and given back at discharge

Practice to Pass

List 10 clues to a client's potential for suicide.

d. The client will be placed on one-to-one observation at all times until the suicide ideation/threats subside

    e. Thereafter, the client then may be placed on checks every 15 minutes depending on agency policy

    f. The nurse will develop a rapport with the client and foster a therapeutic relationship; the nurse will work with the client to develop a safety plan; ongoing safety assessment of the client will continue

    g. The nurse will have ongoing therapeutic communication with the client regarding his or her feelings

    h. The nurse will facilitate the client work toward reengagement with significant others and fulfilling life activities

    i. The nurse should assign the client a roommate when applicable, to reduce solitude

    j. The nurse will ensure that the client swallows (and is not "cheeking") oral medications to hoard for overdose

Practice to Pass

Identify precautions used in ensuring suicidal prevention of a hospitalized client.

    k. The nurse will facilitate the client's participation in a discharge plan that includes a commitment to follow up with psychiatry, therapy, compliance with medications, contact with support systems, emergency contact, and a safety plan

    l. The nurse will understand that, despite use of all proper precautions, a client may still take his or her own life after hospitalization; the ultimate choice for life versus death through suicide is up to the client

E. Evaluations/outcomes for clients contemplating suicide include the following:

    1. The client will remain safe and free from self-directed violence

    2. The client will verbalize the decreased or absence of intensity and severity of suicidal ideations

    3. The client will verbalize a desire to live and state reasons for living

    4. The client will maintain a "no self-harm contract" with staff when indicated

    5. The client will identify a specific safety plan should suicidal ideation worsen and/or reoccur

    6. The client will meet other individualized treatment plan goals as identified

VI. PSYCHOPHARMACOLOGY AS TREATMENT TO PREVENT SUICIDE

A. Pharmacologic intervention used in the presence of suicidal ideations is aimed at treating the underlying anxiety, anxiety disorder, mood disorder, and/or psychotic disorder

B. Mood disorders and suicide

    1. A high correlation exists between mood disorders and suicide, so appropriate treatment of the mood disorders is essential in the treatment of clients at risk for suicide

    2. Federal Drug Administration (FDA) has ruled a warning placed on antidepressants that states after initiation of the medication, an increase in suicidal ideation may exist (see Chapter 4: Mood Disorders, for specifics on antidepressants and mood stabilizers)

C. Serotonin selective reuptake inhibitors (SSRIs) are first-line drugs used for treatment of depression due to mild side effects

    1. Citalopram (Celexa)

    2. Paroxetine (Paxil)

    3. Fluoxetine (Prozac)

    4. Sertraline (Zoloft)

    5. Escitalopram (Lexapro)

D. Tricyclics are not the first-line treatment, due to potential high lethality; when used, the quantity of tablets/capsules dispensed should be prescribed at a minimum and may need to be managed by a family member since the medication can be used for intentional overdose

    1. Amitriptyline (Elavil)

    2. Clomipramine (Anafranil)

       3. Desipramine (Norpramin)

       4. Doxepin (Sinequan)

       5. Imipramine (Tofranil)

       6. Nortriptyline (Pamelor)

E. Other antidepressants such as tetracyclics and serotonin norepinephrine reuptake inhibitors (SNRIs) are prescribed to treat depressive disorders; examples include the following:

       1. Bupropion (Wellbutrin) (psychotherapeutic antidepressant)

       2. Nefazadone (Serzone) (SNRI)

       3. Trazadone (Desyrel) (SNRI)

       4. Venlafaxine (Effexor) (SNRI)

       5. Mirtazipine (Remeron) (tetracyclic, anxiolytic)—often prescribed for clients who cannot gain weight (side effect is weight gain)

       6. Duloxetine (Cymbalta) (SNRI)

F. Monoamine oxidase inhibitors (MAOIs) are not first-line treatment in depressive disorders; clients must comply with a strict tyramine-free diet or a serious and life-threatening disorder called *hypertensive crisis* can occur; MAOIs include the following:

       1. Tranylcypromine (Parnate)

       2. Phenelzine (Nardil)

       3. Isocarboxazid (Marplan)

G. Mood stabilizers are used to treat bipolar disorder, which is characterized by cycling of moods with episodes of mania and depression, and are also associated with suicide; they are treated with two classes of drugs both recognized as mood stabilizers, lithium and antiepileptics

       1. Lithium (Eskalith)

       2. Valproic acid (Depakote)

       3. Lamotrigine (Lamictal) (antiepileptic)

       4. Carbamazepine (Tegretol) (antiepileptic)

Case Study

A 15-year-old male client is transferred from the medical-surgical unit to the pediatric psychiatric unit for a psychiatric evaluation after being stabilized from ingesting an unknown amount of oxycontin. A psychosocial history indicates the client's parents are currently going through a divorce. The family moved from another state one year ago. The teenager has poor attendance at school, declining grades, and has dropped out of football. His mother states he recently has been withdrawing from family and friends and using alcohol and marijuana. A suicide assessment indicates high risk and he is admitted to a pediatric psychiatric hospital.

1. Identify three to five risk factors for suicide for this client.

2. List the top three nursing diagnoses for this client.

3. List at least five nursing interventions for suicidal clients.

4. Identify at least two outcome expectations for this client.

5. What are precautions the nurse should take to ensure the client is safe?

For suggested responses, see page 296.

POSTTEST

1 The client presents in a crisis center saying, "They didn't warn me. After 20 years, my boss just walks in and says I no longer have a job." The client's therapist is ill and unavailable, and the client's immediate family is away and unreachable by telephone. The nurse will interpret that which of the following is the most significant reason that this client is in crisis?

1. The client is misperceiving the event.
2. The client feels confusion and shock about the event.
3. The client cannot process the event with the usual support network.
4. The client is not making sufficient attempts to cope with the event.

2 An unlicensed mental health worker asks the nurse to explain how crisis intervention works. The nurse responds that crisis intervention helps the client to do which of the following?

1. Uncover unconscious processes and early life experiences.
2. Find solutions to an immediate and overwhelming problem.
3. Use new ways of coping with an unexpected major problem.
4. Become aware of personal limitations that led to the crisis state.

3 The client in a crisis state is having difficulty asking for help from significant others. The nurse explains to caregivers that it is important to role model asking for help because, in addition to being anxious and overwhelmed, clients in crisis often exhibit which trait?

1. Uncertainty about how to communicate personal needs
2. Resistant to verbal suggestions about how problems can be approached
3. Hesitant to depend on others for assistance with problem resolution
4. Guarded and protective about talking about anxiety and other feelings

4 A client seeks help in a crisis clinic secondary to having several family members involved in a serious automobile accident. The client speaks in a loud, disorganized manner with frequent changes of subject. Which nursing approach is most likely to be effective?

1. Encourage the client to identify family members involved in the accident.
2. Assist the client locate the chapel or another quiet area.
3. Help the client to identify the problem and possible ways to manage it.
4. Arrange for one-time anxiolytic medication for the client.

5 A client whose life partner recently died from complications of AIDS has learned he has also converted to HIV-positive status. The attending physician's office referred the client to the crisis unit because the client "shut down" emotionally after receiving the lab results. In the initial assessment interview, the nurse's priority is to determine if the client has which of the following?

1. Ideas of self-harm
2. Altered thought processes
3. An available social support network
4. Financial means to obtain medications

6 A young adult client frequently engages in high-risk behaviors, including driving at high speed, drinking excessively, and engaging in high-risk sexual behaviors. The nurse assessing this client should recognize that there is a high probability that which of the following is occurring?

1. Unhealthy grieving is occurring.
2. Unconscious thoughts of suicide are present.
3. Arrested maturation is impairing judgment.
4. Antisocial personality traits are causing disregard for life.

7 A client is admitted to the inpatient unit with a new diagnosis of bipolar disorder, most recent episode mania. The client's history indicates she recently experienced an unresolved crisis; her sister died from a heroin overdose three months ago. The client has been so busy raising her children by herself, and working full time, that she repressed feelings related to the event. The client currently manifests delusions, severe anxiety, and suicidal ideation. The nurse would anticipate which of the following becoming part of her treatment plan? Select all that apply.

1. The client will be placed on one-on-one observation.
2. The client will be placed on a serotonin selective reuptake inhibitor (SSRI).
3. The client will be placed on a mood stabilizer.
4. The client will be placed on an antipsychotic.
5. The client will be placed on an anxiolytic ordered as needed (prn).

8 Five days ago, a client was admitted to the hospital with major depression and suicidal ideations. The suicidal ideations are absent now. Therefore, the client is now preparing for discharge. Which client statement made to the nurse about going home demonstrates that an important outcome/evaluation measure has been met?

1. "I'll finally be able to get some sleep."
2. "I'll be able to take care of my plants again."
3. "I have a list of people that I can call if I need to."
4. "I'll cook for myself."

9 When working with a depressed client who has suicidal ideation, the nurse anticipates that the client may be overwhelmed by personal problems. With this in mind, the nurse should take which action to best assist the client to cope more effectively?

1. Encourage the client to make a list of problems from most urgent to least urgent.
2. Support the client's decision to put off problem solving until outpatient therapy has begun.
3. Encourage the client to work on problems only in group therapy.
4. Take a directive approach and advise the client how to prioritize personal problems.

10 The client has suicidal ideations with a vague plan for suicide. When teaching the family how to care for the person at home, what should the nurse emphasize? Select all that apply.

1. Suicide occurring within the family environment indicates family dysfunction.
2. Warning signs, even if indirect, generally are present before a suicidal attempt.
3. When the client no longer talks about suicide, the risk of suicide has decreased.
4. If a person makes a suicidal attempt and fails, the risk for future suicidal attempts is increased.
5. Family members are responsible for preventing future suicidal attempts.

➤ *See pages 45–47 for Answers and Rationales.*

ANSWERS & RATIONALES

Pretest

1 **Answer: 3** **Rationale:** A situational crisis is one that is often unexpected and unavoidable and causes an acute state of emotional disequilibrium. The stressful event threatens a person's physical, emotional, and/or social integrity. The person feels anxious, overwhelmed, and confused. This

experience is accompanied by a sense of disorganization and an inability to make effective decisions. An adventitious crisis occurs following a major catastrophic event, such as earthquake, hurricane, or war. This type of crisis represents one in which others experiencing the same or comparable event would react similarly. This question describes a unique, personal situation and a response that cannot be generalized to a larger population of individuals. A maturational crisis occurs as part of the person's normal development and maturation. Such crises are predictable and can be expected to occur as individuals age and progress through life events, changes, and stages, such as adolescence and older adulthood. A cultural crisis is a response that occurs while a person is adapting to a new culture or returning to a previous culture after having assimilated into another. There is no indication that this client is in a culturally challenging situation. **Cognitive Level:** Applying **Client Need:** Psychosocial Integrity **Integrated Process:** Nursing Process: Diagnosis **Content Area:** Mental Health **Strategy:** Recall types of crisis responses. Notice that the precipitant event was unexpected and the event applies only to this client. **Reference:** Varcarolis, E., & Halter, M. (2010). *Foundations of psychiatric mental health nursing: A clinical approach* (6th ed.). St. Louis, MO: Saunders Elsevier, pp. 217–221, 457–458.

2 **Answer: 1, 2** **Rationale:** Current feelings and the realistic nature of the event are correct. It is helpful for the client to identify and ventilate personal feelings being experienced. This relieves anxiety, allows the client to feel validated, and prepares the nurse and client to progress to other steps in crisis resolution. The client's perception of the situation should occur very early in crisis intervention. The nurse must have a clear idea of what the problem represents to the client and also be able to identify the current reality the crisis presents for the client. Then action plans can be developed. The focus of crisis intervention is on the individual who is experiencing the crisis response, not on others. The goal is to assist the person in crisis to reestablish equilibrium by using previously effective coping techniques. It is premature to develop an action plan at this time. Complete assessment and analysis of the problem must occur before proceeding to develop an action plan. Past emotional traumas are not explored in crisis intervention. Intervention should focus on the current problem and facilitating the client's coping in order that a return to precrisis baseline may be accomplished. If past emotional traumas become apparent during a crisis, referral for counseling at a later time would be appropriate. **Cognitive Level:** Applying **Client Need:** Psychosocial Integrity **Integrated Process:** Nursing Process: Implementation **Content Area:** Mental Health **Strategy:** Remember that crisis intervention focuses on a current problem and the "here and now." **Reference:** Kneisl, C., Wilson, H., & Trigoboff, E. (2009). *Contemporary psychiatric–mental health nursing.* Upper Saddle River, NJ: Prentice Hall, pp. 794–796.

3 **Answer: 3, 4** **Rationale:** Risk for Suicide related to hopelessness and Social Isolation related to the loss of support system are correct. The client's statement directly indicates feelings of hopelessness, as well as more indirect expressions of risk for suicide. The spouse's death has left the client without adequate interpersonal support to cope with and adjust to a significant loss. The client is experiencing a situational crisis. The client may easily be feeling social isolation because of loss of a key

support system. In order to cope effectively in a crisis situation, individuals must identify and be able to rely on others in their world to support them emotionally both during and after the crisis. While the client is lonely, there is no indication that the client is helpless. Additionally, the question does not indicate there was an actual suicide attempt. Note also that as the diagnosis is written (Helplessness related to suicidal attempt) it says that the suicidal attempt caused helplessness, which is illogical. The client's statement does not suggest difficulty with decision making, although this can be one of the manifestations of a crisis state. Acute Grief caused from risk for suicide does not follow the "problem related to etiologic factor" format. Notice also that the two parts of the nursing diagnosis are reversed. **Cognitive Level:** Analyzing **Client Need:** Psychosocial Integrity **Integrated Process:** Nursing Process: Diagnosis **Content Area:** Mental Health **Strategy:** Look carefully at what the client is saying. The client directly expresses feelings of being alone and isolated. Additionally, there is an indirect message that could indicate suicidal intent. Make sure that the etiologic factor in the nursing diagnosis is shown in the stem of the question. **Reference:** Kneisl, C., Wilson, H., & Trigoboff, E. (2009). *Contemporary psychiatric–mental health nursing.* Upper Saddle River, NJ: Prentice Hall, pp. 787–788, 790, 849–850.

4 **Answer: 4** **Rationale:** Allowing ventilation of feelings is correct. The client is feeling overwhelmed by feelings associated with the crisis precipitant. Before advancing to other interventions, including exploring habitual coping styles and assisting the client with problem solving, the nurse needs to allow the client to freely express emotions being experienced. There is no evidence to suggest that the client would benefit from a visit from clergy. This may be an effective intervention later, but at this point it is not appropriate. The nurse should not make assumptions about this client's religious or spiritual needs. More complete assessment data is needed. Advising the client to avoid going near the school is incorrect because the nurse's first intervention should be to help the client cope with the precipitant and actual event. Emphasis is on perception of presenting event, past experience in coping, available coping mechanisms, and availability of social supports. The client is in a state of emotional crisis that is considered a normal response to the event. Unless the crisis response intensifies and the client develops severe psychologic or physiologic symptoms, the crisis situation should be treatable in a non-hospital setting (not in the emergency department). **Cognitive Level:** Applying **Client Need:** Psychosocial Integrity **Integrated Process:** Nursing Process: Implementation **Content Area:** Mental Health **Strategy:** Note that this client was exposed to an overwhelming stressor and that symptoms began after exposure to the stressor. Consider how you would feel if you had been involved in this situation. Like most other crisis responses, the client's response to this intense situation is understandable. **Reference:** Kneisl, C., Wilson, H., & Trigoboff, E. (2009). *Contemporary psychiatric–mental health nursing.* Upper Saddle River, NJ: Prentice Hall, p. 795.

5 **Answer: 2** **Rationale:** Remaining focused on the immediate problem is correct. Crisis intervention is viewed as a "here-and-now" type of therapy. The only history that is relevant at this juncture is the recent history of events that led up to the crisis. Obtaining a complete past history at this time would impede the nurse's efforts toward assisting in the effective resolution of the client's crisis state and would not be appropriate. Early life experiences are not examined in crisis intervention. The goal is to reestablish equilibrium and return the individual to the precrisis level of functioning. Examination of early life experiences occurs in more traditional insight-oriented psychotherapy. In crisis intervention, the nurse and the client enter into a relationship where action plans are developed jointly. However, it is appropriate for the nurse to be more directive than in other types of interventions. **Cognitive Level:** Analyzing **Client Need:** Psychosocial Integrity **Integrated Process:** Nursing Process: Implementation **Content Area:** Mental Health **Strategy:** Review the steps in crisis intervention. Think also about what makes sense. If the client is currently feeling overwhelmed, doesn't it seem reasonable for the nurse to focus on now, not then? **Reference:** Kneisl, C., Wilson, H., & Trigoboff, E. (2009). *Contemporary psychiatric–mental health nursing.* Upper Saddle River, NJ: Prentice Hall, p. 794.

6 **Answer: 2** **Rationale:** Each attempt should be taken seriously is correct. The risk of suicide is not reduced because a person makes frequent attempts or threats of suicide. Instead, the risk for successful suicide is greater once a single attempt has been carried out. Persons who make verbal threats or attempts are conveying their desperateness and need for assistance in controlling their own impulses for self-harm. Clients with certain personality disorders, including borderline personality disorder, are actually at higher risk for suicide, not lower risk. These individuals are easily overwhelmed and tend to react dramatically to events that others would find more tolerable. The nurse is obligated to provide protection to the client in a suicidal crisis. In every suicidal situation, the nurse must objectively explore the nature, frequency, and specificity of the suicidal thoughts. Talking about this, and determining whether a plan and a means for suicide are present, is a standard part of nursing intervention with the suicidal client. Talking about suicide does not increase the risk for suicide, which is a commonly held myth among non-professionals. There is not enough information to know whether the client will be admitted to an inpatient unit. If a sufficient action plan is developed that will provide for the client's safety outside the hospital, it is possible that the client can be discharged from the emergency department. **Cognitive Level:** Analyzing **Client Need:** Management of Care **Integrated Process:** Teaching

and Learning **Content Area:** Mental Health **Strategy:** Notice that the client has made three suicidal attempts within one month's time. Even if you didn't know that the client had borderline personality disorder, focus on the probability that the client must have a certain sense of desperation to aid in making a selection. **Reference:** Kneisl, C., Wilson, H., & Trigoboff, E. (2009). *Contemporary psychiatric–mental health nursing.* Upper Saddle River, NJ: Prentice Hall, p. 534.

7 **Answer: 1, 3, 4** **Rationale:** A priority goal for the client, once safety has been assured, is to explore life events leading to the decision to die. This can be followed by reviewing current feelings and determining whether the client still has active suicidal urges. If so, the client must be adequately protected while in the inpatient psychiatric setting. When determining potential lethality in a situation with a suicidal client, it is useful to know whether the person has made previous attempts (discussing past suicidal ideations and behavior). If so, this increases the potential lethality of the situation. One of the most effective ways of providing for safety of the suicidal client is to have the client agree (or contract) with the nurse to notify a staff member if the urge to act on suicidal ideas occurs. If the client cannot agree to this, or if the client is very ambivalent or hesitant about agreeing, the nurse should recognize that the risk for self-injury remains very high. It is the nurse's responsibility to initiate contact with the client and to determine whether the risk for suicide is still present; the nurse should not rely on the client to interact spontaneously. The priority should be on continually assessing client's suicidality and keeping the client safe in the present environment, as opposed to identifying post-discharge living arrangements. While discharge planning is important, it is premature at this time. **Cognitive Level:** Analyzing **Client Need:** Psychosocial Integrity **Integrated Process:** Nursing Process: Planning **Content Area:** Mental Health **Strategy:** Recall principles of lethality assessment. The SAD Persons scale would be useful. **Reference:** Varcarolis, E., & Halter, M. (2010). *Foundations of psychiatric mental health nursing: A clinical approach* (6th ed.). St. Louis, MO: Saunders Elsevier, pp. 478–481.

8 **Answer: 3** **Rationale:** The nurse should look beyond the words that the client uses and determine what the underlying meaning is; the client may still be at significant risk for suicide. Improvement in mood and energy often occurs just before the suicidal person carries out a suicidal act. Once a suicidal plan has been made, it is as if the individual feels relieved of a great burden. While the client's words may suggest that the risk of suicide is lessened, the hidden or indirectly expressed message is different. The nurse should recognize that this client may be describing a feeling of relief often experienced by a suicidal client after making a plan to end his or her life. The client may need to be put on heightened suicide precautions and is not ready for discharge. The nurse should realize the client's verbalizations indicate an actual plan to end life may have been made and could be carried out after discharge. Improvement in affect and energy is often observed in suicidal clients right after a suicide plan is made and right before the suicidal client carries it out, so the risk for self-harm is still present. **Cognitive Level:** Analyzing **Client Need:** Safety and Infection Control **Integrated Process:** Nursing Process: Diagnosis **Content Area:** Mental Health **Strategy:** Notice the words *at peace*. Does it seem likely that someone so recently admitted to a psychiatric–mental health unit would feel peaceful? Recognize this as a "red flag" statement. **Reference:** Varcarolis, E., & Halter, M. (2010). *Foundations of psychiatric mental health nursing: A clinical approach* (6th ed.). St. Louis, MO: Saunders Elsevier, pp. 477–479.

9 **Answer: 1, 3, 4, 5 Rationale:** Four options are correct. Resilience is the ability to not only survive, but bounce back from traumatic experiences, and also grow emotionally and psychologically beyond a precrisis state. Hardiness is the individual's level of commitment (control) when confronted with stressful situations. Internal locus of control means the individual believes that her destiny is guided by her own actions. Persons with an internal locus of control tend to do better in crisis situations then those with an external locus of control. An appraisal of stressor is the subjective meaning of how an individual perceives the stressful event. The client sees it as being manageable. **Cognitive Level:** Analyzing **Client Need:** Psychosocial Integrity **Integrated Process:** Nursing Process: Assessment **Content Area:** Mental Health **Strategy:** Listen carefully to what the client is telling you in terms of coping mechanisms that have worked for her in the past. Recall definitions of these mechanisms that often facilitate positive outcomes. **Reference:** Stuart, G. W. (2009). *Principles and practice of psychiatric nursing* (9th ed.). Mosby, Elsevier: St. Louis, p. 246.

10 **Answer: 1 Rationale:** Acknowledging the client's feelings of frustration and reaffirming the need for safety is the priority. The nurse should remain calm and matter-of-fact in this situation while tolerating the client's verbal outburst and allowing for expression of feelings. The nurse's response should include validation of client's feelings and information about the intent of the one-to-one observation, which is to keep the client safe. During one-to-one observation, the nurse must remain at arm's length from the client at all times, including during toileting activities. "Being angry and uncooperative won't change anything…" lacks compassion and is demeaning. While it suggests some awareness of safety considerations and procedure, it fails to express concern for this client's safety. **Cognitive Level:** Applying **Client Need:** Safety and Infection Control **Integrated Process:** Caring **Content Area:** Mental Health **Strategy:** Keep in mind the need to be compassionate and calm while providing for the client's safety. Recognize that what the client is feeling and saying is common and very understandable in situations involving one-to-one care. **Reference:** Fontaine, K. (2009). *Mental health nursing* (6th ed.). Upper Saddle River, NJ: Prentice Hall, p. 604.

Posttest

1 **Answer: 3 Rationale:** This question is asking for the nurse to recognize that availability of social support, one of the balancing factors that determines whether one will enter into a crisis state, is absent. Balancing factors include how the person perceives the event, past experience in coping, available coping mechanisms, and availability of people who can be supportive. There is no indication that the client is misperceiving the event. Feelings of confusion and shock indicate a normal or expected response to an unexpected loss. While the nurse will observe the present state of confusion and shock in assessing the client, this factor does not address why the client is in a crisis state at this time. Going to the crisis clinic for assistance indicates that the client is making a serious attempt at coping. The client is feeling overwhelmed and does not have access to the normal support system. **Cognitive Level:** Applying **Client Need:** Health Promotion and Maintenance **Integrated Process:** Nursing Process: Diagnosis **Content Area:** Mental Health **Strategy:** Recall theory about balancing factors in crisis situations. Determine which of the balancing factors is/are absent. **Reference:** Kneisl, C., Wilson, H., & Trigoboff, E. (2009). *Contemporary psychiatric–mental health nursing.* Upper Saddle River, NJ: Prentice Hall, p. 786.

2 **Answer: 2 Rationale:** Crisis intervention assists a client in resolving an immediate problem that the client perceives as overwhelming. Issues from early life experiences and the client's unconscious processes are not dealt with during crisis intervention. Crisis intervention focuses on the immediate situation and presenting problem. Other issues are dealt with in other therapy modalities and would not be addressed until the presenting crisis is resolved. In early crisis intervention, rather than teaching the client to develop new coping techniques, the client is encouraged to use previously successful coping skills. The emphasis of crisis intervention is on strengths and coping skills of the individual, not on personal limitations. **Cognitive Level:** Applying **Client Need:** Health Promotion and Maintenance **Integrated Process:** Teaching and Learning **Content Area:** Mental Health **Strategy:** To select the correct response, translate more complex theoretical concepts into easily understood language. **Reference:** Kneisl, C., Wilson, H., & Trigoboff, E. (2009). *Contemporary psychiatric–mental health nursing.* Upper Saddle River, NJ: Prentice Hall, p. 791.

3 **Answer: 1 Rationale:** It is natural for clients in crisis to feel isolated and withdrawn. Clients frequently need help communicating with others directly, especially if they place a high value on independence. Role modeling by the nurse helps the client to learn this skill. Being resistant to verbal suggestions is in opposition to a common characteristic of the client in crisis, which is openness to suggestions. Being hesitant is also in opposition to a common characteristic of the client in crisis: readiness to depend on others for assistance with decision making. Most clients in crisis are not guarded and protected; instead, they give free and direct expression to their feelings of anxiety. Severe and panic levels of anxiety are common to crisis states. **Cognitive Level:** Applying **Client Need:** Psychosocial Integrity **Integrated Process:** Communication and Documentation **Content Area:** Mental Health **Strategy:** Realize the client has experienced a crisis. Analyze each option and put yourself in the client's position. Select the option that characterizes how you would expect to act in a crisis situation. **Reference:** Varcarolis, E., & Halter, M. (2010). *Foundations of psychiatric mental health nursing: A clinical approach* (6th ed.). St. Louis, MO: Saunders Elsevier, p. 463.

4 **Answer: 3** **Rationale:** The focus of crisis intervention is on the present, not the past. Particular attention is given to allowing ventilation of current feelings, helping the client with coping mechanisms, and identifying social supports. The focus of the nurse should be on the client, not identifying family members involved. The nurse should keep the client focused and provide direction to avoid fragmentation of the client's efforts. Sending the client to a chapel is not appropriate. The client's behavior and the circumstances require that the nurse respond directly to the client. The client needs to ventilate feelings in order to begin to feel less anxious. Nonpharmacological strategies should be attempted prior to pharmacological strategies (one-time anxiolytic medication). **Cognitive Level:** Analyzing **Client Need:** Psychosocial Integrity **Integrated Process:** Nursing Process: Planning **Content Area:** Mental Health **Strategy:** Apply the principles of presence and support. Also reflect back on the behaviors you observed in a client who was in a crisis state. Consider commonly used crisis intervention techniques and eliminate options that are not included among such techniques. **Reference:** Kneisl, C., Wilson, H., & Trigoboff, E. (2009). *Contemporary psychiatric–mental health nursing.* Upper Saddle River, NJ: Prentice Hall, p. 791.

5 **Answer: 1** **Rationale:** The nurse should recognize that ideas of self-harm are very common in situations of this type. While some clients will not introduce thoughts of self-harm, they will usually talk about suicidal thoughts when asked. The nurse should ask if the client has a plan and the means for suicide. Safety is the priority, and suicidal clients should not be left alone. Altered thought process, availability of social support, and ability to afford medication are important assessment areas after the client's safety has been ensured. **Cognitive Level:** Analyzing **Client Need:** Safety and Infection Control **Integrated Process:** Nursing Process: Assessment **Content Area:** Mental Health **Strategy:** Recognize that this client has just heard news that many people would consider a death sentence. In such situations, suicide as a means of remaining in control is not uncommon. **Reference:** Varcarolis, E., & Halter, M. (2010). *Foundations of psychiatric mental health nursing: A clinical approach* (6th ed.). St. Louis, MO: Saunders Elsevier, p. 461.

6 **Answer: 2** **Rationale:** The nurse should recognize that all the behaviors cited in the stem of the question could result in loss of life. They are therefore considered indicators of

indirect self-destructive behavior. There is no indication of a loss that would have precipitated grieving. While it is true that the client is young and is making unwise choices, there is no indication that the client's development has been arrested. Disregard for the life and needs of others is seen in persons with antisocial personality disorders, but there is no indication in the stem that the client is disregarding or abusing the life of others. **Cognitive Level:** Applying **Client Need:** Psychosocial Integrity **Integrated Process:** Nursing Process: Diagnosis **Content Area:** Mental Health **Strategy:** Look for an option that recognizes the intensity and dangerousness of the client's behaviors. **Reference:** Kneisl, C., Wilson, H., & Trigoboff, E. (2009). *Contemporary psychiatric–mental health nursing.* Upper Saddle River, NJ: Prentice Hall, p. 529.

7 **Answer: 1, 3, 4, 5** **Rationale:** Four options are correct. If left alone the client could harm herself. A high correlation between the presence of suicide and mood disorders exists. It is essential that the mania be stabilized with initiation of a mood stabilizer. The client would benefit from an antipsychotic to treat the delusions. The client needs an anxiolytic to treat the severe anxiety. The client does not need an antidepressant; no signs and symptoms of depression exist. **Cognitive Level:** Analysis **Client Need:** Psychosocial Integrity **Integrated Process:** Nursing Process: Assessment **Content Area:** Mental Health **Strategy:** Assess client's mental status behaviors, identify treatments to keep client safe, and treat target psychiatric symptoms. **Reference:** Stuart, G. W. (2009). *Principles and practice of psychiatric nursing* (9th ed.). Mosby, Inc., pp. 302–304, 327.

8 **Answer: 3** **Rationale:** When a client has been suicidal, it is essential that discharge preparations include a plan for safety including social support contacts that can be used after discharge. This is particularly so if the client has acted on suicidal urges, rather than just having had suicidal impulses. The statement about getting some sleep does not clarify what the client's sleep pattern has been. Additionally, the nurse should remember that disturbed sleep could indicate continuing depressed mood. The statements about caring for the plants and cooking suggest that the client is feeling more energetic and optimistic, which are of course signs of progress. They are, however, not as urgently important as having a post-discharge safety plan. **Cognitive Level:** Analyzing **Client Need:** Safety and Infection Control **Integrated Process:** Nursing Process: Evaluation **Content Area:** Mental Health **Strategy:** Remember that a danger period for suicide among depressed clients is the point at which they begin to improve and have more energy. **Reference:** Varcarolis, E., & Halter, M. (2010). *Foundations of psychiatric mental health nursing: A clinical approach* (6th ed.). St. Louis, MO: Saunders Elsevier, p. 486.

9 **Answer: 1** **Rationale:** Encouraging the client to make a list of problems ranked by urgency is correct. Nurses help reduce the client's feelings of being overwhelmed by helping the client to prioritize concerns and problems. Supporting the client to put off problem solving is not advisable. Working on problem solving within a group setting is one of many ways to solve problems. Being directive and setting the priorities for the client should be avoided. **Cognitive Level:** Applying **Client Need:** Health Promotion and Maintenance **Integrated Process:** Nursing Process: Implementation **Content Area:** Mental Health **Strategy:** Note that the client is feeling overwhelmed by personal problems. Isn't it reasonable to think that if these problems can be managed, the client will no longer feel suicidal? **Reference:** Fontaine, K. (2009). *Mental health nursing* (6th ed.). Upper Saddle River, NJ: Prentice-Hall, p. 604.

10 **Answer: 2, 4** **Rationale:** Warning signs of suicide generally exist but they may not be recognized until after a suicidal attempt or suicidal death. Since almost all suicidal persons are ambivalent about dying, they either consciously or unconsciously communicate their intent to others hoping to be rescued from their own impulses. The nurse should recognize that the risk for future attempts always increases once a person has made an unsuccessful attempt. This means that the nurse should always inquire about past suicidal behaviors and attempts, including those that occurred in the distant past. Suicide is a very individual act that does not necessarily reflect negative relationships in the family. The idea that if the client no longer talks about suicide the risk has decreased reflects a commonly held myth about suicide. Sometimes the person does not talk about suicide because he or she has made a specific plan and has the means to carry it out. Not talking about suicide can be a warning sign, and the nurse and family members need to know this. Family members are not responsible for preventing future suicidal attempts. They should be encouraged to create safe interpersonal and physical environments, but in spite of their best efforts, they may not be able to prevent their family member from ultimate self-destruction. Telling the family members that they are responsible for preventing future suicidal attempts will lead to an increased sense of guilt if their family member successfully suicides at a later time. **Cognitive Level:** Analyzing **Client Need:** Safety and Infection Control **Integrated Process:** Nursing Process: Diagnosis **Content Area:** Mental Health **Strategy:** Look for myths and facts about suicide. Recognize the importance of teaching facts before dispelling myths. **Reference:** Varcarolis, E., & Halter, M. (2010). *Foundations of psychiatric mental health nursing: A clinical approach* (6th ed.). St. Louis, MO: Saunders Elsevier, pp. 477–479.

References

American Psychiatric Association (2000). *Diagnostic and statistical manual of mental disorders* (4th ed. text revision). Washington, DC: American Psychiatric Association.

Center for Disease Control (2011). *Injury prevention and control: Data and statistics.* Retrieved on February 14, 2011, from www.cdc.gov/wisquars/leading causes.html

Center for Disease Control (2011). *Injury prevention and control: Violence prevention.* Retrieved on February 14, 2011, from www.cdc.gov/ViolencePrevention/suicide/

Fontaine, K. (2009). *Mental health nursing* (6th ed.). Upper Saddle River, NJ: Pearson Education.

Fortinash, K., & Holoday-Worret, P. (2008). *Psychiatric–mental health nursing* (4th ed.). St. Louis: Mosby.

Kniesl, C., Wilson, H., & Trigoboff, E. (2009). *Contemporary psychiatric–mental health nursing* (2nd ed.). Upper Saddle River, NJ: Pearson Education.

National Institute of Mental Illness (2011). *Leading causes of death.* Retrieved on January 30, 2011, from www.nimh.nih.gov/statistics/3AGES185.shtml

National Institute of Mental Illness (2011). *Leading causes of death ages 18–65.* Retrieved on January 30, 2011, from www.nimh.nih.gov/statistics/3AGES 1865.shtml

National Institute of Mental Illness (2011). *Reporting on suicide.* Retrieved on January 30, 2011, from www.nimh.nih.gov/health/topics/suicide-prevention/recommendations-for-reporting-on-suicide.shtml

Seyle, H. (1956). *The stress of life.* New York, NY: McGraw-Hill.

Stuart, G. (2009). *Principles and practice of psychiatric nursing* (9th ed.). St. Louis: Elsevier Science.

Townsend, M. (2011). *Essentials of psychiatric–mental health nursing* (5th ed.). Philadelphia, PA: F. A. Davis.

Ursano, R. J., Goldenberg M., Lei, Z., Carlton, J., Fullerton, C. S., Li, H., & Johnson L., et al. (2010). Posttraumatic stress disorder and traumatic stress: from bench to bedside, from war to disaster. *Annals of the New York Academy of Sciences. Psychiatric and Neurologic Aspects of War 1208,* 72–81. Retrieved on February 1, 2011, from www.ncbi.nlm.nih.gov.libproxy.unm.edu//pubmed/20955328

Varcarolis, E. & Halter, M. (2010). *Foundations of psychiatric mental health nursing: A clinical approach* (6th ed.). Philadelphia: Saunders.

3

Infancy, Childhood, Adolescence, and Developmental Disabilities

Chapter Outline

Overview
Potential Causative
  Factors

Assessment
Nursing Diagnoses/
  Analysis

Planning and Implementation
Evaluation
Specific Disorders

NCLEX-RN® Test Prep

Use the accompanying online resource, NursingReviewsandRationales, to test yourself with hundreds of NCLEX®-style practice questions.

Objectives

➤ Identify at least three causative factors pertaining to disorders of infancy, childhood, and adolescence.
➤ Differentiate assessment techniques used in evaluating infants, children, and adolescents.
➤ List four nursing diagnoses associated with psychiatric disorders in infancy, childhood, and adolescence.
➤ Formulate four intervention strategies unique to disorders of infancy, childhood, and adolescence.
➤ Identify five characteristics commonly seen in developmental disorders.
➤ Explain the dynamics of autistic behavior.
➤ Formulate four intervention strategies frequently used for children with developmental disorders.
➤ Describe at least five factors that may contribute to development of an eating disorder.
➤ Differentiate between anorexia nervosa and bulimia nervosa.

Review at a Glance

anorexia nervosa an eating disorder in which a person attempts to lose weight by dramatically decreasing food intake and increasing physical exercise
autistic disorder a focus inward, excluding the external environment

binge eating episodes of continuous eating even when not hungry
bulimia nervosa an eating disorder in which a person attempts to manage weight through dieting, binge eating, and purging

encopresis fecal incontinence
enuresis incontinence of urine, especially nocturnal bedwetting
purging the act of self-induced vomiting to empty the stomach after eating
tic a sudden, repetitive movement, gesture, or utterance

1 The nurse is evaluating the progress of an adolescent bulimic client who is being treated as an outpatient. Which client behavior would indicate that the client is making positive progress?

1. The client asks the nurse many details about the nutritional content of foods.
2. The client shows the nurse a completed food and emotion diary.
3. The client reports enjoying spending time alone after meals.
4. The client describes eating at times other than when the family members eat.

2 A 13-year-old child is brought to the clinic with a history of conduct disorder. The nursing history reveals several facts about the family. Which parent-related factor is most likely to have contributed to the child's conduct problems?

1. Have very high expectations of the child
2. Employ harsh discipline and inconsistent limit setting
3. Are excessively involved in the everyday life of the child
4. Have no other children

3 The parent of a child with attention deficit hyperactivity disorder (ADHD) tells the nurse that the child doesn't follow instructions well. Which strategy should the nurse recommend to the parent?

1. "Teach your child to be less aggressive and more assertive."
2. "Consider developing a predictable daily routine."
3. "It could be helpful to assign a time out if instructions aren't followed."
4. "Try having your child repeat what was said before starting the task."

4 Which primary interventions should the nurse plan for when a child has conduct disorder and is impulsive and aggressive?

1. Limit setting and consistency
2. Open communication and a flexible approach
3. Open expression of feelings
4. Assertiveness training

5 The school nurse is teaching parents of six- and seven-year-old students about anxiety disorders in early school-age children. Which disorder should the nurse emphasize in the discussion?

1. Obsessive-compulsive disorder
2. Depression
3. Separation anxiety disorder
4. Posttraumatic stress disorder (PTSD)

6 When planning the care of a six-year-old child with oppositional defiant disorder, the psychiatric nurse should include which of the following?

1. Reminiscence therapy
2. Emotive therapy
3. Behavior modification
4. Cognitive reframing

7 A three-year-old client has been diagnosed with attention deficit hyperactivity disorder (ADHD). The child's parents report that a friend told them that the child will likely receive "lots of drugs." The nurse should reply that the child will most likely be prescribed which of the following drugs? Select all that apply.

1. Amitriptyline (Elavil)
2. Paroxetine (Paxil)
3. Amphetamine and dextroamphetamine (Adderall)
4. Haloperidol (Haldol)
5. Atomoxetine (Strattera)

8 The nurse employs play therapy with a small group of six-year-old clients. The primary expected outcome is for the clients to do which of the following?

1. Act out feelings in a constructive manner.
2. Learn to talk openly about themselves.
3. Learn how to give and receive feedback.
4. Learn problem-solving skills.

9 The parent of a child recently diagnosed with opposi-tional defiant disorder (ODD) asks the nurse to explain what behaviors are associated with the condi-tion. Which information should the nurse include in an answer? Select all that apply.

1. Cruelty
2. Stealing
3. Argumentativeness
4. Irritability
5. Arson

10 The school nurse is planning a community education program about childhood mental health problems that appear to be genetically transmitted. While conducting the program, the nurse will emphasize information about which problem?

1. Anxiety states
2. Sleepwalking
3. Enuresis
4. Oppositional defiance disorder

➤ *See pages 58–59 for Answers and Rationales.*

I. OVERVIEW

A. **Although children and adolescents** may experience some of the same mental disorders as adults, their symptoms are often determined by their developmental level; other disorders may arise in childhood and continue on through adulthood

B. **In evaluating disorders in children and adolescents,** it is important to keep these points in mind:
   1. The diagnosis does not define the person
   2. All behavior has meaning
   3. Behavior does not define the person
   4. Identify the source of the primary problem
      a. The person being assessed (infant, child, or adolescent)
      b. The caregiver (parent or family)
   5. What need the behavior is fulfilling
      a. Attention from significant other(s) (parent, family, caregiver)
      b. Avoidance of task or situation
      c. Expression of some "inexpressible" thing (something the client has no words for)
         1) Pain
         2) Fear
         3) Hunger
         4) Cold/hot
         5) Upper respiratory tract infection, urinary tract infection, constipation
         6) Response to internal stimuli
         7) Withdrawal from "reality"
   6. Whether the behavior is dangerous to self or other
   7. Maladaptive behavior(s) are learned and take time to "unlearn" or replace with socially acceptable behavior(s)

II. POTENTIAL CAUSATIVE FACTORS

A. **Newborns/infants**
   1. Genetic: inborn anomalies passed from parent to newborn/infant
   2. Medical
      a. Perinatal exposure to viruses
      b. Injury during the birth process

3. Environmental
   a. Income status, living situation
   b. Access to health care
   c. Level of education of parent/family
   d. Prenatal and/or perinatal exposure to drugs and/or alcohol or other toxins
B. **Children:** in addition to all of the previously noted factors:
   1. Postnatal injury
   2. Postnatal exposure to chemicals/toxins
C. **Adolescents:** in addition to all of the previously noted factors:
   1. Self-medication
   2. Substance abuse
D. **Developmental theory** is basic to the understanding of infant, childhood, and adolescent disorders; deviation from developmental norms is an important assessment screen and a sign of potential problems

III. ASSESSMENT

A. **Bio-psycho-social-spiritual assessment of client is imperative**
B. **Bio**: biological assessment
   1. Complete medical workup
   2. Medication used in the past, successful or not
   3. Onset of or worsening of symptoms
   4. Description of symptoms
   5. Allergies
   6. Cyclical quality to symptoms
   7. Family history of medical illnesses/substance abuse
   8. Goal of intervention for client
   9. Goal of intervention for parent/family
C. **Psycho**: psychological or psychiatric assessment
   1. Understanding of the disorder
   2. Medications used in the past, successful or not
   3. Family history of psychiatric disorder(s)/substance abuse
   4. Coping mechanisms present and past (successful or not)
   5. Support system
   6. Onset of or worsening of symptoms
   7. Psychiatric evaluation/mental status assessment
   8. Cyclical quality to symptoms
   9. Goal of intervention for client
   10. Goal of intervention for parent/family
D. **Social**: social setting, social network, and social interactions assessment
   1. Support system
   2. Family constellation
   3. Social contacts for client
   4. Social contacts for parent/family
E. **Spiritual**: spiritual assessment (not necessarily religious)
   1. What is important to client
   2. What gives meaning to life of client
   3. What is important to parent/family
   4. What gives meaning to life of parent/family

IV. NURSING DIAGNOSES/ANALYSIS

A. Anxiety related to separation from parents; school phobia; unrealistic concerns over past behaviors and future events

B. Fear related to unfamiliar people and situations

C. Impaired social interactions related to problems with peers; antisocial behaviors

D. Low self-esteem related to low achievement in school; beliefs that others do not understand them; frequent criticism from self and others

E. High risk for violence directed at others related to aggression; antisocial behaviors

F. High risk for self-directed violence related to poor impulse control leading to accidents; repetitive behavior such as head banging; risk-taking behaviors; poor judgment and poor concentration; suicide or self-inflicted harm

G. Impaired physical mobility related to unusual motor behavior

H. Impaired thought processes related to loose association; poor concentration

I. Impaired verbal communication related to an inability to formulate words; labile mood

J. Impaired family processes related to intensified parent–child conflict; dysfunctional family communication

V. PLANNING AND IMPLEMENTATION

A. Psychopharmacological interventions

Practice to Pass

Which medication is most often prescribed for ADHD and why?

1. Children suffering from major depression may be prescribed selective serotonin reuptake inhibitors (SSRIs); however, no SSRIs are approved for treatment of major depression in children; FDA also has ruled that a warning label be placed on all antidepressants, indicating that suicidal thinking may increase with drug therapy

2. Mood stabilizers such as lithium, valproic acid (Depakote), lamotrigine (Lamictal), and atypical antipsychotics may be used to manage symptoms of bipolar disorder

3. Children experiencing ADHD usually are prescribed methylphenidate (Ritalin), dextroamphetamine (Dexedrine), or amphetamine salts (Adderall); pemoline (Cyclert) is prescribed less often because it takes six to eight weeks to become effective

B. Multidisciplinary interventions

1. Play therapy is used to establish rapport with children, reveal feelings they are unable to verbalize, enable them to act out their feelings in a constructive manner, understand their relationships and interactions with others, and teach adaptive socialization skills

2. Group therapy gives children and adolescents the opportunity to learn to talk openly about themselves, practice active listening, give and receive feedback, learn to help others, and learn new ways of relating to others

3. Parents may be involved in a parallel group to learn growth and development stages, give and receive support, increase parenting skills, and explore their own needs and problems

4. Art therapy is a way for children to express what is contained in the unconscious

5. Guided imagery or visualization can facilitate coping and increase sense of self-esteem

6. Behavior modification identifies behaviors that are unacceptable, those that are acceptable, and consequences for undesirable behavior

7. Community-based programs to improve mental health of children and adolescents include adult mentor plans, youth organizations, and peer-assistance programs

8. Family therapy can facilitate healthy functioning in the family

Practice to Pass

What are some common side effects and toxic effects of CNS stimulants?

C. Nursing interventions

1. Avoid asking multiple questions of children and adolescents; they respond better to active listening and undivided attention
2. Focusing on positive characteristics and behaviors will assist clients to improve their self-esteem
3. Social skills training includes self-expression skills, using support systems, seeing the perspective of others, helping others, assertiveness techniques, and social problem-solving techniques
4. Through the use of problem solving, older children and adolescents can locate information, design solutions, predict consequences, implement strategies, and confirm the outcomes
5. Homework assignments increase clients' active participation in the therapeutic process

VI. EVALUATION

A. **Successfully meeting the outcome criteria** depends on individualizing strategies according to cognitive level, emotional and social development, and physical abilities
B. **Plan and discuss termination of the nurse–client relationship in advance**

VII. SPECIFIC DISORDERS

A. **Obsessive-compulsive disorder (OCD)**: like adults with OCD, children with OCD try to hide symptoms from others
B. **Younger children with posttraumatic stress disorder (PTSD)** may repeatedly act out specific themes of the trauma
C. **General anxiety disorder (GAD)**: characterized by unrealistic concerns over past behavior, future events, and personal competency
  1. Social phobia is a persistent fear of such things as formal speaking, eating in front of others, using public restrooms, and speaking to authorities
  2. Separation anxiety is more common in children than in adolescents; the child may need to remain close to the parent(s), and the child's worries focus on separation themes
  3. Selective mutism is the steady failure to speak in specific social situations where speaking is expected
D. **Depression**
  1. Depression in infants may be exhibited with frozen facial expression, weepy and withdrawn behaviors, weight loss or failure to thrive, and an increased incidence of infections
  2. Depression in toddlers may be noted by a sad or expressionless face; they may experience delays or regression in developmental skills; they may become apathetic or clingier; and may have an increase in nightmares
  3. Depression in preschoolers may be exhibited by a loss of interest in newly acquired skills, frequent negative self-statements, thoughts of self-harm, **enuresis** (incontinence of urine, especially nocturnal bed wetting), **encopresis** (fecal incontinence), anorexia, or binge eating
  4. School-age children who are depressed may have problems with depressed, irritable, or aggressive moods; academic difficulties; eating and sleeping disturbances; self-criticism; and suicidal ideation and plans
  5. Adolescents who are depressed exhibit antisocial behavior, aggression, intense labile moods, difficulties at school, withdrawal, hypersomnia, and very low self-esteem
  6. Seasonal affective disorder (SAD) is more frequent after puberty, especially in girls
  7. Bipolar disorder is frequently misdiagnosed as ADHD, conduct disorder, or schizophrenia when it occurs in adolescents

Practice to Pass

What are some problem behaviors associated with mood disorders in school-age children?

Practice to Pass

What are some problem behaviors associated with mood disorders in adolescents?

E. **Attention-deficit hyperactivity disorder (ADHD)**
   1. Children with ADHD have impulsive behavior and seek immediate gratification
   2. Children with ADHD have labile emotions, and they have difficulty maintaining interpersonal relationships
   3. They have an extremely short attention span, which may be accompanied by learning disabilities
   4. The exact cause of ADHD is unknown, but it likely involves genetic factors, anatomical abnormalities, neurotransmission problems, and environmental factors
F. **Oppositional defiant disorder (ODD) and conduct disorder (CD)**
   1. Children with ODD are disruptive, argumentative, hostile, and irritable; they have social problems with peers and adults and impaired academic functioning
   2. Children with CD engage in antisocial behavior that violates the rights of others: physical aggression, cruelty, stealing, robbing, arson; relationships with peers and adults are manipulative and used for personal advantage
G. *Autistic disorder*
   1. Children with autistic disorder spend hours in repetitive behavior, have bizarre motor and stereotypical behaviors, have severely impaired communication, poor social skills, and are often mentally retarded
   2. Age at onset is usually prior to age three (most frequently noted between 18 and 36 months); it is a lifelong disorder
   3. Parents often report the infant does not want to cuddle, makes no eye contact, is indifferent to affection or touch, and has little change in facial expression
   4. Other associated behavioral problems may include hyperactivity, aggressiveness, temper tantrums, hypersensitivity to touch or hyposensitivity to pain, and self-injuring behaviors such as head banging or hand biting
   5. Children with autism will exhibit ritualistic behavior and prefer rigid, unchanging routines, and they are likely to act out if these routines are changed
   6. Communication with others is greatly impaired because client may be mute, may utter sounds only, or may repeat words or phrases over and over
   7. Thus, these children fail to develop interpersonal relationships, which leads to social isolation that is heightened by difficulties with communication and possible mood disorder
H. **Asperger's disorder**
   1. Impaired social interactions
   2. Repetitive behaviors that interfere with areas of functioning
   3. No significant delays in areas other than social interactions
I. **Tic disorders**
   1. **Tic** disorders involve sudden, rapid, recurrent, stereotyped movements and/or sounds
   2. They are more noticeable or severe during times of stress but are less pronounced or reduced in intensity when focused intently on an activity, such as watching television, reading, or playing a video game
   3. They can be classified into one of three disorders
      a. Tourette disorder is characterized by multiple motor tics and one or more vocal tics that occur either simultaneously or at different times; there is not a tic-free period for more than three months; the diagnosis implies that symptoms have occurred for at least one year or more
      b. Chronic motor or vocal tics involve either vocal or motor tics, but not both; the diagnosis implies that symptoms have occurred for at least one year or more
      c. Transient tic disorder: a tic disorder that does not last longer than 12 months
   4. Generally the severity and frequency of symptoms decline as the child progresses through adolescence into adulthood

J. Eating disorders

1. People with anorexia lose weight by dramatically decreasing their food intake and/or sharply increasing their amount of physical exercise

2. People with bulimia remain at near-normal weight and develop a cycle of minimal food intake, followed by binge eating, and then purging

3. The two disorders have many features in common, and a person can revert from one disorder to the other

4. Obesity
    a. Psychosocial factors contributing to the development of obesity include learned patterns of eating, overeating to manage negative feelings, and viewing food as a reward
    b. Leptin, produced by a gene for obesity, travels to the brain, where it affects appetite and metabolic rate
    c. Obese people are no more prone to emotional problems than are people of normal weight; it is the internalization of the culture's hatred and rejection that contributes to the psychological problems of obese people

5. **Anorexia and bulimia**
    a. **Anorexia nervosa** is an eating disorder in which a person attempts to lose weight by dramatically decreasing food intake and increasing physical exercise
    b. **Bulima nervosa** is an eating disorder in which a person attempts to manage weight through dieting, binge eating, and purging
    c. Behaviors associated with anorexia and bulimia are compulsions and rituals about food and exercise, phobic responses to food, **binge eating** (eating a large portion of food in short time [fewer than two hours], and the associated sense of loss of control), **purging** (the act of self-induced vomiting to empty the stomach after eating), and the abuse of laxatives and diuretics
    d. Affective characteristics include multiple fears, dependency, and a high need for acceptance and approval from others
    e. Cognitive characteristics include selective abstraction, overgeneralization, magnification, personalization, superstitious thinking, dichotomous thinking, distorted body image, self-depreciation, and perfectionist standard of behavior
    f. In U.S. society, thinness is equated with attractiveness, success, and happiness; this is a contributing factor to eating disorders
    g. Eating disorders are considered to be culture-reactive syndromes in the Western world
    h. Physiological characteristics include fluid and electrolyte imbalances, decreased blood volume, cardiac arrhythmias, elevated BUN, constipation, esophagitis, potential rupture of the esophagus or stomach, tooth loss, dental enamel erosion, swollen salivary glands, Russell sign, menstrual problems, and weight loss
    i. Concomitant disorders include depression, social phobias, panic attacks, obsessive-compulsive symptoms, and substance abuse
    j. Neurobiological factors in the development of eating disorders include 5-HT dysregulation, low levels of endorphins, and a genetic predisposition
    k. Intrapersonal theorists consider low self-esteem, problems with identity formation, anxiety intolerance, and maturational problems to be factors in the development of eating disorders
    l. Cognitive theorists believe that cognitive distortions and dysfunctional thoughts contribute to disordered eating patterns
    m. The family system of a person with an eating disorder may be enmeshed; family members may have difficulty with conflict resolution and have high ambitions for achievement and performance

Practice to Pass

What are two appropriate nursing diagnoses for clients with eating disorders?

n. Feminist theorists consider that women's preoccupation with their bodies results from the cultural ideal of thinness, and that their identity and self-esteem depend on physical appearance

o. Antidepressant medication (SSRI) is more helpful in treating bulimia than anorexia

Case Study

You are working in a community mental health center. A mother reports that her 10-year-old boy has become unmanageable, and she no longer knows how to cope with his behavior. At home, the boy is a bully, insisting on having his way. He takes toys from his siblings, causing arguments and crying, but seldom plays with the toy for more than a few minutes. He has difficulty staying in his chair at school, misses important information, and disrupts other children while they are working.

1. What data would be helpful to you in making an accurate assessment of the boy's problem?

2. What questions would you ask the mother to learn more about the child's bullying behaviors?

3. What indications do you have that the boy is not suffering from a pervasive development disorder, such as autistic disorder?

4. If the boy's practitioner placed him on a CNS stimulant for ADHD, what outcome would you expect of the medication?

5. Select two interventions that you think could be helpful in managing the child's behaviors.

For suggested responses, see page 296.

POSTTEST

❶ The nurse is caring for a four-year-old child. To elicit information about the child's feelings, the nurse offers the child a series of pictures showing facial expressions and asks the child to point to the picture that shows the child's own feelings. The nurse bases these actions on which developmental concept?

1. Sullivan's concept of dynamism
2. Piaget's concept of preoperational thinking
3. Freud's concept of mechanisms of the ego
4. Erickson's concept of industry versus inferiority

❷ The nurse is providing community education about autism to a group of parents. The nurse concludes that teaching has been effective if the parents describe which of the following as common behavioral signs of autism?

1. Highly creative, imaginative play
2. Early development of language
3. Overly affectionate behavior toward parents
4. Indifference to being held or hugged

❸ Which of the following is the highest priority intervention for the nurse who is working with a child with a phobia?

1. Have the child face his or her fear.
2. Decrease fear and anxiety.
3. Protect the child from fears.
4. Allow the child to express fears.

4 The nurse is conducting a community education session about preventing deaths in adolescents. Place in order from most frequent to least frequent the causes of preventable adolescent deaths that the nurse needs to include in the presentation.

1. Accidents
2. Suicide
3. Homicide
4. Acquired immunodeficiency syndrome (AIDS)

5 The nurse is teaching a group of young adolescents about eating disorders. The nurse would consider the sessions effective if the participants state that anorexia nervosa is best defined as an eating disorder that occurs in which individuals?

1. Only in young girls who are depressed
2. Mainly in young girls who perceive themselves to be grossly overweight
3. Primarily in young girls who live in chaotic families
4. In young boys and girls alike

6 The nurse is conducting an in-service education session about the relationship between anxiety and bulimia nervosa. The nurse best describes the relationship by stating when a client has bulimia nervosa, an increase in the anxiety level will generally result in which of the following?

1. Rigidly controlling what he or she eats
2. Binging and purging
3. Overeating
4. Consuming alcohol

7 When assessing an adolescent client for depression, it is most important for the nurse to recognize that depression in adolescents is often which of the following?

1. Similar in presentation to depression in adult clients
2. Masked by aggressive behaviors
3. Situational and not as serious as depression in adults
4. An indication of family dysfunction

8 The school nurse is conducting an assessment to determine if a client has anorexia nervosa. Which statement(s) by the client will most suggest that the client may indeed have anorexia nervosa? Select all that apply.

1. "I don't have periods anymore. I'm glad."
2. "People say I'm skinny, but I'm fat and repulsive."
3. "I want to be a chef and cook for other people."
4. "The idea of eating makes me nauseated."
5. "I know that I have a problem with eating."

9 In order to be admitted to an inpatient treatment program, clients with anorexia nervosa must meet the admission criterion of having experienced at least a 30% weight loss over the immediate past six months. The client currently weighs 84 pounds. The nurse calculates that six months ago, this client weighed at least _____ pounds. Record your number rounding to a whole number.

Fill in your answer below:
_____ pounds

10 The adolescent client is depressed. The client's ordered medication is fluoxetine (Prozac). What is the best response by the nurse when the client says, "What will this medicine do inside my brain?"

1. "It will help you feel less depressed."
2. "It will regulate a neurotransmitter called serotonin."
3. "It will raise your level of the brain hormone norepinephrine."
4. "It will balance blood glucose and dopamine levels."

POSTTEST

➤ *See pages 60–61 for Answers and Rationales.*

ANSWERS & RATIONALES

Pretest

1 Answer: 2 Rationale: It is important for the client with an eating disorder to be able to connect emotion to the relief-seeking behavior: bulimia, anorexia, or binging without purging. Completing such a diary in an honest manner will assist the client to recognize that the eating behavior is an unhealthy attempt to deal with uncomfortable feelings. Individuals with eating disorders are often preoccupied with food and its nutritional content, although they do not eat normally. The client's remaining focus of attention in this area does not suggest that therapeutic progress is being made. Persons with bulimia generally isolate themselves from others before, during, and after eating. They eat in secret, ingest unusually large quantities of food while alone, and purge themselves as soon as possible after the meal. One of the means of discouraging purging is to have the individual remain in the presence of others for at least an hour after eating. Also, the client is an adolescent and should continue to function as a member of the family, even if family discord is present (which is often the case in families with bulimic members). **Cognitive Level:** Analyzing **Client Need:** Psychosocial Integrity **Integrated Process:** Nursing Process: Evaluation **Content Area:** Mental Health **Strategy:** Recall that underlying psychological problems and emotions exist in clients with eating disorders. **Reference:** Varcarolis, E., & Halter, M. (2010). *Foundations of psychiatric mental health nursing: A clinical approach* (6th ed.). St. Louis, MO: Saunders Elsevier, p. 357.

2 Answer: 2 Rationale: Harsh discipline and inconsistent limit setting is correct. Conduct problems are considered manifestations of acting out behaviors. Inconsistent limit setting with very harsh discipline is often characteristic of families with children suffering from conduct disorders. Imposing high expectations on the child may cause the child to be anxious, but this parental behavior is not generally thought to be directly related to conduct disorders. Being excessively involved in the child's life may indeed make the child anxious, but it is not directly related to conduct disorders. Conduct disorders occur in one-child and multichild families. **Cognitive Level:** Analyzing **Client Need:** Psychosocial Integrity **Integrated Process:** Nursing Process: Diagnosis **Content Area:** Mental Health **Strategy:** Look carefully at the options. Notice that limit setting is the only one that deals with behaviors, or conduct. **Reference:** Fontaine, K. (2009). *Mental health nursing* (6th ed.). Upper Saddle River, NJ: Prentice Hall, p. 437.

3 Answer: 4 Rationale: The child with ADHD has difficulty concentrating and maintaining a focus. Behavior that is seen as resistant may actually result from the child's not having properly understood what has been said. If the child repeats what was heard, the parent will be able to know if the intended message was actually received. If not, the message can be sent again in simple, concrete language. It is also helpful for the parent to know that giving only one instruction at a time is likely to be more effective than giving a complex set of instructions at the same time. The other options are useful techniques to employ when the child has ADHD, but they address an area of functioning that is not shown in the parent's statement. **Cognitive Level:** Analyzing **Client Need:** Health Promotion and Maintenance **Integrated Process:** Nursing Process: Implementation **Content Area:** Mental Health **Strategy:** Look exactly at the parent's statement. The child does not follow instructions. Ask yourself if any of the other options show a relationship to that behavior. **Reference:** Fontaine, K. (2009). *Mental health nursing* (6th ed.). Upper Saddle River, NJ: Prentice Hall, pp. 475–476.

4 Answer: 1 Rationale: Limit setting and consistency is correct. Behavior modification is an effective strategy with children and adolescents. The child is told exactly what behaviors are expected, what is not acceptable, and the consequences for specific undesirable behaviors. These strategies use limit setting and require consistency for correct implementation. Open communication is effective, but a flexible approach to acceptable behavior may be confusing to the child because a flexible approach may be equated with inconsistency. Open expression of feelings and assertiveness training are useful techniques; however, they are more effective within a controlled environment and will not necessarily address impulsive and aggressive behavior. **Cognitive Level:** Applying **Client Need:** Psychosocial Integrity **Integrated Process:** Nursing Process: Planning **Content Area:** Mental Health **Strategy:** Notice that the client has conduct disorder and that specific problematic behaviors are cited. Then select the option that is most directly related to changing behavior. **Reference:** Varcarolis, E., & Halter, M. (2009). *Foundations of psychiatric mental health nursing: A clinical approach* (6th ed.). St. Louis, MO: Saunders Elsevier, pp. 645–646.

5 Answer: 3 Rationale: Separation anxiety disorder is correct. Separation anxiety disorder may develop at any age, although it is most common in children, with the peak onset between seven and nine years old. When it does occur, the child generally has performance and attendance difficulties in school. Obsessive-compulsive disorder is not common in children, although obsessive compulsive personality traits may be present in children this age. While the incidence of depression in children is increasing, it is not as common a problem in this age group as is separation anxiety. Posttraumatic stress disorder can occur in persons of any age, but it is not as common as separation anxiety. As with adults, PTSD in children occurs following some intensely emotionally painful event, which is not an average occurrence for children. However, separation anxiety is considered more common. **Cognitive Level:** Applying **Client Need:** Psychosocial Integrity **Integrated Process:** Nursing Process: Planning **Content Area:** Mental Health **Strategy:** Recall statistics about normal growth and development and mental health disorders in children. **Reference:** Fontaine, K. (2009). *Mental health nursing* (6th ed.). Upper Saddle River, NJ: Prentice Hall, p. 248.

6 **Answer: 3** **Rationale:** Behavior modification is correct. Behavior modification is quite effective with young children and adolescents. The child is told what is expected, what is not acceptable, and what the consequences will be for undesirable behavior. The child is rewarded for changes in behavior. Reminiscence therapy is indicated for clients who have memory deficits. It is often used with the geriatric population, particularly individuals with dementia. Emotive therapy is more effective in older children. The young child with oppositional defiant behavior is often very emotive, but in an inappropriate way. While cognitive reframing can be used with young children, the first approach should be to modify the behavior. Once the child is behaving more acceptably, other interventions such as cognitive reframing can be used. **Cognitive Level:** Analyzing **Client Need:** Psychosocial Integrity **Integrated Process:** Nursing Process: Planning **Content Area:** Mental Health **Strategy:** Notice that this child's problem is related to conduct, or inappropriate behaviors. Choose the option that is expected to have the most immediate effect on modifying behavior. **Reference:** Fontaine, K. (2009). *Mental health nursing* (6th ed.). Upper Saddle River, NJ: Prentice Hall, pp. 475–476.

7 **Answer: 3, 5** **Rationale:** Amphetamine and dextroamphetamine (Adderall) and atomoxetine (Strattera) are correct. Central nervous system stimulants such as methylphenidate (Ritalin), amphetamine and dextroamphetamine (Adderall) and atomoxetine (Strattera) are the most frequently used medications for ADHD. These medications increase the ability to focus attention by blocking out irrelevant thoughts and impulses. Antidepressants are not typically prescribed for the treatment of ADHD. When they are used for depression, venlafaxine (Effexor) and fluoxetine (Prozac) seem to be the most effective. Haloperidol (Haldol) is an antipsychotic drug that is useful in treating children and adolescents with Tourette's syndrome. It is not commonly prescribed for clients with ADHD. When it is, the nurse must be particularly observant for the occurrence of extrapyramidal side effects (EPS). **Cognitive Level:** Applying **Client Need:** Pharmacological and Parenteral Therapies **Integrated Process:** Teaching and Learning **Content Area:** Mental Health **Strategy:** Consider the classifications of each drug. Recall that children often have paradoxical responses to drugs. Think about recent controversies in the public media about giving stimulant

drugs to children. **Reference:** Fontaine, K. (2009). *Mental health nursing* (6th ed.). Upper Saddle River, NJ: Prentice Hall, p. 468.

8 **Answer: 1** **Rationale:** Acting out feelings in a constructive manner is correct. Play therapy is especially useful for children under 12 because their developmental level makes them less able to verbalize thoughts and feelings. Learning to talk openly about themselves, learning how to give and receive feedback, and learning problem-solving skills are not the intended goals of play therapy. These options require more structured group and individual activities than six-year-olds are able to master. Play therapy provides an opportunity for children to express their feelings through play, without the need for advanced verbal or social skill sets. **Cognitive Level:** Applying **Client Need:** Psychosocial Integrity **Integrated Process:** Nursing Process: Planning **Content Area:** Mental Health **Strategy:** Recall developmentally appropriate behaviors of six-year-old children. Think perhaps about six-year-old children you have known or worked with in clinical settings. **Reference:** Fontaine, K. (2009). *Mental health nursing* (6th ed.). Upper Saddle River, NJ: Prentice Hall, pp. 175–176.

9 **Answer: 3, 4** **Rationale:** Argumentativeness and irritability are correct. Recall that children with ODD are disruptive, argumentative, hostile, and irritable. These children also have social problems with peers and adults and have impaired academic functioning. Stealing, along with cruelty and arson, are included in the antisocial behaviors seen in children with conduct disorder. On the other hand, children with ODD are primarily disruptive, argumentative, hostile, and irritable. **Cognitive Level:** Analyzing **Client Need:** Health Promotion and Maintenance **Integrated Process:** Teaching and Learning **Content Area:** Mental Health **Strategy:** Recall behaviors associated with ODD. Look for behaviors that are oppositional, but not dangerous or antisocial. **Reference:** Varcarolis, E., & Halter, M. (2009). *Foundations of psychiatric mental health nursing: A clinical approach* (6th ed.). St. Louis, MO: Saunders Elsevier, p. 643.

10 **Answer: 3** **Rationale:** Enuresis is correct. Childhood disorders that appear to be genetically transmitted include enuresis, autism, mental retardation, some language disorders, Tourette's syndrome, and attention-deficit hyperactivity disorder (ADHD). Of these, autism is the more pervasive disorder. Anxiety, sleepwalking, and oppositional defiance disorder (ODD) do not appear to be genetically transmitted. **Cognitive Level:** Applying **Client Need:** Health Promotion and Maintenance **Integrated Process:** Teaching and Learning **Content Area:** Mental Health **Strategy:** Notice that autism is a more pervasive problem than the other three options. Recall statistics about childhood mental health disorders to make a selection. **Reference:** Kneisl, C., Wilson, H., & Trigoboff, E. (2009). *Contemporary psychiatric–mental health nursing* (2nd ed.). Upper Saddle River, NJ: Prentice Hall, pp. 700–701.

Posttest

1 **Answer: 2** **Rationale:** In Piaget's concept of preoperational thinking the child can use symbols to represent objects and has the ability to pretend. The child does not think logically. Sullivan describes dynamisms as habits that highlight personality traits. Freud's theory regarding defense mechanisms of the ego is that they are unconsciously motivated ways of dealing with anxiety. According to Erickson's theory, these developmental tasks are appropriate to middle childhood (six to eleven years). **Cognitive Level:** Applying **Client Need:** Health Promotion and Maintenance **Integrated Process:** Nursing Process: Diagnosis **Content Area:** Mental Health **Strategy:** Note the age of the child. Recall the main age-related concepts of the different theorists. **Reference:** Fontaine, K. (2009). *Mental health nursing* (6th ed.). Upper Saddle River, NJ: Prentice Hall, pp. 18–19.

2 **Answer: 4** **Rationale:** Indifference to being held or hugged is correct. Children with autistic disorders are highly indifferent to shows of affection by anyone and do not relate well with others. The way autistic children play is generally ritualistic and repetitive, rather than creative and imaginative and involves inanimate objects rather than people. Rather than having early speech development many autistic children have delayed development of language and mental retardation. Children with autistic disorders are not overly affectionate. They instead are remote and uninvolved emotionally, usually resisting shows of affection by the parents. **Cognitive Level:** Analyzing **Client Need:** Psychosocial Integrity **Integrated Process:** Teaching and Learning **Content Area:** Mental Health **Strategy:** Recall the basic characteristics of autism, particularly the ones that relate to social skills, interest in others, and ability to connect with others. **Reference:** Fontaine, K. (2009). *Mental health nursing* (6th ed.). Upper Saddle River, NJ: Prentice Hall, p. 465.

3 **Answer: 2** **Rationale:** Decreasing fear and anxiety is correct. The primary focus of treating anxiety disorders in children is to decrease fear and anxiety. The most useful techniques for reducing phobias and the anxiety and fear associated with them are desensitization, reciprocal inhibition, and cognitive restructuring. These techniques can be used with any age group. Having the child face his or her fear is often unrealistic because of the developmental level of the child. Children are easily overwhelmed when forced to face fears directly. The primary focus of treating anxiety disorders in children is to decrease fear and anxiety. Decreasing the fear, not protecting from fear, is the aim of treatment. Allowing the child to express his or her fears may be useful but does not necessarily lead to decreased anxiety or fears. **Cognitive Level:** Analyzing **Client Need:** Physiological Adaptation **Integrated Process:** Nursing Process: Implementation **Content Area:** Mental Health **Strategy:** Consider the primary effect associated with phobias. Look for an option that would minimize that effect. **Reference:** Kneisl, C., Wilson, H., & Trigoboff, E. (2009). *Contemporary psychiatric–mental health nursing* (2nd ed.). Upper Saddle River, NJ: Prentice Hall, p. 457.

4 **Answer: 1, 3, 2, 4** **Rationale:** Accidents are the leading cause of death in people from 15–24 years of age. For people 15–24 years of age, homicide is the second leading cause of death behind accidents. Suicide is third; because of their lack of maturation and the developmental issues they face, many adolescents have a fatalistic perspective of the future and view suicide as the only option to manage their pain or problems. Deaths caused by AIDS are least common among the listed causes. **Cognitive Level:** Analyzing **Client Need:** Psychosocial Integrity **Integrated Process:** Teaching and Learning **Content Area:** Mental Health **Strategy:** Rank in the order of frequency, beginning with 1 as the most frequent. Specific knowledge is needed to answer the question. **Reference:** Kneisl, C., Wilson, H., & Trigoboff, E. (2009). *Contemporary psychiatric–mental health nursing* (2nd ed.). Upper Saddle River, NJ: Prentice Hall, p. 746.

5 **Answer: 2** **Rationale:** Mainly in young girls who perceive themselves to be grossly overweight is correct. Anorexia nervosa and other eating disorders are considered to be manifestations of underlying psychological issues, such as control, power, and denied sexuality. If untreated or inadequately treated, complications of anorexia nervosa can lead to death. Anorexia occurs most often in young girls, but increasing numbers of boys and adult women and men are affected as well. Depression often coexists with anorexia, and antidepressants are often given to the client who is anorexic. Anorexia nervosa occurs more often in girls whose families are perfectionistic and rigid. If they develop an eating disorder, girls whose families are more chaotic and impulsive tend to have bulimia nervosa. Anorexia nervosa is not seen exclusively in young boys and girls. Increasing numbers of adult males and females are developing this problem. **Cognitive Level:** Analyzing **Client Need:** Health Promotion and Maintenance **Integrated Process:** Teaching and Learning **Content Area:** Mental Health **Strategy:** Disregard any options that are exclusive and include or infer the word only. **Reference:** Kneisl, C., Wilson, H., & Trigoboff, E. (2009). *Contemporary psychiatric–mental health nursing* (2nd ed.). Upper Saddle River, NJ: Prentice Hall, p. 551.

6 **Answer: 2** **Rationale:** Binging and purging is correct. Bingeing (excessive overeating) and purging (intentionally ridding one's body of food ingested) are characteristics of bulimia nervosa. These behaviors represent unhealthy attempts to cope and increase in frequency as anxiety increases. At the beginning of a bingeing episode, the client loses all self-control and ingests enormous quantities of food in a short period of time. The purging activity temporarily—and falsely—restores the sense of control. Rigid control of what one eats is characteristic of anorexia nervosa. The person with bulimia actually loses all self-control when beginning a bingeing episode and subsequently ingests enormous quantities of food. When the client has bulimia nervosa, overeating does occur, but it is followed by purging, which is used as a relief behavior.

Overeating in the absence of purging is not considered to be a typical behavior associated with bulimia nervosa. Since the client with an eating disorder is using food-related behaviors as an unhealthy means of coping with stress, the client is also likely to use other unhealthy coping methods, such as excessive alcohol intake. However, bulimia nervosa is characterized by bingeing and purging food, not alcoholic beverages. **Cognitive Level:** Applying **Client Need:** Psychosocial Integrity **Integrated Process:** Teaching and Learning **Content Area:** Mental Health **Strategy:** Mentally compare and contrast usual signs and symptoms of the eating disorders. Select the answer that is most specific to bulimia nervosa. **Reference:** Kneisl, C., Wilson, H., & Trigoboff, E. (2009). *Contemporary psychiatric–mental health nursing* (2nd ed.). Upper Saddle River, NJ: Prentice Hall, pp. 552–553.

7 **Answer: 2 Rationale:** Masked by aggressive behaviors is correct. Depression in adolescents is often masked by aggressive and/or behavioral problems. Symptoms are usually different from adults in that adolescents often exhibit intense mood swings, academic difficulties, antisocial behavior, and hypersomnia. While the *DSM-IV-TR* criteria for depression are the same for adults, children, and adolescents, the clinical presentation may be different in the different age groups. Depression in adolescents can have the same consequences as in adults and should be treated seriously. Family dysfunction may or may not be present when the adolescent client is depressed. As with adults who are depressed, there is evidence that depression in adolescence is highly associated with psychobiologic changes, especially in neuroendocrine functioning. **Cognitive Level:** Applying **Client Need:** Psychosocial Integrity **Integrated Process:** Nursing Process: Assessment **Content Area:** Mental Health **Strategy:** Consider normal or expected adolescent behavior. Ask yourself what relationship exists between this developmental level and the way in which the adolescent experiences depression. **Reference:** Fontaine, K. (2009). *Mental health nursing* (6th ed.). Upper Saddle River, NJ: Prentice Hall, pp. 317–319.

8 **Answer: 1, 2, 3, 4 Rationale:** The client that indicates that she no longer has periods is experiencing amenorrhea. *DSM-IV-TR* criteria for anorexia nervosa include the absence of at least three menstrual cycles when there is not another medical reason for this, including pregnancy. Others perceiving the client as skinny but the client perceiving herself as fat indicates that the client has disturbed body image and an unrealistic perception of own body appearance. A client suffering from anorexia nervosa has a weight loss of 15% or greater of normal body weight because of self-imposed dietary restrictions and/or excessive exercise regimes. Even when dangerously underweight and in physiologic peril, the anorexic client will continue to believe that more weight should be lost. The desire to be a chef indicates a serious interest in food, but not in eating it. Persons with anorexia

are indeed often preoccupied with food, but they refuse to allow it into their bodies. It is not uncommon for them to prepare food for others but not to partake of it. Feelings of nausea related to eating indicates a severe revulsion to food, which is common to persons who have anorexia nervosa. It does not suggest that the client will self-stimulate nausea, as would the bulimic individual. Acknowledgment of having an eating problem is not a correct statement. In addition to denying the reality of their extreme thinness, clients with anorexia deny that they have an eating problem. **Cognitive Level:** Analyzing **Client Need:** Psychosocial Integrity **Integrated Process:** Nursing Process: Assessment **Content Area:** Mental Health **Strategy:** Consider *DSM-IV-TR* criteria for anorexia nervosa. Apply them to the client's statements. **Reference:** Varcarolis, E., & Halter, M. (2009). *Foundations of psychiatric mental health nursing: A clinical approach* (6th ed.). St. Louis, MO: Saunders Elsevier, pp. 349–351.

9 **Answer: 120 Rationale:** Set this up as a ratio and proportion problem.
Step 1 (Basic ratio) 84 pounds: 70% = $\times$: 100%
Step 2 (Cross-multiply) .70 $\times$ = 84 pounds
Step 3 (Divide by .70) $\times$ = 120 pounds **Cognitive Level:** Applying **Client Need:** Physiological Adaptation **Integrated Process:** Nursing Process: Assessment **Content Area:** Mental Health **Strategy:** Review basic information about ratio and proportion. No equivalencies are necessary for this calculation, which is based on basic mathematical and algebraic principles. **Reference:** Deglin, A., & Vallerand, A. (2011). *Davis' drug guide for nurses* (12th ed.). Philadelphia: F.A. Davis, version 14.0.2/2011.02.18 Skyscape.

10 **Answer: 2 Rationale:** Regulating serotonin is correct. It is important for the nurse to answer this question in an accurate and factual way that the adolescent can understand. The nurse should know that fluoxetine (Prozac) is classified as a selective serotonin reuptake inhibitor (SSRI) and that it is one of the antidepressants fully approved for treating children and adolescents. By stating it makes one less depressed, the nurse is not responding to what the client has asked. This is a non-answer, and the adolescent is likely to feel demeaned and belittled by it, feeling that the nurse is treating the client like a child. Unlike tricyclic antidepressants, it is not associated with changes in norepinephrine levels and is not known to have a direct effect on blood glucose and dopamine levels. **Cognitive Level:** Applying **Client Need:** Pharmacological and Parenteral Therapies **Integrated Process:** Teaching and Learning **Content Area:** Mental Health **Strategy:** Review basic information about neurotransmitters and antidepressants. **Reference:** Varcarolis, E., & Halter, M. (2010). *Foundations of psychiatric mental health nursing: A clinical approach* (6th ed.). St. Louis, MO: Saunders Elsevier, pp. 64–65.

ANSWERS & RATIONALES

References

American Psychiatric Association (2000). *Diagnostic and statistical manual of mental disorders* (4th ed. text revision). Washington, DC: American Psychiatric Association.

Fontaine, K. L. (2009). *Mental health nursing* (6th ed.). Upper Saddle River, NJ: Pearson Education.

Kneisl, C. R., Wilson, H. S., & Trigoboff, E. (2009). *Contemporary psychiatric–mental health nursing* (2nd ed.). Upper Saddle River, NJ: Pearson Education, Inc.

North American Nursing Diagnosis Association (2008). *Nursing diagnosis: Definitions and classification 2009–2011.* Indianapolis, IN: Wiley-Blackwell.

Stuart, G. W., & Laraia, M. T. (2009). *Principles and practice of psychiatric nursing* (9th ed.). St. Louis, MO: Mosby.

Townsend, M. (2011). *Essentials in psychiatric mental health nursing* (5th ed.). Philadelphia: F. A. Davis.

Varcarolis, E., & Halter, M. (2010). *Foundations of psychiatric mental health nursing: A clinical approach* (5th ed.). St. Louis, MO: Saunders Elsevier.

Chapter Outline

Overview/Classification
Etiology
Assessment

Nursing Diagnoses/Analysis
Planning and
  Implementation

Evaluation/Outcomes
Specific Mood Disorders

Objectives

➤ Discuss at least three etiological theories of mood disorders.
➤ Differentiate between the primary behavioral characteristics of depressive disorders and manic disorders.
➤ Identify four specific treatment modalities used in the treatment of mood disorders.
➤ State examples of at least five nursing diagnoses frequently used in the management of clients experiencing mood disorders.

NCLEX-RN® Test Prep

Use the accompanying online resource, NursingReviewsandRationales, to test yourself with hundreds of NCLEX®-style practice questions.

Review at a Glance

alogia restricted thought or speech
affect the outward expression of emotions ranging from joy, sorrow, anger, etc.
ambivalence experiencing two opposing feelings, thoughts, drives, or intentions at the same time
anergia lack of activity
anhedonia loss of pleasure; loss of interest in pleasurable activities previously enjoyed
avolition lack of goal-oriented behavior
bipolar disorder a mood disorder characterized by variations in mood between depression and elation; also called manic-depressive disorder
bipolar I disorder a mood disorder characterized by a single manic episode with a possible history of major depressive episodes

bipolar II disorder a mood disorder characterized by at least one major depressive episode and past hypomanic episodes but not a full manic episode
catastrophize to exaggerate all failure in one's life
circadian rhythms correlation of a person's activities, behaviors, and external environmental stimuli for a 24-hour period
cyclothymic disorder a mood disorder characterized by a mood range from moderate depression to hypomania, which may or may not include periods of normal mood
dysthymic disorder a mood disorder similar to major depression but remaining mild or moderate in severity
electroconvulsive therapy (ECT) introduction of an electric current through one or two electrodes

attached to the temple; used primarily to treat major depression
flight of ideas fragmented ideas expressed through a rapid shift in speech
grandiosity belief or idea that one has great and/or special powers
group therapy persons coming together to receive psychotherapy
hypomania mild mania
illusions sensory stimulus is perceived in a false perspective
labile rapid shift in mood/affect from one to another
loose associations ideas and thoughts expressed through speech that do not have a logical relationship
major depression a mood disorder characterized by a loss of interest in life events or situations; usually lasts at least two weeks; also known as unipolar disorder

manic-depressive disorder a mood disorder characterized by variations in mood between depression and elation; also called bipolar disorder

mood an individual's state of mind that is exhibited through feelings and emotions

negative symptoms flat affect, anhedonia, alogia, asociality, avolition, apathy, attention impairment, poverty of speech: speech lacks language, depth, and/or meaning

positive symptoms delusions, hallucinations, disorganized speech, bizarre behavior

pressured speech very rapid speech, as seen in mania

schizoaffective disorder a combination of the signs and symptoms of schizophrenia and those of the mood disorders

schizophrenia a psychotic disorder whereby a person has hallucinations,

delusions, disorganized thought and behavior

seasonal affective disorder (SAD) depression that occurs in the fall and winter months, while during the spring and summer the client experiences normal mood or hypomania

unipolar disorder a loss of interest in life and a depressed mood that moves from mild to severe and lasts at least two weeks; also known as major depression

PRETEST

1 The client is scheduled for electroconvulsive therapy (ECT). When teaching the client about what to expect in the post-ECT period, which statements should the nurse make? Select all that apply.

1. "You should expect that you will be able to remember recent events more clearly than you did before you started receiving ECT."
2. "It may hard for you to remember everything that happens during the days and weeks you receive ECT."
3. "It is common for persons who receive ECT to lose all painful memories of early life."
4. "If you notice that you are having changes in your memory, let a staff member know immediately."
5. "Even though modifications have been made in ECT over the years, you may have some disorientation briefly upon awakening from the procedure."

2 The client has bipolar I disorder. Lithium carbonate (Eskalith) 300 mg four times daily has been prescribed. After three days of lithium therapy, the client says, "What's wrong? My hands are shaking a little." What is the best response by the nurse?

1. "Minor hand trembling often happens for a few days after lithium is started. It usually stops in one to two weeks."
2. "There's no reason to worry about that. We won't, unless it lasts longer than a couple of weeks."
3. "Just in case your blood level is too high, I am not going to give you your next dose of lithium."
4. "I wouldn't worry about it if I were you. It's a small tremor that doesn't interfere with your functioning."

3 The client is being admitted to the inpatient psychiatric unit with a diagnosis of major depression. During the initial nursing assessment, the nurse anticipates that the client will acknowledge which of the following? Select all that apply.

1. Suicidal thoughts or plans of suicide over at least the last two weeks
2. History of one depressive episode within the last two years
3. Loss of appetite for approximately three days
4. Loss of interest in previously enjoyed activities
5. Presence of hallucinations for at least three days

4 A client hospitalized with bipolar disorder is in a state of mania. The client, who was admitted on a formal voluntary status, demands immediate discharge from the facility. What should the nurse do first?

1. Notify the police of the client's intention.
2. Inform the client's spouse of the request of the client.
3. Offer the client a contract for safety.
4. Notify the supervisor on the nursing unit.

5 The nurse needs to teach a client about newly prescribed sertraline (Zoloft). Which information is essential to include in the teaching? Select all that apply.

1. Sertraline is most often taken as a morning dose.
2. Constipation is a common side effect of sertraline.
3. Fever and flu-like symptoms are bothersome but not dangerous side effects of sertraline.
4. Clients taking sertraline will usually recognize improvement within one week.
5. It is possible that sexual side effects will occur.

6 A client who had coronary bypass surgery six days ago reports having no appetite and feeling very sad. The client further complains of having difficulty falling asleep. The nurse concludes that it is likely that this client is experiencing which of the following?

1. Disturbed body image
2. Activity intolerance
3. Depressed mood
4. Delayed surgical recovery

7 The client diagnosed with dysthymia asks the nurse to explain what the diagnosis means. When responding to the client, the nurse should state that before dysthymia can be diagnosed, depressed mood needs to be present for at least how long?

1. Two weeks
2. Four weeks
3. One year
4. Two years

8 The hospitalized client is in the acute stage of mania. What is an appropriate client goal for the client to work toward?

1. Spend at least 30 minutes per hour watching TV in the activity room.
2. Participate actively in the psychodrama group each day.
3. Lead other clients in group physical exercises each morning.
4. Maintain distance of two to three feet at all times when interacting with others.

9 The family members of a client in an acute state of mania relate that the client has not slept for four nights. They further report that the client climbed up and down the stairs of a nearby sports stadium for at least six hours without stopping. The client now has blisters on the feet and is perspiring profusely. When planning care for this client, the nurse should give priority to which of the following problems?

1. Risk for Deficient Fluid Volume
2. Ineffective Coping
3. Impaired Skin Integrity
4. Impaired Adjustment

10 The nurse assesses that a client in a state of elevated affect is at risk for self-harm. The nurse then places high priority on including which of the following in the plan of care?

1. A room that is observable from the nurses' station
2. Constant supervision of the client
3. Administration of all medications intramuscularly rather than orally
4. A quiet, non-stimulating private room for the client

➤ *See pages 93–95 for Answers and Rationales.*

I. OVERVIEW/CLASSIFICATION

A. *Mood*

 1. The client's subjective report of his or her emotional state that impacts the current life situation
 2. A change of mood is a normal and expected life occurrence; each individual feels a range of emotions during life, such as anger, depression, hopelessness, happiness, euphoria, and anxiety

B. *Affect*

 1. The emotional tone the client projects may be manifested by the client's statements of his or her mood
 2. Individuals give both verbal and nonverbal cues that reflect how they feel, and what their mood is in their present emotional state
 3. Examples of affect commonly observed in mood disorders are flat, labile, and incongruent

C. When either the mood is fixed or changes in mood are too pronounced and/or interfere with social, academic, and/or occupational functioning, then the individual may be experiencing a psychiatric problem known as a mood disorder

D. Mood disorders are characterized by changes in mood that range from depression to elation and/or mixed (see Figure 4-1); the prevalence of mood disorders annually in the United States is 9.5% of the adult population; severe cases comprise 4.3% of these cases; females are 50% more likely to have a mood disorder

 1. Major depression (unipolar disorder)
    a. A mood disorder whereby a person experiences a loss of interest in life and manifests a depressed mood that shifts from mild to severe; the depressed mood must have occurred for a minimum of two weeks, and coexist with at least four other symptoms
    b. Other key features of major depression can include decreased pleasure in activities, significant weight loss or weight gain, sleep disturbances, psychomotor retardation or agitation, feelings of guilt and/or worthlessness, problems with cognition, and/or social withdrawal
    c. Individuals may also experience thoughts of death and/or suicidal ideation/threats

Figure 4-1

Mood disorders and ranges

Mood Range

Depressed   Normal   Manic

Severe Moderate Mild   Hypomanic   Euphoric

Bipolar disorder

Cyclothymic disorder

Major depression (unipolar disorder)

Dysthymic disorder

    d. If an individual with major depressive disorder experiences delusions and/or hallucinations then a diagnosis of major depressive disorder with psychosis is made

2. **Dysthymic disorder**
   a. A mood disorder that is misclassified as chronic
   b. There is a depressed mood that fluctuates with a normal mood
   c. The depressed mood must last for the duration of a minimum of two years before a diagnosis is made (in children the duration is one year)
   d. The depressed symptoms in dysthymic disorder are less severe than in major depressive disorder

3. **Bipolar disorder** (also called **manic-depressive disorder**)
   a. A mood disorder whereby an individual experiences moods that alternate between depression and elation
   b. The categories of bipolar disorder are defined as follows:
      1) **Bipolar I disorder** is characterized by the occurrence of one or more manic, depressed, and/or mixed episodes
      2) A mixed state is when the individual has rapidly alternating moods between depression and mania
      3) **Bipolar II disorder** is characterized by the occurrence of one or more hypomanic episodes along with one or more major depressive episodes
      4) Depressed moods may be characterized by any of the following: decreased pleasure in activities, significant weight loss or weight gain, sleep disturbances, psychomotor retardation or agitation, feelings of guilt and/or worthlessness, problems with cognition
      5) Manic moods may be characterized by: elation, euphoria, humorousness, flight of ideas, illusions, **grandiosity** (belief that one has great and/or special powers), hyperactivity, sexual overactivity, provocativeness, verbosity, excessive spending, loose associations, pressured speech, decreased food and fluid intake
      6) If an individual with bipolar I disorder or bipolar II disorder manifests delusions and/or hallucinations he or she may be diagnosed as having bipolar (I, II, or mixed) disorder with psychosis

4. **Cyclothymic disorder**
   a. Is a mood disorder with mild to moderate intensity of symptoms
   b. The client demonstrates a range of mood changes that fluctuate between moderate depression and hypomaniac
   c. The hypomanic and depressed moods are not of the sufficiency, severity, duration, or pervasiveness to meet the criteria for major depressive disorder or bipolar disorder

5. **Seasonal affective disorder (SAD)**
   a. Client exhibits a depressed mood that occurs specifically during the fall and winter months only
   b. During the spring and summer the client experiences a normal mood or hypomania
   c. There is a direct correlation with light and the production of melatonin in clients with SAD

6. **Schizoaffective disorder**
   a. Is a psychotic disorder whereby the signs and symptoms of the psychotic disorder **schizophrenia** coexist with those of a mood disorder (i.e., depression, mania, or mixed)
   b. Symptoms

           1) Positive symptoms include delusions, hallucinations, disorganized speech, and/or disorganized behavior

           2) Negative symptoms include flat affect, **anergia**, asociality, **alogia**, **avoliton** and/or apathy, **ambivalence** (experiencing two opposing feelings, thoughts, drives, or intentions at the same time)

           3) Mood symptoms include depressive, manic, or mixed symptoms

7. Co-occurring disorders

  a. Persons who suffer from mood disorders may also suffer from physical and/or psychological co-morbid disorders

  b. Examples of physical disorders include pain, physical illness, stroke, dementia, diabetes, coronary artery disease, cancer, chronic fatigue syndrome, and fibromyalgia

  c. Examples of coexisting psychiatric disorders seen in persons with mood disorders include substance abuse disorders, anxiety disorders (i.e., panic, obsessive compulsive), eating disorders (i.e., anorexia nervosa), somatization disorders, and/or personality disorders

8. Suicide and mood disorders

  a. 15% of the population who experiences major depressive disorder dies by suicide

  b. Epidemiological evidence suggests that there is a fourfold increase in death rates in individuals who suffer from a major depressive disorder and are over age 55

  c. Individuals with major depressive disorder admitted to nursing homes are said to be more likely to commit suicide during the first year after admission

9. In the United States, many individuals with mood disorders go undiagnosed or are misdiagnosed because their symptoms are seen as part of a medical disorder and/or a manifestation of substance abuse

> ### Practice to Pass
>
> A client with major depressive disorder is on suicide precautions. She states she does not want anyone with her when she is taking a shower. What would be your best therapeutic response?

II. ETIOLOGY

A. Biological causative theories of mood disorders

1. Alterations in neurochemical functioning

  a. Have been very prominent in the literature in the past few years

  b. During the "Decade of the Brain" (1990s) researchers studied correlations between the central nervous system's neurotransmitter levels and mood disorders

  c. The neurotransmitters most often identified as relevant in depression and bipolar disorder are serotonin, norepinephrine, dopamine, acetylcholine, and gamma aminobutyric acid (GABA)

  d. Studies investigating these neurotransmitters have found that there can be an alteration in the amount of specific neurotransmitters or a change in neurosynaptic receptor sites in the brain

  e. The result of these changes can be a significant change in mood on a continuum from depression to mania

2. Familial/genetic predisposition

  a. Familial/genetics are a significant contributor to depression; first-degree biological relatives of individuals who have suffered from major depression are at increased risk

  b. Studies conducted with twins show significantly high incidences of depression when one or both parents have been diagnosed with major depression

  c. Familial/genetics are a significant contributor to bipolar disorders; first degree biological relatives of individuals who have suffered from major depressive disorder, bipolar I, and bipolar II are at increased risk

3. Endocrine or hormonal change

  a. Strongly affect an individual's mood and emotions

  b. Irregularities in the thyroid (such as insufficient secretion of thyroxin) are seen as especially important in relation to major depressive disorder

    c. There is also evidence of a strong correlation with depression and the hypothalamic-pituitary-adrenal (HPA) axis that mediates the stress response; studies indicate that malfunction of this system leads to hypersecretion of cortisol and subsequent increase in depressive symptoms

4. Circadian rhythms

    a. Individuals exhibiting changes in circadian rhythms are at increased risk for developing depressive symptoms and mood disorders

    b. Circadian rhythms are responsible for an individual's daily regulation of sleep–wake cycles, arousal and activity patterns, and hormonal secretions

    c. In depressed individuals, these regulatory mechanisms are altered, which can generate alterations in sleep–wake patterns, changes in rapid eye movement (REM), sleep and dreaming patterns as manifested by insomnia, frequent waking, and/or more intensified dreaming; these alterations may be caused by several factors including changes in overall biological functioning, nutritional status, and/or hormones

B. Psychological theories

1. Are derived from the psychoanalytic, cognitive, interpersonal, and behavioral perspectives

2. Psychoanalytic perspective

    a. Freud believed depression occurs because of an ego or object loss in early life

    b. He also believed the loss had a profound effect on the development of mental difficulties in later life

    c. Freud explained depression as an anger turned inward

    d. The loss of a person or object was usually the *trigger* of the depression

    e. In order to help clients regain or attain an improved mental health status, Freud developed psychoanalysis to help the client gain insight into the meaning of thoughts, feelings, and actions

    f. Freud believed insight could help the person gain/regain his or her mentally healthy state

3. Cognitive perspective

    a. The cognitive theorists believe that depression is the outcome when an individual perceives all stressful situations as negative

    b. The person sees most situations in a negative light because of early life experiences of loss of significant people in his or her life and spends most of life believing that life is negative

    c. Cognitive therapy aims to help individuals learn how to perceive the world in a positive light and teaches them how to relearn thinking and decision making based on positive rather than negative cognitive processing

    d. The process of relearning is slow but has an outcome that helps the individual change his or her moment-to-moment thinking from a negative frame of reference to a positive outlook

    e. In essence, the client expels negative perceptions and distortions and replaces them with positive experiences and tools, called *thought stopping*

4. Behavioral perspective

    a. The behavioral therapists believe that individuals develop depression when feelings of helplessness, unworthiness, and powerlessness are the norm during the developmental years

    b. Once learned, these attitudes are used by individuals to evaluate and respond to life situations whereby the individual finds the majority of life outcomes to be negative

5. Sociological perspective

    a. The sociological theorists use the medical, social learning, stress, and antipsychiatric models to explain the development of depression

       b. The medical model theorists believe that depression is treatable using psychotropics, changes in nutrition, and in some cases electroconvulsive therapy (ECT) treatments

       c. The social learning theorists believe that the individual becomes depressed because of repetitively reinforced learned negative attitudes and outlook

       d. Variations of the learned theory include stress theory and antipsychiatric theory

          1) The stress theorists believe that the individual becomes depressed because of an inability to incorporate life experiences, perceptions, social support, biopsychosocial powerlessness, and occurrences of stress into life; this outlook is partially based on problems in interpersonal relationships from attachment figures and other significant persons in one's life

          2) Seyle's stress theory states that persons have a limited amount of resources to cope with stress; stress overload places a person in stages of alarm, resistance, and exhaustion

          3) The antipsychiatric theorists believe that depression is not an abnormal state but rather a reaction to oppression and socioeconomic inequality

III. ASSESSMENT

A. Overview of assessment: intake assessment of individuals with a mood disorder should be conducted in 15- to 20-minute segments so as to allow for rest periods, allow for time to refocus, and allow for a decrease in anxiety and/or psychomotor agitation

    1. Individuals with depression may have insufficient energy to talk, psychomotor retardation, difficulty concentrating, and/or withdrawal symptoms

    2. Individuals with mania may have **pressured speech**, psychomotor agitation, anxiety or irritability, difficulty concentrating, and/or **flight of ideas**

    3. An intake assessment helps the clinician formulate a diagnosis based on the *DSM-IV-TR* criteria, while differentiating other problems/diagnoses such as a medical disorders, substance abuse problems, normal grief/bereavement (symptoms may mimic depression), and attention deficit disorder (symptoms may mimic mania)

B. The initial assessment should include *priority* examination of biological, psychological, and social components of the client's state; physical assessment is completed first to rule out a pathophysiological basis for the symptoms; the initial assessment is then followed by a comprehensive mental status exam, physiological assessment, and assessment of any social/cultural factors

    1. A history of onset of symptoms: when did they begin, are symptoms intermittent, chronic?

    2. A history/physical and head to toe assessment completed by the nurse, followed by a history and physical examination by the health care provider

    3. Current or past history of alcohol or other drug use

    4. Drug screening (serum or urinalysis)

    5. Anxiety level: ask client what his or her anxiety level is on a scale of 1–10 (impulsivity related to increased anxiety levels may be an indicator of suicidal risk)

    6. Current use of prescription, over-the-counter, and/or complimentary/alternative medicines

    7. Levels of suicidality and/or homicidal ideation

    8. Available support systems in the client's life

    9. Level of physiological and psychological stressors currently perceived by the client

    10. Current or past history of trauma and or neglect/abuse

C. The mental status examination is completed on all persons suspected of having a psychiatric disorder, and includes the following:

    1. Appearance: observe age, dress, posture, hygiene, gait, facial expressions, overall nutritional status, and overall health status (persons who are manic or depressed

Practice to Pass

A client states, "I can't believe my mother gave me bipolar disorder; I was adopted!" Is this statement accurate, and what is your best therapeutic response to the client?

may neglect self-care); some persons with mania may be dressed in colorful clothing and/or excessive make up (when female) with a high emphasis on appearance

2. **Speech**: assess volume, rate, amount, and any other distinct features (i.e., slurred, stuttering), slowed speech (as seen in depression), pressured speech (as seen in mania)

3. **Motor activity**: examine level of activity, restless, agitation, grimaces, tics, tremors, psychomotor retardation (as seen in depressive disorders), psychomotor agitation (as seen in depression and mania) compulsions, and signs of extrapyramidal movements (possible medication side effects)

4. **Mood**: ask the client how he or she is feeling; examples related to mania include labile, angry, irritable, euphoric, and examples related to depression include hopelessness, helplessness, depressed, sad, fearful; anxiety may be expressed in both manic and depressed states

5. **Affect**: objectively assess the client's expression of mood; observe both verbal and nonverbal cues; a flat affect is seen in people with depressive disorders; a **labile** affect may be observed in people with mania

6. **Perceptions**: observe for signs of auditory and/or visual hallucinations, **illusions** (ask the client if he or she is hearing voices/seeing anything/anybody); the client may have psychotic features secondary to bipolar or major depressive disorder with psychosis; also observe for any tactile, olfactory, or gustatory hallucinations (can help differentiate organic versus inorganic causes of psychosis)

7. **Thought content**: reflects the thinking inside the client's head; ask the client about obsessions, compulsions, delusions, phobias; the client may manifest some of these psychotic features secondary to bipolar or major depressive disorder with psychosis

8. **Thought process**: this is observed through the client's speech; examples of distortions in thought process include tangentiality, circumstantiality (may be symptomatic of paranoia), word salad, thought blocking, perseveration, neologisms, **loose associations** (as seen in mania), and flight of ideas (as seen in mania)

9. **Level of consciousness**: is the client awake, alert, lethargic, or stuporous; ask the client if he or she is oriented to person, place, and time; disorientation and confusion can occur in both mania and depression; persons who are depressed may be lethargic

10. **Memory**: assess short- and long-term memory (people with any mood disorder may have impairment in both areas)

D. **Physiological assessment**

1. Is based on Maslow's hierarchy of needs theory; indicates priority needs for human survival

2. **Assess nutrition**: (any increase or decrease), inquire if any weight loss/weight gain in last several months, and whether it was purposeful; persons with depressed symptoms may have recent weight loss or weight gain; persons with mania may have recent weight loss (too "on the go" to eat)

3. **Assess hydration**: assess skin turgor, mucous membranes, and specifically ask the client about fluid intake in a 24-hour period; inquire about urinary output; persons with depressed or manic symptoms may be fluid deprived

4. **Assess sleep patterns**: (amount, quality, duration); ask specifically how many hours of sleep the client has per night (if any), when was the last time he or she slept, and if he or she has interrupted sleep; is the client taking any over-the-counter, herbal, or prescribed sleep aids; persons with depressed mood may have a decreased, increased, or interrupted sleep; persons with mania may have not slept for days

5. **Assess bowel patterns**: when was the last bowel movement, and what was the size; any constipation or diarrhea; persons with depression may have constipation secondary to slowed gastrointestinal system

Practice to Pass

Assessment of a client with a mood disorder is often done in 15- to 20-minute segments. Discuss the rationale for this for a client with bipolar disorder, most recent episode mania. Compare the rationale for a client with major depressive disorder.

E. Social assessment

1. Examine the individual's ability to interact and participate in life activities such as work, social interactions, ongoing interpersonal relationships, and the ability to have intimate relationship(s)
2. Clients with mania may demonstrate boundary violations in relationships, and/or have increased social activity
3. Clients with depression may be withdrawn and/or socially isolated; social assessment also includes identifying social support systems

F. Cultural assessment

1. It is the examination of the client's cultural norms and how the present psychiatric characteristics may be viewed in the context of a particular culture
2. Some cultures recognize depression as a moral weakness, or an invasion of the body by evil spirits
3. If the individual displays psychiatric behaviors out of norm of the subgroup, then cultural stigma may place the person at a higher risk for increased devastation, powerlessness, and/or hopelessness
4. Some persons are stoic in nature, and not willing to seek psychiatric help, support systems, and/or resources; they feel shame and guilt if they do not internalize/externalize hardiness and resilience
5. These cultural burdens can contribute to, and complicate the client's already compromised physiological and psychological health

G. Examples of screening tools used to help determine a diagnosis of mood disorders are as follows:

1. Beck Depression Inventory
2. Geriatric Depression Scale
3. Zung Self-Rating Depression Scale
4. Schedule for Affective Disorders and Schizophrenia
5. Manic State Rating Scale

IV. NURSING DIAGNOSES/ANALYSIS

A. Risk for Violence, Self-Directed related to depressed mood, feelings of worthlessness, hopelessness, suicide threats and ideation

1. The client's safety is the nurse's number one priority
2. History of violence to the self is *always* important in determining seriousness of the client's current risk factors for self-harm
3. The client often displays ambivalence or expresses sadness, dejection, hopelessness, or loss of pleasure or purpose in life
4. The nurse must be constantly alert for overt signs of hopelessness
   a. Refusal to eat
   b. Withdrawal from the milieu
   c. Resisting or refusing medications
   d. Cheeks and hoards medications (to overdose later)
   e. Demonstrates self-harm behaviors (attempts to hang self, self-mutilation)
   f. Inability to envision the future
   g. Gives personal and meaningful possessions away
5. The danger for self-harm is elevated as the client begins to regain strength and hope; therefore, frequent and ongoing assessment of the client's levels of hopefulness/hopelessness, self-esteem, mood, affect, and suicidality is essential

6. Antidepressants may begin to take effect in two to four weeks; this may contribute to the client's increased risk for self-harm due to the regaining of strength (may now how the energy to make and/or initiate a suicidal plan)

7. The nurse must be alert for overt signs of hopelessness: refusal to eat; withdrawal from the milieu; resisting or refusing medications; inability to see future for self; suddenly gives away possessions; refusal to sign a "no self-harm" contract

B. **Risk for Violence, Directed at Others** related to poor impulse control and labile affect

1. Clients with bipolar disorder may exhibit emotional difficulties, irritability, impulsive behavior, delusional thinking (including paranoid thinking), and angry responses when ideas are refuted and requests are denied

   a. The client's safety is the nurse's most important priority

   b. Assist client to identify alternative behaviors that are acceptable to client and staff

   c. Encourage client, during calm moments, to recognize antecedents/precipitants to agitation and loss of control

   d. Always give realistic feedback to the client; set limits when necessary

   e. Give positive feedback, when applicable, to the client

2. The danger of risk to harm others is always present in a client who is in a manic state

   a. Some of the more prominent risk factors include the following:

      1) History of harm to self/others during the manic phase

      2) History of another's death as a result of the client's abuse

      3) History of substance use/abuse

      4) Overt attempts to harm self or others

      5) Demonstrated aggressive behavior such as hitting, kicking objects, clenched fists, rigid posture, angry facial features

      6) Impulsive actions

      7) Subjective statements of feeling confined, trapped, or crowded

   b. Nursing interventions to prevent violent behavior include the following:

      1) Place client on one-to-one observation when necessary

      2) Work at establishing trust through the use of therapeutic communication and caring behaviors

      3) Always communicate with client in a dignified, respectful, non-judgmental manner

      4) Decrease environmental stimuli when psychomotor behavior begins to escalate

      5) Continually monitor client's ability to tolerate frustration and/or individual situations

      6) Provide a safe environment by removing objects and/or barriers to prevent accidental or purposeful injury to self or others

      7) When agitation decreases, gradually increase environmental stimuli

      8) Offer alternatives when client requests something that is not available (e.g., "There is no coffee available; how about a glass of juice?")

      9) Be aware of verbal and non-verbal cues that indicate increased agitation, medicate client as necessary *before* client is out of control

      10) Set limits on aggressive behaviors in an assertive, respectful, non-judgmental manner

      11) Initiate seclusion, physical/chemical restraints in the least restricted manner when applicable and as per agency policy and law

C. Ineffective Individual Coping related to lack of energy, inability to concentrate or make decisions, impaired judgment and insight, social isolation, and/or faulty thinking

   1. Clients with mood disorders who have difficulty coping

   a. May be unable to accomplish activities of daily living such as failing to meet basic grooming and hygiene needs

   b. May be unable to concentrate, become easily overwhelmed, and/or have problems remaining in the present

   c. May be unable to problem solve; and may demonstrate problem grouping (stating several problems at once)

   d. May have minimal or no energy to accomplish tasks (i.e., finishing a meal, staying in a group, or completing an activity)

   e. May make known their needs by verbal expression of inability to cope by making statements such as "I can't do this"; and/or the client may have frequent outbursts of crying for no evident reason

   f. May demonstrate impaired judgment and insight and manifest this through statements such as "I was doing okay before I came in here"

   g. May completely isolate themselves from other clients on the unit, staff, visitors, and or may refuse to attend group activities

   h. May verbalize self-depreciating thoughts such as "I'm no good"

   i. May have faulty thinking or delusions as evidenced by statements such as "I will die soon" or "I don't deserve to live"

   2. Nursing interventions for clients with mood disorders who demonstrate inability to cope are as follows:

   a. Provide a safe environment for the client

   b. Observe the client closely; after the antidepressant medication begins to elevate the client's mood, the client may now have the energy to plan and complete a suicide

   c. Assess the client closely when any sudden and dramatic behavioral change occurs

   d. Observe the client closely during unstructured time on the unit

   e. Facilitate the client to focus on strengths rather than weaknesses

   f. Encourage the client to identify meaningful and supportive persons in their lives

   g. Teach the client to learn cognitive and behavioral strategies that facilitate positive thinking and positive self-talk

   h. Teach the client guided imagery to replace negative thoughts with positive thoughts

   i. Encourage the client to express all feelings (untoward or positive) and any needs

   j. Inform family/caregivers and significant others that the client may displace anger on them; reinforce to these persons that the client is learning effective strategies to deal with the anger

   k. Gradually assist the client to become involved in various group activities (i.e., art, exercise, spirituality, psychoeducation) that are offered on the unit

   l. Encourage the client to socialize in an appropriate manner with staff, other clients on the unit, and family members

D. Imbalanced Nutrition: Less/More Than Body Requirements related to inappropriate nutritional intake to meet metabolic needs; lack of interest in eating/food or choosing nutritional foods; aversion to eating; dysfunctional eating pattern (e.g., eating in response to internal cues other than hunger)

   1. For clients with mania this nursing diagnosis can be vital to the overall physiological/psychological well-being and recovery

   a. A client in the manic phase may be preoccupied with racing thoughts, anxious feelings, and/or ineffective coping related to internal or external stimuli

     b. A client in the manic phase may have a general decrease in appetite and/or desire for fluid intake

     c. A client in the manic phase may have psychomotor hyperactivity that interferes with the ability to sit still or take time out to eat or drink fluids

     d. A client in a manic state with psychosis may have an aversion to eating due to paranoid ideation (i.e., food is contaminated or poisoned)

     e. All of these factors can lead to significant and serious weight loss

2. Some of the frequent nutritionally related signs and symptoms associated with the manic state include the following:

     a. At least 20% loss of ideal body weight

     b. Easily distracted from eating or while eating

     c. Psychomotor hyperactivity so does not take time to eat

     d. Appears wary or frightened when offered food

     e. Pale, dry mucous membranes and conjunctivae

     f. Decreased capillary refill

     g. Loose, dry skin; poor skin turgor

     h. Decreased subcutaneous fat; poor muscle tone

     i. Fluid and electrolytes imbalances

     j. Hyperactive bowel sounds

     k. Nausea and vomiting if increased or toxic lithium levels

3. Nursing interventions for nutritional deficits during manic episodes

     a. Weigh client daily, calculate BMI

     b. Calculate client's daily caloric intake when applicable

     c. Offer small frequent meals rich in carbohydrates and protein (six small meals if client cannot tolerate three large meals per day)

     d. Offer nutritious finger foods such as sandwiches, crackers, cheese, and fruit

     e. Offer easy-to-carry drinks that are high in vitamins, minerals, and electrolytes

     f. Assess fluid and electrolyte status

     g. Monitor urinary output every eight hours

     h. Monitor laboratory studies as indicated for dehydration: blood urea nitrogen (BUN), creatinine, hematocrit, and lithium levels

     i. Monitor laboratory studies as indicated for nutritional balance: pre-albumin, albumin, ferritin, hemoglobin, and hematocrit levels

     j. Assess bowel movements daily for frequency and consistency; obtain order for laxatives or stimulants when indicated

     k. Assess for abdominal pain or discomfort

     l. Administer high-fiber foods unless contraindicated

     m. Offer frequent fluids to maintain hydration; encourage 2000 mL in 24 hours unless contraindicated

     n. Monitor and record daily input and output

4. Clients with depression demonstrate a nutritional pattern specific to the depressed mood and/or anxiety; persons with depression may have decreased or increased appetite as manifested by (weight loss or weight gain)

     a. Lack of interest in eating; poor or no appetite

     b. Overeating, binge eating

     c. Aversion to food

     d. Dysfunctional eating patterns

     e. Poor choices of food

     f. Recent weight loss or gain

     g. Poor muscle tone

     h. Decreased or increased subcutaneous fat/muscle mass

     i. Pale conjunctivae and mucous membranes (if dehydrated)

5. Nursing interventions for nutritional deficits during depression
   a. Monitor and record daily intake and output
   b. Explain to client the importance of maintaining an adequate intake of food and fluids to prevent malnutrition
   c. Calculate client's daily caloric intake when applicable
   d. Monitor body weight; depending on the seriousness of the depression and weight problem and response to being weighed, calculate BMI
   e. When possible, obtain and offer client desirable small amounts of food frequently throughout the day (when client is under eating)
   f. Monitor laboratory studies as indicated nutritional balance: pre-albumin and albumin levels
   g. Monitor laboratory studies as indicated for dehydration: blood urea nitrogen, hematocrit
   h. Collaborate with dietician

E. **Disturbed Sleep Pattern** related to biochemical alterations (decreased serotonin) or psychological stress, lack of recognition of fatigue/need to sleep, hyperactivity
   1. Mania
      a. In clients with mania, sleep disturbances can be evidenced by a denial by the client of a need to sleep
      b. The client can also demonstrate changes in behavior and performance, increasing irritability, restlessness, and dark circles under the eyes
      c. The client may experience interrupted nighttime sleep or one or more nights without sleep
      d. Nursing interventions
         1) Identify with client the environmental stimuli that might prevent or interrupt sleep
         2) Restrict intake of caffeine
         3) Offer small snack/warm milk at bedtime or when awake during the night
         4) Encourage activities in morning and early afternoon, and restrict activities during the evening and prior to bedtime
         5) Encourage routine bedtime relaxation techniques
         6) Collaboratively administer medications hypnotics/sedatives as indicated
         7) Record client sleep patterns in chart
   2. Depression
      a. In clients with depression, sleep problems may include difficulty falling asleep, staying asleep, early morning awakening, and sleeping in later then desired; many persons with depression take excessive naps and/or do not have the energy/motivation to get out of bed
      b. The client may indicate not feeling rested, demonstrate hypersomnia, or use sleep as an escape
      c. Nursing interventions
         1) Identify nature of sleep disturbance and variations from usual pattern (difficulty falling asleep, difficulty remaining asleep, early morning awakening, and/or inability to fall back asleep)
         2) Assess what client does when awakened or unable to fall asleep; collaborate with client to make a plan that facilitates healthy sleep patterns
         3) Identify previous nighttime rituals that may have been effective and reestablish them when possible
         4) Decrease intake of caffeine especially later in afternoon or in the early evening
         5) Restrict evening fluids; have client void before sleeping
         6) Provide a light bedtime snack such as warm milk, if not contraindicated

7) Encourage use of bedtime relaxation techniques

8) Reduce environmental stimuli (i.e., lights, noises, television, radios, computer, and cell phones)

9) Encourage use of alternative therapies as client recovers to make available more effective illness-prevention techniques

10) Collaboratively administer hypnotic or sedative medications when other methods fail

11) Record sleep patterns in chart

F. **Spiritual distress** related to a sense of no purpose or joy in life; lack of connectedness to others; misperceived shame and guilt

1. Spiritual distress is a disruption in the life principle that pervades a person's entire being and that integrates and transcends his or her biological and psychosocial nature

2. The client demonstrates a sense of despair and reports feelings of abandonment by God/and or higher power, and may choose not to practice religious/spiritual rituals

3. The client may report ambivalent feelings (doubts) about beliefs, express a sense of spiritual emptiness, and exhibit signs of emotional detachment from self and others

4. Nursing interventions

   a. Allow the client to express feelings and thoughts about religious/spiritual doubt or fears of abandonment

   b. Explore with the client religious/spiritual practices or rituals that have been effective in the past

   c. Refer client to chaplain/spiritual counselor when applicable

   d. Encourage client to attend any spiritual groups on unit if available

Practice to Pass

You are formulating a nursing care plan for a female client who is recovering from a manic episode with a nursing diagnosis of Ineffective Individual Coping. Identify five short-term goals (while inpatient) and five long-term goals for her once she is discharged into the community.

V. PLANNING AND IMPLEMENTATION

A. **Specific treatment modalities**

1. **Electroconvulsive therapy (ECT)**

   a. ECT is used for the treatment of depression; multiple studies have reported it to be highly effective in improving outcomes in clients with severe depression who are resistant to other types of treatment (i.e., antidepressants)

   b. The effects of ECT are effective in many of the cases of depression

   c. The procedure involves the application of electrical energy to bilateral, unilateral, or bifrontal areas of the head; the amount of energy is sufficient to induce a brief grand mal seizure; anxiolytics are held the night before the procedure; the procedure is done under anesthesia; clients are premedicated with an anticholinergic (to decrease saliva) and succinylcholine (a muscle relaxant) to decrease tonic/clonic effects of the seizure

   d. The series of ECT is individualized to the client's needs; 6 to 12 treatments administered three times a week is a common course of treatment

   e. Electroencephalogram (EEG), vital signs including blood pressure, and pulse oximetry monitoring is done during the procedure; electrocardiogram (EKG) is done routinely due to the potential for cardiovascular complications

   f. The potential untoward side effects include headaches, nausea, drowsiness, confusion immediately after the procedure, memory loss (may be temporary or permanent), and in some cases cardiovascular complications; deaths have been reported but are rare; risks related to anesthesia are present

2. Antidepressant medications

   a. Table 4-1 presents an overview of antidepressants, their usual dosage ranges, common adverse effects, and associated nursing responsibilities

Table 4-1   **Medications Commonly Used to Treat Depression**

Drug Class and Name: Generic (Trade)	Usual Adult Dosage Range (mg/day)	Most Common Adverse Effects*	Nursing Responsibilities
Tricyclic antidepressants (TCAs)			
Amitriptyline (Elavil)	75–300	1 (++), 2 (++++), 3 (++++), 4 (++++), 5 (+++)	• Educate the client early about potential side effects
Clomipramine (Anafranil)	75–300	1 (++), 2 (++++), 3 (++++), 4 (++++), 5 (++++)	• Inform client that side effects will diminish with time and, if necessary, there are management alternatives that can be implemented
Desipramine (Norpramin)	75–300	1 (++), 2 (++), 3 (++), 4 (+++), 5 (++)	• Advise client that response will take some time and continued efficacy is essential
Doxepin (Senequin)	75–300	1 (++), 2 (+++), 3 (++++), 4 (++), 5 (++)	• Inform client that first-time treatment for major depression should continue for 6 to 12 months
Imipramine (Tofranil)	50–150	1 (+++), 2 (+++), 3 (+++), 4 (++++), 5 (++)	• Warn client of a possible significant weight gain
Maprotiline (Ludiomil)	50–100	1 (++), 2 (+++), 3 (+++), 4 (+++), 5 (+++)	• Monitor for improvement. If no change or minimum change after two to four weeks it may be necessary to change the medication
Nortriptyline (Pamelor)	25–100	1 (+), 2 (++), 3 (+++), 4 (+++), 5 (++)	• Assess for increased suicidal thoughts
Protriptyline (Vivactil)	10–60	1 (++), 2 (+++), 3 (+), 4 (++++), 5 (++)	
Trimipramine (Surmontil)	50–150	1 (+++), 2 (+++), 3 (++++), 4 (++++), 5 (++)	
Selective serotonin reuptake inhibitors (SSRIs)			
Fluoxetine (Prozac)	20–80	Stimulation, skin rash, weight loss, anticholinergic effects (++), nausea and vomiting, insomnia, and headache; monitor liver function early in treatment	• Inform client to take medication as prescribed; abrupt discontinuation of the drug is contraindicated • Continuously monitor client for side effects or adverse effects, particularly in the area of sexual dysfunction; client may be reluctant to discuss
Paroxetine (Paxil)	20–50	Can cause headache and weight gain, or mild stimulation	
Sertraline (Zoloft)	50–200	Can cause headache, tremor, stimulation, lethargy or insomnia, agitation, anxiety, nausea, diarrhea, constipation, and sexual dysfunction	
Citalopra (Celexa)	20–60		
Escitalopram (Lexapro)	10–20		

Table 4-1	Medications Commonly Used to Treat Depression (Continued)		
Drug Class and Name: Generic (Trade)	**Usual Adult Dosage Range (mg/day)**	**Most Common Adverse Effects***	**Nursing Responsibilities**
Monoamine oxidase inhibitors (MAOIs)			
Phenelzine (Nardil)	45–75	1 (++), 3 (+), 6 (even mania), 8	• Educate client concerning a tyramine restricted diet • Caution client about side effects and adverse effects of the MAOIs • Educate client about careful use of over-the-counter or other prescription medications and be sure client understands the seriousness of the effects • Monitor efficacy of drugs and continuously reeducate client concerning abrupt discontinuation of medication or not taking medications as prescribed
Tranylcypromine (Parnate)	20–30	1 (++), 8 and can cause stimulation	
Atypical antidepressants			
Bupropion (Wellbutrin)	150–450	1 (+), 2 (++), 3 (produces stimulation not sedation), 4 (+), 5 (++++)	• Instruct client about the side effects and adverse effects of the medication, especially seizure risks at higher drug doses • Instruct client concerning the importance of taking this and all medication as prescribed
Trazodone (Desyrel)	50–300	1 (+++), 3 (+++), 4(+), 5 (+), priapism (painful and continuous penile erection)	• Instruct client to take medication as prescribed and monitor for any adverse or side effects • Instruct client to report any signs of sexual dysfunction, especially priapism, immediately
Serotonin norepinephrine reuptake inhibitors (SNRIs)			
Venlafaxine (Effexor SR)	75–300	Both can cause dose-related hypertension, as well as nausea, headache, nightmares, increased anxiety, insomnia, and sweating	• Report adverse effects to prescriber
Duloxetine (Cymbalta)	30–60		

*See Table 4-2 for details.

Note: (+) indicates mild reaction and (++++) indicates severe reaction.

    b. Tricyclic antidepressants (TCAs)
        1) Imipramine (Tofranil), the first antidepressant medication used to treat depression, was introduced in the late 1950s and is still used effectively in the treatment of depressive disorders
        2) TCAs block monoamine (norepinephrine and serotonin) reuptake, thus intensifying the effects of the norepinephrine and serotonin
        3) TCAs can elevate mood, increase activity and alertness, decrease a client's preoccupation with morbidity, improve appetite, and regulate sleep patterns

4) The *initial* mechanism of the TCAs is said to take about one to three weeks to develop while the maximum response is achieved in approximately six to eight weeks

5) Dosing with TCAs is individualized and based *on clinical response* or *plasma drug levels*

6) The normal route for administration of TCAs is oral; amitriptyline and imipramine may be given by intramuscular (IM) injection

7) Nine TCAs, all equally effective, are available in the United States

8) Major differences among these preparations can be found in their side effects; for example, doxepin has sedative effects and could be more effectively used with clients who experience insomnia

9) Other uses for the TCAs are to treat clients with chronic insomnia, panic disorder, and obsessive-compulsive disorder (OCD)

10) Clients who are elderly, have glaucoma or constipation, or have prostatic hypertrophy (males) can be especially sensitive to anticholinergic effects, making desipramine (a TCA with weak anticholinergic effects) more appropriate for use with these clients

11) Although dosing is individualized, TCAs generally have long half-lives; thus, they can be taken daily at bedtime in a single dose

12) Once-daily dosing at bedtime has several advantages, including ease of taking as part of daily routine, promotion of sleep-through sedative effect, and reduced intensity of the daytime side effects

13) Table 4-2 lists the most common adverse effects from TCAs and other antidepressant medications

Table 4-2	Most Common Adverse Effects from Antidepressant Medications	
Effect	**Identifiers**	**Notes**
1. Orthostatic hypotension*	Major decrease in blood pressure with body position changes	The most serious of the common adverse responses to TCAs Advise client to rise slowly, in stages
2. Anticholinergic*	Block muscarinic cholinergic receptors, which produces the following: • Dry mouth • Blurred vision • Photophobia • Constipation • Urinary hesitancy/retention • Tachycardia	Advise client to use sugarless mints, ice chips for dry mouth Advise client to drink adequate fluid, eat bulk-forming foods, and get exercise to prevent constipation Monitor clients with benign prostatic hyperplasia for increased difficulty with urination
3. Sedation*	A common response to TCAs; the cause is blockade of histamine receptors in the CNS	Clients should be advised to avoid hazardous activities if sedation is present
4. Cardiac toxicity*	TCAs can adversely effect the heart's function: Decreasing vagal influence (secondary to muscarinic blockade) Acting directly on the Bundle of His to slow conduction	Rare occurrences Clients over 40 or who have a family history of heart disease should have baseline ECG periodically during treatment
5. Seizures*	Lower seizure threshold	Caution must be taken with clients who have seizure disorders
6. Hypomania*	Mild mania can occur	If hypomania develops, client should be evaluated for drug adverse effects or symptoms of bipolar disorder

Table 4-2	Most Common Adverse Effects from Antidepressant Medications (Continued)	
Effect	**Identifiers**	**Notes**
7. Sexual dysfunction	• Anorgasm • Delayed ejaculation • Decreased libido	Occurs in about 70% of men and women
8. Hypertensive crisis from dietary tyramine	Although MAOIs normally produce hypotension, these drugs can be the cause of severe hypertension if client eats tyramine-rich foods	Always caution clients using MAOIs of the many and serious adverse effects indicated with this class of drugs
9. Drug interactions	Always teach clients the importance of preventing adverse drug effects/drug interactions; see individual classification in Table 4-1 for specific nursing responsibilities	Instruct client to *always* take medications as directed Take over-the-counter medications *only after consulting an appropriate health care professional* Always teach clients of *any* specific instructions for medications they are taking

Reported in Table 4-1 as a +, where (+) indicates mild and (++++) indicates more severe reactions reported.

14) A major consideration for clients at risk for suicide who are taking TCA medications is availability of large amounts of TCA medication; clients taking TCAs should always be hospitalized until the danger of suicide has been ruled out, and they should not have access to a large quantity of the medication

c. Selective serotonin reuptake inhibitors (SSRIs)
   1) Are considered first-line treatment for many cases of depression
   2) This class of antidepressant medications has the same efficacy as the TCAs, causes fewer side effects than the TCAs or MAO inhibitors, and has a decreased time between the time of initial dose and the reporting of initial reduction (two to four weeks) of the signs and symptoms of the depression
   3) SSRIs do not cause hypotension, sedation, or anticholinergic effects, as do the TCAs; the only side effects usually reported are nausea, insomnia, and sexual dysfunction (refer again to Table 4-2 for specific sexual dysfunctions and other mild side effects for each drug)
   4) All of the SSRIs have been found to be effective in the treatment of obsessive-compulsive disorder (OCD)
   5) The mechanism of action for SSRIs is to block the reuptake of serotonin and intensify the transmission at serotonergic synapses; the effects can usually be seen after one to three weeks and are equivalent to those produced from TCAs
   6) The SSRIs are administered orally in liquid or pills; for elderly clients or clients with impaired renal function, low doses are given and increases are done cautiously
   7) Evaluate clients frequently for safety and desired effect of medication

d. Neither selective nor epinephrine reuptake inhibitors (SNRIs) may also be administered for depression
   1) Two examples are venlafaxine (Effexor SR) and duloxetine (Cymbalta), which block reuptake of serotonin and norepinephrine; can precipitate hypertension at higher doses
   2) Potential untoward side effects are similar to those of the SSRIs, but hypertension may occur, so B/P must be closely monitored

e. Monoamine oxidase inhibitors (MAOIs)
   1) MAOIs are still used to treat major depression but only as a second or third choice (when depression is refractive to treatment)
   2) There is also a danger if taking MAOIs at the same time as other antidepressant medications (refer to Tables 4-1 and 4-2 for details)

          3) MAOIs decrease the amount of monoamine oxidase in the liver, which breaks down the amino acids tyramine and tryptophan

          4) This class of medications has some very dangerous adverse effects such as hypertensive crisis when clients ingest tyramine-rich foods

          5) So, clients must maintain a tyramine-free diet when on this medication (see Box 4-1 for a listing of foods to avoid or use cautiously while taking MAOIs)

     f. Atypical antidepressants

          1) Bupropion (Wellbutrin) blocks reuptake of dopamine; can suppress appetite; is without the usual cardiotoxic, anticholinergic, and antiadrenergic side effects (therefore can be used more readily with elderly clients); the most common adverse effects are as listed in Tables 4-1 and 4-2; daily dose should be limited to 450 mg/day to reduce risk of seizures at higher doses

          2) Trazodone (Desyrel) is a second-line agent for the treatment of depression; is usually used in combination with another antidepressant agent; usually is prescribed for treatment of insomnia because of its very pronounced sedative effect; refer to Tables 4-1 and Table 4-2 for common side effects

3. Mood stabilizer medications

     a. Lithium is used for controlling manic episodes in clients with bipolar disorder; is also used for long-term prophylaxis against recurrent mania and depression

          1) Is an inorganic ion that carries a single positive charge; occurs naturally in animal tissues but has no known physiologic functions

          2) Is well absorbed following oral administration and distributes evenly to all tissues and body fluids; mechanism of action is not known

          3) Has a short half-life and high toxicity; is excreted by the kidneys

          4) Instruct clients to maintain a constant sodium intake; sodium depletion will *decrease* renal excretion of lithium, which will cause the drug to accumulate and lead to lithium toxicity

---

Box 4-1

Foods to Avoid with Monoamine Oxidase Inhibitors (can cause hypertensive crisis)

Foods to Avoid
- Dairy products: all cheeses except those listed below; yogurt
- Meats and fish: pickled herring, dried fish, fermented fish, sausage (bologna, salami, pepperoni, and summer sausage), hoisin sauce (fermented oyster sauce for oriental dishes)
- Fruits and vegetables: broad bean pods, tofu, soybean extracts, and fava beans
- Alcohol: draft beer, Chianti wine, aged wines, imported and aged beers, sherry
- Combination foods: pizza, lasagna, soufflés, macaroni and cheese, quiche, liver pate, Caesar salads, eggplant parmigiana
- Other: sauerkraut, soy sauce, yeast products, soups (especially miso), marmite, vegemite, Bovril
- Medications: other antidepressant drugs; nasal and sinus decongestants and cold remedies; allergy, hayfever, and asthma remedies; narcotics (especially meperidine); epinephrine; stimulants; cocaine; amphetamines (weight reduction/anti-appetite)

Consume with Caution
- Cheeses: mozzarella, cottage, ricotta, cream, processed American
- Fruits and vegetables: raisins, prunes, plums, raspberries, bananas, small amounts only of avocado, spinach, canned figs
- Alcohol: red wine, domestic beer, and ales (note: alcohol is a depressant and generally should be omitted from diet of client with depression)
- Other: monosodium glutamate, consume only small amounts of chocolate, caffeine, colas, and nuts
- Medications: insulin, oral hypoglycemics, oral anticoagulants, thiazide diuretics, anticholinergic agents, muscle relaxants

5) It is essential that serum lithium be monitored frequently to detect lithium toxicity, since the *therapeutic level* and the *toxic levels* are very close; the therapeutic range is 0.6 to 1.2 mEq/L, while the toxic level is 1.5 mEq/L or greater

6) In clients with mania, lithium reduces euphoria, hyperactivity, and other symptoms but does not cause sedation; antimanic effects are usually seen five to seven days after initial doses, although the full effect does not usually occur for two to three weeks

7) For many clients, adjunctive therapy with a benzodiazepine can be used to provide the sedation clients need

8) Antipsychotic medications can also be used short term to rapidly decrease the symptoms of psychoses

9) Some adverse effects that have been reported at therapeutic drug levels are fine hand tremors, gastrointestinal upset, thirst, and muscle weakness

10) At toxic levels, more adverse effects are seen, such as persistent GI upset, coarse hand tremor, confusion, hyperirritability of muscles, ECG changes, sedation, and incoordination; at levels in the blood above 2.5 mEq/L, death has resulted

b. Valproic acid (Depakote), carbamazepine (Tegretol), and lamotrigine (Lamictal)

1) Were originally developed and marketed for treatment of seizure disorders (as anti-epileptic drugs)

2) Valproic acid (Depakote) has become a first-line treatment for bipolar disorder, but it can cause hepatotoxicity and thrombocytopenia (risk of bleeding)

3) Carbamazepine (Tegretol) can cause agranulocytosis with increased risk of infection

4) Lamotrigine (Lamictal) can cause Stevens-Johnson syndrome

5) Gabapentin (Neurontin) is commonly prescribed for bipolar disorder

6) Treatment protocols include antiepileptic medication alone, lithium alone, or antiepileptic and lithium, depending on client response and side effects

c. Atypical antipsychotics

1) Include olanzapine (Zyprexa), risperidone (Risperdal), quetiapine (Seroquel), ziprasidone (Geodon), and aripiprazole (Abilify)

2) All of the above are approved for treatment of bipolar disorder

3) Use caution secondary to weight gain and subsequent development of metabolic syndrome

4. Group and individual therapies

a. Have proven to be very effective treatment methodologies for mood disorders; can be done with or without adjunct use of psychopharmacologic agents

b. Some methodologies that have been used to treat mood disorders and associated psychosocial issues include cognitive, behavioral, interpersonal relationship, psychodynamic, family, and group therapy

c. Cognitive therapy

1) Was introduced in the late 1960s

2) The therapist helps the client address negative cognitive processing

3) Once the underlying cognitive schemata and specific distortions in thinking are identified, the client is asked to identify automatic thoughts, silent assumptions, and arbitrary inferences so that negative thoughts and assumptions can be examined logically, challenged against realistic attributes, and subsequently validated or refuted

4) Cognitive therapy has been effective in treating clients with unipolar mild to moderate depression

     d. Behavioral therapy
       1) Is often successfully used in conjunction with cognitive therapy for the treatment of mild to moderately depressed outpatients
       2) Is an effective treatment for depression, comparing favorably with medication and cognitive therapy
       3) There is less information about its effectiveness with clients experiencing mania
       4) Behavioral therapy is based on learning theory
       5) Abnormal or negative behaviors, such as the symptoms of depression and mania, represent behaviors acquired as a result of negative environmental events that are reinforced
       6) The behavioral therapist works with clients to determine specific behaviors to be modified and identify factors that evoke and reinforce these behaviors
       7) Using role-modeling, role-playing, and situational analysis, clients learn and practice different adaptive behaviors that elicit positive environmental reinforcement

     e. Interpersonal therapy
       1) Is based on beliefs that depression develops from pathologic early interpersonal relationship patterns that continue to be repeated in adulthood
       2) The emphasis for this therapy is on relationships and social functioning
       3) The goal of the therapy is to understand the social context of current problems based on earlier relationships and to provide symptomatic relief by solving or managing current interpersonal problems
       4) It has been demonstrated to be effective for clients with mild to moderate depression, although not more so than other types of psychotherapy

     f. Psychodynamic therapy
       1) Is derived from Freud's psychoanalytic model
       2) Depression is derived from early childhood loss of a significant object
       3) There is ambivalence about the object, which then affects the libido and produces an intrapsychic conflict during the oral or anal stage of psychosexual development
       4) The client's self-esteem is damaged, and there is a repetition of the primary loss pattern occurring throughout life
       5) The psychodynamic therapist establishes a relationship with the client and helps uncover repressed experiences, which then leads the client to experience a catharsis of feelings, confront defenses, interpret current behavior, and work through early loss and cravings for love

     g. Family therapy
       1) Is an assessment, intervention, and evaluation of family functional and dysfunctional patterns of behavior and relating
       2) There is a need to examine interactions between parents/adults and children
       3) The goal is to help family members identify and change behaviors that maintain depression and dependence among the family members
       4) This form of therapy is a specialized area of care and the psychiatric nurse needs additional education in order to practice this type of therapy
       5) Family should be referred to National Alliance of Mentally Ill (NAMI), a national organization that provides for decreased stigma, client and family support, advocacy, education, peer training, and research

     h. Group therapy
       1) Consists of persons coming together to receive psychotherapy; provides a safe environment where clients can receive feedback, share coping skills, resources, and problem solving
       2) The phases of group work are orientation, working, and termination

        3) Whatever the kind of group, virtually all groups go through phases identical to those described in relation to the nurse–patient relationship

  i. Examples of various types of groups include support, self-help, psychoeducational, psychotherapeutic, socialization, and peer support groups

  j. The psychiatric mental health nurse has the skills and the license to assess and provide care for clients utilizing group process in many settings; frequently combines expertise in group process, therapeutic nurse–patient relationship skills, experience in client education, and personal creativity to establish and manage supportive groups

5. Phototherapy

  a. A treatment that has effectively been used to lessen symptoms of recurrent seasonal affective disorder

  b. The exact mechanism of action remains unclear, although it is believed that exposure to morning light causes a circadian rhythm shift that regulates the normal relationships between sleep and circadian rhythms

  c. Phototherapy treatment consists of a minimum of 2500 lux of light usually administered on waking in the morning; the clients can be exposed for 30 minutes to several hours, depending on the strength of the light source

  d. An antidepressant effect is usually seen within two to four days and is complete after two weeks

  e. Maintenance treatment usually consists of 30 minutes of exposure each day; side effects are usually minimal

B. Nursing modalities

1. Planning and implementation of nursing care for clients with mood disorders is based on an established nursing theoretical foundation

2. The nursing process combines scientific principles with the most desirable elements of the art of nursing and with the appropriate systems theory

3. This theoretical foundation should be based on criteria such as found in *A Statement on Psychiatric–Mental Health Clinical Nursing Practice* and *Standards of Psychiatric–Mental Health Clinical Nursing Practice* (ANA, 1994)

4. These standards have provided the impetus and support for individualized and appropriate nursing care to psychiatric mental health clients in all types of settings

5. The nurse establishes a cost-effective, timely plan of care based on client's abilities, needs, resources, and outcome criteria, and identifies the appropriate nursing diagnoses, prioritizes interventions, and selects desired outcomes

6. The care plan documents prioritized nursing interventions based on the interdisciplinary resource data including diagnostic studies, support systems available to the client, response to treatment, financial abilities/restraints, and client's abilities/need

7. The nurse collaborates with an interdisciplinary team that includes psychiatrist, psychologist, social worker, occupational therapist, and in some cases art therapist and spiritual counselor

Practice to Pass

A client with major depressive disorder is not responding to antidepressants. She will be going for ECT tomorrow morning. What will you tell her regarding the procedure in terms of medications she will be receiving? Will you administer the prescribed Ativan this evening? Why or why not? What will you tell her in terms of potential untoward effects of ECT?

VI. EVALUATION/OUTCOMES

A. Outcome criteria for clients suffering from mood disorders include long- and short-term behaviors and responses that indicate improved functioning

B. These are based on nursing diagnoses and are achieved through the implementation of specific nursing interventions

C. Outcome criteria provide the nurse with direction for evaluating the client's response to treatment and nursing care

D. **Short- and long-term goals** for clients with mood disorders
   1. The client will remain safe and free from harm
   2. The client will verbalize suicidal threats and suicidal ideations and agree to seek help when indicated
   3. The client will verbalize absence of suicidal or homicidal intent or plan
   4. The client will express a desire to live and not to harm self or others
   5. The client will establish a pattern of rest/activity/sleep that enables fulfillment of role and self-care demands
   6. The client will establish a pattern of nutritional and hydration needs
   7. The client will initiate social interactions with others, and attend groups
   8. The client will verbalizes understanding of psychoeducation regarding the disorder, psychopharmacology, and other treatments
   9. The client will identify triggers for relapse and preventive measures put in place for relapse prevention
   10. The client will demonstrate increased communication skills and problem-solving strategies between self and significant others
   11. The client will verbalize reinstatement of religious/spiritual practices when applicable
E. **The nurse evaluates the client's progress** by measuring achievement of identified outcomes
F. **The data for evaluation** is derived from the nurses' interactions with client, observations of client's behavior changes over time, client's verbalization of feelings, and client's changes in mood, affect, thought content, thought process, judgment, and behavior
G. **Once the client is transitioned** from the inpatient setting to the community (i.e., outpatient treatment, case manager, home care), the nurse will evaluate the client's progress at a community level
H. **Due to decreased lengths of stay** inpatient unit nurses, regardless of health care settings, must continue to evaluate and reevaluate prioritized short- and long-term goals for the client; the nurse must do the following:
   1. Continue to observe clear progress related to absence of imminent suicidal intent and a plan for addressing the potential return of suicidal ideation after discharge
   2. Monitor clients with depression for evidence of improvement in the ability to perform self-care activities, and manifestation of decreased neurovegetative symptoms (i.e., irregular patterns of sleep, loss of or increased appetite, fatigue, psychomotor retardation, social withdrawal)
   3. Monitor clients with mania for evidence of alleviation of the symptoms of mania (i.e., hyperactivity, pressured speech, poor judgment, promiscuity), client should demonstrate improvement in cognitive and communicative functioning; the client should verbalize the need to understand symptoms of exacerbation of the disorder, necessary treatment, and self-care management; some persons with bipolar disorder do not like to take the mood stabilizers because they enjoy the mania
   4. Monitor compliance of all clients with mood disorders whether they are attending regular visits to a psychiatrists, therapists, family/group therapy, day-treatment programs, case management, and/or other community mental health agencies
   5. Assess for improvement in long-term outcomes such as a reduction in negative thinking, increase in self-esteem, application of new coping strategies, improvement in socialization/occupational and/or academic function, and return to routine of activities of daily living (ADLs)
   6. Improvement in long-term outcomes is individualized and can take weeks to months; some clients experience complete relapse, while others may manifest exacerbation of symptoms
   7. Assess clients frequently for depressive episodes, especially in clients who have recently been in a state of mania (they may flip to depression after mania)
   8. Provide careful follow-up after discharge into the community

VII. SPECIFIC DISORDERS

A. Bipolar disorders (12-month prevalence in the United States is 2.6% of adult populations; severe cases comprise 2.2% of these cases)

1. Are characterized by moods alternating between episodes of depression and episodes of mania or hypomania, and/or mixed

2. Are defined by the pattern of manic, hypomanic, and depressed episodes over time

3. For a diagnosis to occur, the depressed and manic episodes cannot be etiologically based on the effects of a substance (i.e., alcohol, prescribed, over-the-counter medication, illicit drug use, ECT, and/or light therapy)

4. For a diagnosis to occur, the depressed and manic episodes cannot be etiologically based on the pathology of a medical illness

5. Various theories have been proposed concerning the cause of mood disorders, but the precise etiology still remains unknown

6. Bipolar disorders can be further described as any of the following (*DSM-IV-TR*):

   a. Bipolar I disorder can occur when there is only a single manic episode and no past major depressive episodes

   b. Bipolar I episodes can be defined with the most recent episode being a hypomanic episode where the client has experienced at least one previous manic episode

   c. Bipolar I, the most recent episode, is manic and at least one previous depressive, hypomanic, or manic episode has occurred

   d. Bipolar I, the most recent episode, is mixed and at least one past major depressive or hypomanic episode has occurred

   e. Bipolar I, the most recent episode, is depressed mood and the client has experienced at least one past manic episode

   f. Bipolar II disorder is assigned when the client has never exhibited a full manic episode but has experienced at least one prior major depressive and one prior hypomanic episode

7. Manic episodes are episodes of elation where there is an abnormally and persistently elevated, expansive, or irritable mood for at least one week; in addition to the mood experience, before a diagnosis can be made, at least three of the following must occur:

   a. Grandiosity or inflated self-esteem

   b. Decreased need for sleep (feels good after three hours of sleep)

   c. Excessive talkativeness, pressured speech

   d. Racing thoughts, flight of ideas

   e. Distractibility, poor attention span

   f. Increase in goal-directed activity (may be sexual, social) and/or psychomotor agitation

   g. Excessive involvement in pleasurable activities (i.e., spending, sexual behaviors, poor business investments)

8. **Hypomania** is described as an elevation in mood with increases in activity but not as severe elation as in mania

9. Recent data suggest that the lifetime prevalence of bipolar disorder is about equal for men and women

B. Major depressive disorder (12-month prevalence in the United States is 6.7%; of these cases 2% is classified as severe; women are 70% more apt to experience depression then men)

1. Is characterized by loss of interest in life and a depressed mood, which moves from mild to severe and lasts at least two weeks

2. For a diagnosis to occur, the depression cannot be etiologically based on the effects of a substance (i.e., alcohol, prescribed, illicit drug use)

3. For a diagnosis to occur, the depression cannot be etiologically based on medical illness

4. Other major features include marked disturbance in occupational, academic, and/or social functioning
5. Most individuals with major depression become less socially active over time and may completely withdraw
6. In addition to the loss of interest in life and a depressed mood, five of the following must occur for a diagnosis to be made:
   a. Depressed mood present for most of the day, nearly every day, as indicated by subjective or objective data
   b. Markedly decreased pleasure or interest in all or almost all activities most of the day, nearly every day (**anhedonia**)
   c. Significant weight loss (when not dieting) or weight gain
   d. Sleep disturbances as manifested by hypersomnia or insomnia
   e. Manifests on nearly a daily basis psychomotor agitation or retardation
   f. Manifests on nearly a daily basis loss of energy
   g. Feelings of irrational guilt (may be delusional), feelings of worthlessness
   h. Decreased ability to concentrate, think indecisiveness
   i. Recurrent thoughts of death; suicidal ideation with or without a specific plan, or a suicide attempt
7. The symptoms do not meet criteria for a mixed episode
8. The symptoms are not better accounted for by grief or bereavement

C. **Dysthymic disorder** differs from major depression in that it is a chronic, low-level depression; (12 month prevalence in the United States is 1.5 of adults; of these cases 0.8% is considered severe) *DSM-IV-TR* criteria that must be present for this diagnosis include the following:
   1. Must have had depressed mood and at least three of the following symptoms for most of the day, nearly every day, for at least two years: poor appetite/overeating; insomnia/hypersomnia; low energy; low self-esteem; poor concentration/difficulty making decisions; and feelings of hopelessness
   2. There cannot have been a manic or hypomanic episode
   3. There may have been an episode of major depression before the onset of dysthymia, provided there were at least six months with no signs or symptoms of depression
   4. After two years, the client may be diagnosed with dysthymia; the client may be diagnosed with major depression superimposed on dysthymia if symptoms increase in severity
   5. The disorder cannot be caused by the effects of a substance or medical condition
   6. There are usually no psychotic features present in this disorder

D. **Comparing and contrasting major depressive disorder with mania in bipolar disorder**
   1. Behavioral characteristic differences
      a. Major depressive disorder manifests with a progression from a decreased desire to engage in social, work, and school activities to an absence of participation in most activities of daily living
         1) There is a progressive loss of self-esteem; the individual feels increased incompetence and decreased motivation
         2) Statements such as, "Why bother, I can't anyway" or "I don't want to live anymore" are common
      b. In contrast, the manic episode of bipolar disorder manifest with excessive high energy levels and initially productivity
         1) Sometimes there is positive feedback from others (i.e., productivity, or people may enjoy being around a "happy" manic)
         2) With progression of disease, there is decreased ability to concentrate, make judgments, or participate in everyday activities, and hence decreased productivity; this can lead to frustration and increased efforts to regain control

        3) Frustration and irritability continue to escalate, adjoined with a shortened attention span, grandiosity, and poor judgment; day-to-day function becomes impaired

        4) This is exhibited by engagement in spending sprees, making foolish financial investments, and/or high-risk behaviors such as gambling, speeding in the car, excessive spending, or promiscuous sexual behaviors

    c. Relationships and interactions with others are impacted by a mood disorder

        1) Individuals with depression withdraw from family, friends, social activities, and events

        2) Individuals may state they feel lonely but often cannot halt the process of withdrawal and isolation; this further reinforces feelings of social isolation

        3) In contrast, persons with bipolar disorder during a manic state are unable to set boundaries, exhibit incessant talkativeness, and gregarious behavior; often they have feelings of shame and embarrassment about the behavior once their mood is stabilized

2. Affective characteristics

    a. Alterations in affect for individuals with depression are broad and in depth

        1) Initially, there is a vague sense of sadness that gradually becomes more and more pronounced

        2) This can be accompanied by guilt that may be expressed as a vague concern or a specific issue

        3) Cues to these emotions are statements such as, "I have so much to be thankful for; I shouldn't feel this way"

        4) There is also a loss of emotional attachment in depressed individuals that is evidenced by expressions of indifference toward family and friends

    b. In contrast, individuals with bipolar disorder during the manic phase exhibit mood ranges between cheerful and euphoric to irritable and angry

        1) For example, they make statements such as, "I feel great!" or "Life is amazing"

        2) When confronted with external negative stimulus, the individual can become irritable, argumentative, hostile, and even combative

        3) Once the untoward stimulus is removed, there is usually a return to euphoria; this may explain the labile affect

        4) During the manic phase, these individuals usually do not feel a sense of guilt (may be due to poor insight)

        5) They respond to another's feelings of hurt or anger with their own anger, laughter, or indifference

    c. Clients with mild or moderate depression exhibit bouts of crying; those in the severe stages of depression may not have the energy to cry; those with bipolar disorder, to the contrast express feelings of euphoria and "all being wonderful"

    d. Depressed individuals exhibit depressed or sad affect or flat affect, to the contrast individuals with bipolar disorder during the manic phase usually exhibit a cheerful to euphoric presentation; they may also be irritable, angry, and or labile

    e. Clients with major depression exhibit anhedonia or a lack of pleasure; to the contrast individuals who are bipolar may be overly social (to the point of boundary violations) and overparticipate in activities and events during the manic phase

3. Cognitive characteristics

    a. A person's perceptions about personal worth and value contributes to a sense of self-esteem

    b. The client in a manic state does not suffer from low self-esteem; on the contrary, there is a very grandiose belief about self

    c. The client in a depressed state focuses on the negative, with a presentation of self as a failure and totally incompetent

    d. A client with depression will **catastrophize** or exaggerate all of life as a failure; depressed clients will personalize comments made by others, and perceive current and future life as hopeless .

    e. A client in a depressed state overgeneralizes, is self-critical and perfectionistic, and anticipates disapproval from others; in contrast, persons with bipolar disorder while the person in a manic state, exhibits unwarranted positive expectations, are unable to foresee potential negative outcomes, and are irate if criticized by others

    f. The client in the manic state of bipolar disorder manifests the following:
        1) Presents as easily distractible and impulsive
        2) Demonstrates flight of ideas
        3) Maintains a belief in self as being very attractive
        4) Exhibits delusions of grandeur
        5) The experience of hallucinations occur in approximately 15–25% of cases

    g. The client in the depressed state will manifest the following:
        1) Presents with a decreased ability or inability to make decisions
        2) Experiences a decrease in rate and number of thoughts
        3) Maintains a belief about self as being ugly or unattractive
        4) May experience somatic delusions
        5) The experience of hallucinations occurs in approximately 15–25% of cases

4. Sociocultural characteristics associated with the depressed state include a loss of desire in sexual activities; to the contrast persons with bipolar disorder, while in the manic state, manifest increase in promiscuity and sexual activity

5. Physiological characteristics

    a. A client with bipolar disorder in the manic state may have decreased or no appetite due to no desire and/or the inability to physically slow down to sit and eat; on the contrary, the person in the depressed state will have either an increased or decreased appetite; in severe states of depression, a decrease in appetite usually occurs

    b. A client with bipolar disorder in the manic state will sleep one or two hours per night, or may not sleep for days; on the contrary, the person in a mild to moderate depressed state may have either increased or decreased sleep; persons with severe depression typically manifest persistent insomnia

    c. Reported gastrointestinal activity for those in manic and depressed states is usually constipation

    d. Physical appearance of the client with bipolar in a manic state commonly includes bright clothing, frequent changes in clothing, and an exaggerated self-presentation; on the contrary, the person with depression may exhibit an unkempt presentation and the appearance of little attention to self and/or poor hygiene

Case Study

You are admitting a female client to the inpatient unit. The client is in a manic state, and has been diagnosed with bipolar disorder, most recent episode mania, with psychosis. She is exhibiting flight of ideas, loose association, paranoid delusions, poor appetite, irritability, and rapid mood swings between elation and crying spells. The client has been unable to sleep for the past three nights and stays awake pacing the floor.

1. Identify at least five questions you will ask during your initial interview.

2. List three priorities of care for this client. Give a rationale for each priority.

3. What classifications of medications might be prescribed to her? List at least two to three. Explain the reasoning for each prescription.

For suggested responses, see pages 296–297.

4. You assign her a nursing diagnosis of Disturbed Sleep Pattern. List four nursing interventions to promote sleep in this client.

5. You assign her a nursing diagnosis of Imbalanced Nutrition: Less than Body Requirements. List four nursing interventions to promote improved nutritional status in this client.

POSTTEST

1 The inpatient mental health client is being treated for major depression. The client has psychomotor retardation, speaks very little, and is extremely inactive physically. The client takes an antidepressant that causes anticholinergic side effects. The nurse should conclude that this client is at particular risk for developing which of the following? Select all that apply.

1. Dry mouth
2. Vomiting
3. Constipation
4. Diarrhea
5. Weight loss

2 The 26-year-old female hospitalized client is being treated for major depressive disorder. The client participated actively in group therapy during the hour before lunchtime. When it is time for lunch, the client tells the nurse, "I'm not going. I'm going to my room." What is the nurse's best response?

1. Ask the client to sit for a few minutes to discuss this.
2. Ask the client if she is angry.
3. Tell the client that there is a unit schedule that must be followed by everyone.
4. Ask the client if there is a problem with the food.

3 The nurse is conducting discharge teaching for a client taking tranylcypromine (Parnate). The nurse determines that the client understands the instructions given if the client says not to eat which food while taking the medication?

1. Potatoes
2. Salami
3. Baked chicken
4. Apples

4 A client is admitted to a secure psychiatric inpatient unit for the treatment of bipolar I disorder. The nurse begins the intake assessment but the client stands up and begins to walk around the room and shouts, "You can't do this to me! Do you know who I am? I want out of here!!" The best action of the nurse at this time focuses on which of the following?

1. Obtaining the assessment information limited to 20 minutes at a time, allowing for rest periods
2. Providing the client with adequate food and fluids to maintain homeostasis
3. Providing client and self with a safe environment
4. Administering the prescribed prn neuroleptic medication to prevent escalation of behavior

5 The nurse observed that earlier in the afternoon a depressed client visited the coffee shop and sat at a table with two other clients. What is the best positive feedback the nurse can give to the client?

1. "You are doing such a wonderful job interacting with the other clients."
2. "I saw that you sat with others in the coffee shop this afternoon."
3. "How are you feeling after your visit to the coffee shop with other clients today?"
4. "Do you plan to go to the coffee shop again tomorrow?"

6 The hospitalized client is in a manic phase of bipolar I disorder. When developing the nursing care plan for this client, how should the nurse expect the client's behavior to be in social interactions? Select all that apply.

1. Unpredictable
2. Isolative
3. Demanding
4. Competitive
5. Indecisive

7 The nurse observes that a client is pacing in the hallway, talking rapidly, and gesturing dramatically. The nurse concludes that the client is beginning to demonstrate what kind of behavior?

1. Psychomotor retardation
2. Anxiety
3. Psychomotor agitation
4. Depression

8 A client states, "I just want to sleep all the time. I am overweight again. I will go to work and do my grocery shopping, but that's all. My life's a mess." The nurse should conclude that which nursing diagnosis is most relevant?

1. Ineffective Coping
2. Risk for Violence: Self-Directed
3. Activity Intolerance
4. Anxiety

9 The client who has a diagnosis of bipolar I disorder has a new order for carbamazepine (Tegretol). Before beginning to administer the medication, the nurse checks to see that which laboratory results are in the client's record?

1. Blood glucose
2. Liver function studies
3. Bleeding and clotting time
4. Thyroid profile

10 A client in an inpatient unit is awake at one a.m. and tells the nurse, "I can't sleep because of the light in the hall and the noise from the kitchen. I need to have another sleeping pill." What is the most appropriate nursing intervention?

1. Administer a prn sedative.
2. Move the client to a quieter room.
3. Close the door to the client's room.
4. Allow the client to watch television for one hour.

➤ *See pages 95–97 for Answers and Rationales.*

POSTTEST

ANSWERS & RATIONALES

Pretest

1 **Answer: 2, 5** **Rationale:** The client receiving a series of ECTs can be expected to have "patchy" memories of events occurring during the days or weeks of the treatment period. This may or may not resolve as time passes. While modifications in the ECT procedure have increased the level of safety for the client, amnesia and possibly temporary confusion still remain as side effects of the procedure. The client is likely to have amnesia for recent events, especially for events that occurred just before the treatment was administered, so the client will not remember that the treatment has been administered. The memory loss that may occur as a side effect to ECT is not selective. Both positive and negative life events may be forgotten. Memory deficits are common in the client receiving ECT. When they do occur, the client and significant others generally feel alarmed. However, the nurse should recognize this as an expected and non-urgent side effect. **Cognitive Level:** Analyzing **Client Need:** Psychosocial Integrity **Integrated Process:** Teaching and Learning **Content Area:** Mental Health **Strategy:** Recall information about expected side effects of ECT. Present this information to the client in a simple and non-alarming style. **Reference:** Fontaine, K. (2009). *Mental health nursing* (8th ed.). Upper Saddle River, NJ: Prentice Hall, p. 250.

2 **Answer: 1** **Rationale:** The nurse should recognize that the client is experiencing side effects that are normal at this time. That information should be conveyed to the client, as well as information about what to expect in the future. It is important that the client continue to take the medication as prescribed. Serum lithium levels should be monitored frequently in order to determine therapeutic blood levels and prevent lithium toxicity. Minor hand tremors do not indicate lithium toxicity, but they can interfere with writing and other motor skills. Helping the client understand that the tremors can subside or disappear after one or two weeks is reassuring. Reassuring the client not to worry unless the tremor lasts than a couple weeks fails to give the client important information about side effects of lithium. It also fails to respond to the client's concern that something is wrong. Fine hand tremors are expected side effects at this time in the client's treatment. However, the presence of coarse tremors, coupled with such symptoms as gait changes, would suggest possible toxicity, which would require a totally different response from the nurse. Reassuring the client that the tremor is too small to interfere with his or her functioning will likely result in the client feeling demeaned. This response also deprives the client of the opportunity to receive important teaching. **Cognitive Level:** Analyzing

Client Need: Health Promotion and Maintenance **Integrated Process:** Communication and Documentation **Content Area:** Mental Health **Strategy:** Recall normal and expected side effects of lithium. Choose a response that gives that information to the client in simple terms. **Reference:** Fontaine, K. (2009). *Mental health nursing* (6th ed.). Upper Saddle River, NJ: Prentice Hall, p. 196.

3 **Answer: 1, 4** **Rationale:** The nurse should understand that in order for a client to be diagnosed with major depression, *DSM-IV-TR* specifies that symptoms consistent with at least five of nine criteria must have been present for at least two weeks. Suicidal ideations and plans are included in one criterion. The nurse should keep in mind that the presence of suicidal ideations alone would not support the diagnosis of major depression. Another criterion for major depression involves markedly diminished interest or pleasure in all, or almost all, activities. History of one depressive episode within the last two years is incorrect because major depressive symptoms represent a more recent change in functioning, not a single episode within two years. While persons with major depression often have changes in weight and appetite, the relevant *DSM-IV-TR* criterion for major depression does not involve a three-day period. It also allows for either increases or decreases in appetite to have occurred. Hallucinations may occur in psychotic levels of major depression, but they are not part of the diagnostic criteria in *DSM-IV-TR*. **Cognitive Level:** Analyzing **Client Need:** Psychosocial Integrity **Integrated Process:** Nursing Process: Assessment **Content Area:** Mental Health **Strategy:** Compare and contrast usual presenting symptoms and *DSM-IV-TR* criteria for major depression. **Reference:** Varcarolis, E., & Halter, M. (2010). *Foundations of psychiatric mental health nursing: A clinical approach* (6th ed.). St. Louis, MO: Saunders Elsevier, p. 329.

4 **Answer: 3** **Rationale:** The manic client has poor judgment and is impulsive and at risk for injury. The nurse should attend to the safety needs of this client before taking other actions. It is possible that the client will not be able to contract for safety. (At this point the first part of the contract would be for the client to remain in the hospital.) If the client could not do this, the nurse's next action is to explain the terms of the client's admission status. Because the client is being treated on a formal voluntary basis, the nurse cannot comply with the client's demand to be discharged. It is not appropriate to involve the police. While informing the spouse might be an appropriate later action, at this time the nurse should focus attention on the client. It is appropriate for the nurse to report the client's request to the nursing supervisor, but the first response to the client's request should be made to the client. Meeting the client's safety needs is of higher priority than informing the supervisor. **Cognitive Level:** Analyzing **Client Need:** Management of Care **Integrated Process:** Nursing Process: Implementation **Content Area:** Mental Health **Strategy:** Ask yourself if it would be a good idea for this client to be able to leave the hospital at will. Consider the obligation of the nurse to provide safety for all clients. Recall relevant facts about types of psychiatric admissions. **Reference:** Fontaine, K. (2009). *Mental health nursing* (6th ed.). Upper Saddle River, NJ: Prentice Hall, p. 138.

5 **Answer: 1, 5 Rationale:** The nurse should know that one of the common side effects of sertraline (Zoloft) is insomnia. Therefore, most clients are given sertraline (Zoloft) early in the day. Sexual side effects to sertraline (Zoloft) and other SSRIs are common. One way to decrease the likelihood of noncompliance is to inform the client that prompt reporting of such side effects can lead to corrective treatment measures. It is important for the nurse to know that diarrhea is a much more common side effect to sertraline (Zoloft) than is constipation. It is vital for the nurse to know that all persons taking sertraline (Zoloft) or other SSRIs should be taught to recognize early symptoms of possible central serotonin syndrome. Such symptoms include sudden onset fever, sweating, and extrapyramidal side effects (EPS). The development of central serotonin syndrome is a rare medical emergency, but the client will need intensive medical treatment because the mortality rate is very high. The nurse should teach the client that while some reduction in symptoms may occur in a relatively short period of time, it may be several weeks before full therapeutic effects are realized. Without this knowledge, clients often become discouraged and think that the medication is ineffective. **Cognitive Level:** Analyzing **Client Need:** Pharmacological and Parenteral Therapies **Integrated Process:** Nursing Process: Planning **Content Area:** Mental Health **Strategy:** Translate the statements of the nurse into medical terminology and then determine if each option is related to a known side effect of sertraline (Zoloft). **Reference:** Varcarolis, E., & Halter, M. (2010). *Foundations of psychiatric mental health nursing: A clinical approach* (6th ed.). St. Louis, MO: Saunders Elsevier, pp. 344–345.

6 **Answer: 3 Rationale:** The clinical presentation of depressed mood is similar to that of medically diagnosed depression. There is a high incidence of depressed mood and depression among hospitalized clients. Usually the more severe the illness, the more pronounced the symptoms. Clinical depression in the recovery period is relatively common among cardiovascular surgical clients. There is nothing in the client's complaint that suggests body image concerns, although most postsurgical clients have this concern to some degree. The statements of this client instead suggest that the client is experiencing depressed mood, which is similar to the medical diagnosis of

depression. Nothing the client has said indicates that the client is intolerant of activity. Feeling tired is a much more moderate problem than being intolerant of activity. There is no data in the stem of this question to suggest that the client's recovery is delayed. **Cognitive Level:** Analyzing **Client Need:** Psychosocial Integrity **Integrated Process:** Nursing Process: Assessment **Content Area:** Mental Health **Strategy:** Look carefully at the client's words. Think about clinical signs of depression. Remember that depression is a medical diagnosis, not a nursing diagnosis. **Reference:** Fontaine, K. (2009). *Mental health nursing* (6th ed.). Upper Saddle River, NJ: Prentice-Hall, p. 203.

7 **Answer: 4 Rationale:** According to *DSM-IV-TR*, dysthymic disorder cannot be fully diagnosed until the depressed mood has been present for at least two years. Additional criteria are specified to diagnose dysthymic disorder, and once the depressed mood criterion has been met, only some of the other criteria must be met. This is in contrast to the *DSM-IV-TR* criteria for diagnosing major depression. In this case, at least five of nine criteria must be met. **Cognitive Level:** Applying **Client Need:** Psychosocial Integrity **Integrated Process:** Teaching and Learning **Content Area:** Mental Health **Strategy:** Review *DSM-IV-TR* criteria for dysthymia and major depression. **Reference:** Kneisl, C., Wilson, H., & Trigoboff, E. (2009). *Contemporary psychiatric–mental health nursing* (2nd ed.). Upper Saddle River, NJ: Prentice Hall, p. 337.

8 **Answer: 4 Rationale:** The client in the manic state is generally intrusive and insensitive to the needs of others and does not recognize boundaries, whether psychologic or physical. The client also tends to have an intense preoccupation with sexual urges and frequently touches others or positions self in socially inappropriate ways. The nurse must encourage the client to set and maintain boundaries while interacting with others. The person in a manic state is unlikely to be able to conform to the schedule of spending at least 30 minutes per hour watching TV or to sustain attention for this period of time. Additionally, the client is likely to find the activity room more stimulating than a quieter area of the unit. Individuals experiencing manic affect tend toward overreaction and overdramatization in any situation, so participating in such a group would likely increase the client's manic hyperactivity and dramatization. While physical exercising will allow the client to sublimate some of the excessive energy that is felt, the client is likely to be domineering, overbearing, and highly competitive in groups. Further, it is likely that the client's level of mania will increase because of the extra stimulation. **Cognitive Level:** Analyzing **Client Need:** Safety and Infection Control **Integrated Process:** Nursing Process: Planning **Content Area:** Mental Health **Strategy:** Develop a mental picture of how the person with elevated affect is likely to act. "See" this client before you, and the correct answer will be obvious. **Reference:** Varcarolis, E., & Halter, M. (2010). *Foundations of psychiatric mental health nursing: A clinical approach* (6th ed.). St. Louis, MO: Saunders Elsevier, pp. 364–366.

9 **Answer: 1 Rationale:** The nurse must first attend to safety and physiologic needs necessary to sustain life. Considering the prior level of physical activity of the client and that the client is currently perspiring profusely, the nurse should recognize that this client could easily enter into a state of fluid and/or electrolyte imbalance. This at-risk problem will take priority over actual problems that do not involve basic physical needs or safety. Impaired Skin Integrity is incorrect. The nurse should recognize that while this is an actual physical problem, it does not pose the same level of risk that the risk for injury and fluid deficit pose for this client. Like the psychological needs, this problem can be addressed after basic physiologic and safety needs are addressed. Ineffective Coping and Impaired Adjustment are not priority problems at this time. They are psychologic problems that can be addressed after basic physiologic and safety needs are addressed. **Cognitive Level:** Analyzing **Client Need:** Physiological Adaptation **Integrated Process:** Nursing Process: Planning **Content Area:** Mental Health **Strategy:** Develop a mental picture of this client. Notice the perspiration and connect it with the family's report of extreme hyperactivity. Recall basic facts about fluid and electrolyte balance to choose correctly. **Reference:** Varcarolis, E., & Halter, M. (2010). *Foundations of psychiatric mental health nursing: A clinical approach* (6th ed.). St. Louis, MO: Saunders Elsevier, p. 364.

10 **Answer: 2 Rationale:** Clients in a manic state are vulnerable to injure self or others, either through restless hyperactivity and poor judgment or through actions during unpredictable mood swings. Continuous and close nursing supervision of these clients to ensure safety is imperative, regardless of the type of room to which they are assigned. A room near the nurse's station (if it is not too loud) may be advisable for the client with elevated affect, but this will not substitute for constant immediate supervision of the client. Medications should be given orally if possible since the manic client is likely to overreact to any physical contact, either interpreting it as a physical assault or ascribing a sexual intent to it. Being in a quiet, non-stimulating private room is advisable for this client, but it is not as urgent as close personal supervision by the nurse. **Cognitive Level:** Analyzing **Client Need:** Psychosocial Integrity **Integrated Process:** Nursing Process: Planning **Content Area:** Mental Health **Strategy:** Recall behaviors common to the client with elevated mood. Recognize that the nurse's priority is always to provide for the safety of individual clients, as well as groups of clients. **Reference:** Varcarolis, E., & Halter, M. (2010). *Foundations of psychiatric mental health nursing: A clinical approach* (6th ed.). St. Louis, MO: Saunders Elsevier, p. 359.

Posttest

1 **Answer: 1, 3 Rationale:** Anticholinergic effects of the client's medication will decrease motility of the GI tract, specifically the stomach and bowel. The nurse should remember that the client's low level of physical activity increases the risk for constipation. There is nothing to indicate that the client is at high risk for vomiting, although dry mouth is likely. The nurse should recognize that this client not at risk for diarrhea, but is actually at high risk for constipation. Most experts consider weight gain (a common side effect of antipsychotics) to be an anticholinergic side effect. **Cognitive Level:** Analyzing **Client Need:** Physiological Adaptation **Integrated Process:** Nursing Process: Diagnosis **Content Area:** Mental Health **Strategy:** Recall physiologic manifestations of depression and anticholinergic side effects. **Reference:** Kneisl, C., Wilson, H., & Trigoboff, E. (2009). *Contemporary psychiatric–mental health nursing* (2nd ed.). Upper Saddle River, NJ: Prentice Hall, p. 746.

2 **Answer: 1 Rationale:** The client is demonstrating a pattern of behavior that should be investigated. The nurse should take the time to assess the client's feelings, thoughts, and actions. The client may just be tired and have a need to rest, but the nurse needs to be sure that the client is safe and not upset. The nurse should not make assumptions about what the client is feeling (asking if she is angry). Before ascribing a meaning to the client's behavior, the nurse should first talk to the client to determine what feelings she is experiencing. Additionally, the nurse is using a closed-ended question that can be answered with a "yes" or "no." This is not the correct therapeutic technique to use when interviewing a client. Telling the client that there is a unit schedule that everyone must follow does acknowledge the client's change in attitude but does not indicate that the nurse has any concern for the client. Asking the client if there is a problem with the food changes the focus from the client to food in addition to prematurely and inappropriately presuming to understand the meaning of the client's behavior. **Cognitive Level:** Analyzing **Client Need:** Psychosocial Integrity **Integrated Process:** Caring **Content Area:** Mental Health **Strategy:** Notice that the client has not expressed any reasons for wanting to return to her own room. This indicates a need for more information. **Reference:** Fontaine, K. (2009). *Mental health nursing* (6th ed.). Upper Saddle River, NJ: Prentice Hall, p. 380.

3 **Answer: 2 Rationale:** Salami is a cured meat and must be avoided by clients taking tranylcypromine, a monoamine oxidase inhibitor (MAOI). Foods rich in tyramine or tryptophan, such as cured foods, may induce a hypertensive episode in clients taking MAOI medication. Other foods to be avoided include those that have been aged, pickled, fermented, or smoked. Clients taking monoamine oxidase inhibitors (MAOIs) can eat potatoes, baked chicken in reasonable amounts, and apples. **Cognitive Level:** Analyzing **Client Need:** Pharmacological and

Parenteral Therapies **Integrated Process:** Teaching and Learning **Content Area:** Mental Health **Strategy:** Notice that salami is the only food listed that is prepared for a long-term shelf life. **Reference:** Varcarolis, E., & Halter, M. (2010). *Foundations of psychiatric mental health nursing: A clinical approach* (6th ed.). St. Louis, MO: Saunders Elsevier, p. 349.

4 **Answer: 3** **Rationale:** Providing safety for the nurse and the client is the primary concern immediately after admission when the client is in a manic state. This is because the client is likely to be labile, hostile, and uncooperative. The information given in this question suggests that the client's elevated and angry mood poses potential safety hazards for the client and the nurse. While obtaining the intake assessment data is important, this activity can be delayed until safety issues have been addressed. When the client demonstrates an elevated angry mood, it poses a potential safety risk for the client and the nurse. It is this risk that requires the nurse's immediate focus, not nutritional imbalance, even though this is often a nursing diagnosis for a client in a manic episode. There is nothing in the question that indicates that the client's behavior is so extreme that medications must be given. The nurse should remember that prn neuroleptic medication is considered to be a chemical form of restraint. Other less restrictive measures, such as environmental manipulation, must always be used before the nurse administers prn medication. **Cognitive Level:** Analyzing **Client Need:** Safety and Infection Control **Integrated Process:** Nursing Process: Implementation **Content Area:** Mental Health **Strategy:** Notice the aggression of the client and recognize its possible danger to client and others. **Reference:** Kneisl, C., Wilson, H., & Trigoboff, E. (2009). *Contemporary psychiatric–mental health nursing* (2nd ed.). Upper Saddle River, NJ: Prentice Hall, pp. 156–157.

5 **Answer: 2** **Rationale:** "I saw that you sat with others in the coffee shop this afternoon" acknowledges independent and positive actions by the client. Information is reported in a matter-of-fact manner to the client, and no evaluative words are used. While it is probably intended to convey encouragement, the word "wonderful" is very much overstated. Depressed clients do not accept praise easily. The appropriate feedback for the nurse to provide is a matter-of-fact observation that does not include evaluative terms like "wonderful." Asking how the client is feeling after visiting the coffee shop and asking if the client plans to go there again tomorrow uses the technique of exploring. The question that is being asked concerns feedback. Feedback involves the giving of information to the client, rather than getting information from the client. Questions are not asked when feedback is given. **Cognitive Level:** Analyzing **Client Need:** Psychosocial Integrity **Integrated Process:** Communication and Documentation **Content Area:** Mental Health **Strategy:** Notice that the question is asking about feedback and that the client is depressed. Integrate your knowledge of each as

you make your choice. **Reference:** Kneisl, C., Wilson, H., & Trigoboff, E. (2009). *Contemporary psychiatric–mental health nursing* (2nd ed.). Upper Saddle River, NJ: Prentice Hall, pp. 349, 351.

6 **Answer: 1, 3, 4** **Rationale:** Providing nursing care to clients with elevated mood (mania) can be particularly challenging for the nurse. The client will generally be excited, physically hyperactive, labile, and unpredictable. Clients in manic states tend to exhibit behaviors that are controlling, competitive, irritable, aggressive, and domineering in social situations. They are often socially intrusive and inappropriate. When their demands are not met, they can easily become aggressive in ways that are dangerous to self or others. Because of this, the nurse should always consider the person in a manic state to be at risk for injury to self or others especially. Persons experiencing manic states will resist being isolated and act as if they feel compelled to interact with others at all times. Persons in a manic state have unrealistically elevated self-esteem, often feeling that they are the brightest, the wisest, or the most knowledgeable person in the world. They will therefore not hesitate to make decisions, but the decisions are made impulsively and without regard for consequences. **Cognitive Level:** Analyzing **Client Need:** Psychosocial Integrity **Integrated Process:** Nursing Process: Diagnosis **Content Area:** Mental Health **Strategy:** Develop a mental image of the client with elevated mood. As you read an option, "see" the client. Will he or she be likely to carry out this behavior? **Reference:** Kneisl, C., Wilson, H., & Trigoboff, E. (2009). *Contemporary psychiatric–mental health nursing* (2nd ed.). Upper Saddle River, NJ: Prentice Hall, pp. 340–341.

7 **Answer: 3** **Rationale:** Psychomotor agitation is recognized when a person's behavior involves increased physical activity, restless, and/or aggression. The behavioral manifestations will be accompanied by strong affects, such as anxiety, and speeding of physiologic processes. When psychomotor agitation is present, the client and others are at risk for injury. Psychomotor retardation is a term that refers to slowing of physical activities and bodily processes. It is the opposite of what is described in this situation. Anxiety is a feeling, not a behavior. This question calls for the nurse to identify a behavior. The behavior of the client may be indeed be related to anxiety, but there are other possible reasons for the behavior. Depression is a mood state, not a behavior. The behavior of the client may be related to depressed mood, but there are other possible reasons for the behavior. **Cognitive Level:** Applying **Client Need:** Psychosocial Integrity **Integrated Process:** Nursing Process: Assessment **Content Area:** Mental Health **Strategy:** Look for a behavior, not an emotion. **Reference:** Varcarolis, E., & Halter, M. (2010). *Foundations of psychiatric mental health nursing: A clinical approach* (6th ed.). St. Louis, MO: Saunders Elsevier, p. 793.

8 **Answer: 1** **Rationale:** The client is describing symptoms that are consistent with those of a mood disorder, probably dysthymic disorder. The client's life is not well managed, nor does the client experience pleasure, and thus coping is impaired. There is nothing in the client's statement to indicate an immediate risk for self-directed violence. The client is dispirited and dissatisfied, but does not indicate that this is overwhelming enough to cause self-destructive ideas or urges. The client's statement does not suggest inability to tolerate physical activity, but rather fatigue and disinterest. Activity intolerance is much more intense and specific than fatigue. Nothing in the client's statement suggests that acute anxiety is present. Anxiety is a common human emotion, but in order for it to be a nursing diagnosis, there should be clear evidence that the anxiety level is elevated beyond normal. **Cognitive Level:** Analyzing **Client Need:** Psychosocial Integrity **Integrated Process:** Nursing Process: Diagnosis **Content Area:** Mental Health **Strategy:** Ask yourself if this client is managing life very well. **Reference:** Kneisl, C., Wilson, H., & Trigoboff, E. (2009). *Contemporary psychiatric–mental health nursing* (2nd ed.). Upper Saddle River, NJ: Prentice Hall, p. 337.

9 **Answer: 2 Rationale:** The nurse should know that carbamazepine (Tegretol) frequently causes changes in liver enzymes. These changes can result in dangerous or fatal problems for the client. Therefore, baseline laboratory results must be available before the first dose of the drug is administered. Subsequent results are then compared to this set of baseline data as the prescriber makes decisions about future doses. Changes in blood glucose are not commonly associated with carbamazepine. Instead, there is a strong relationship to blood glucose changes and certain second generation antipsychotics, such as olanzepine (Zyprexa). While it is true that bleeding problems can be associated with

carbamazepine, baseline bleed/clotting times are not required before the drug is administered. If the client were being given lithium, baseline information about thyroid functioning would be required. **Cognitive Level:** Applying **Client Need:** Pharmacological and Parenteral Therapies **Integrated Process:** Nursing Process: Assessment **Content Area:** Mental Health **Strategy:** Read the question carefully and draw on knowledge of pharmacology and common adverse drug effects. **Reference:** Varcarolis, E. & Halter, M. (2010). *Foundations of psychiatric mental health nursing: A clinical approach* (6th ed.). St. Louis, MO: Saunders Elsevier, p. 53.

10 **Answer: 3 Rationale:** The client has indicated that environmental noise and activity are preventing sleep. The nurse should first attempt to minimize environmental stimuli. Simply closing the client's door is a noninvasive, non-stimulating strategy that may work, assuming that it will not pose a safety hazard for the client. Before administering a prn sedative, the nurse should attempt other non-pharmacological options. It is not necessary to move the client to a quieter room when closing the door can produce a noninvasive strategy. However, the door should not be closed if this would pose a risk for the client's safety. Turning on the television will increase the amount of noise in the environment and could further stimulate the client and/or others. **Cognitive Level:** Analyzing **Client Need:** Safety and Infection Control **Integrated Process:** Nursing Process: Implementation **Content Area:** Mental Health **Strategy:** Pay attention to the client's words. They define the exact nature of the problem. **Reference:** Varcarolis, E., & Halter, M. (2010). *Foundations of psychiatric mental health nursing: A clinical approach* (6th ed.). St. Louis, MO: Saunders Elsevier, p. 670.

References

American Psychiatric Association (2000). *Diagnostic and statistical manual of mental disorders* (4th ed., text revision [*DSM-IV-TR*]). Washington, DC: American Psychiatric Association, pp. 345–428.

Carpenito, L. J. (2011). *Nursing diagnosis: Application to clinical practice* (13th ed.). Philadelphia, PA: Lippincott Williams & Wilkins.

Fontaine, K. L. (2009). *Mental health nursing* (6th ed.). Upper Saddle River, NJ: Pearson Education.

Kneisl, C. R., Wilson, H. S., & Trigoboff, E. (2009). *Contemporary psychiatric mental health nursing* (2nd ed.). Upper Saddle River, NJ: Prentice Hall, pp. 404–432.

Sajatovic, M., & Ramirez, L. F. (2006). *Rating scales in mental health* (2nd ed.). Hudson, OH: Lexi-Comp, Inc., pp. 36, 47, 55, 66.

National Alliance of the Mentally Ill (2011). *Inform yourself*. Retrieved on February 10, 2011, from www.nami.org/template.cfm?section=inform_yourself

National Institute of Mental Health (2011). *Any mood disorder*. Retrieved on February 2, 2011, from www.nimh.nih.gov/statistics/1ANYMOODDIS_ADULT.shtml

National Institute of Mental Health (2011). *Bipolar disorders among adults*. Retrieved on February 2, 2011, from http://nimh.nih.gov/statistics/1BIPOLAR_ADULT.shtml

National Institute of Mental Health (2011). *Dysthymic disorder among adults*. Retrieved on February 2, 2011, from http://nimh.nih.gov/statistics/1DD_ADULT.shtml

National Institute of Mental Health (2011). *Major depressive disorders among adults*. Retrieved on February 2, 2011, from http://nimh.nih.gov/statistics/1MDD_ADULT.shtml

Seyle, H. (1956). *The stress of life*. New York, NY: McGraw Hill.

Stuart, G. W., & Laraia, M. T. (2009). *Principles and practice of psychiatric nursing* (9th ed.). St. Louis, MO: Mosby, Inc., pp. 282–310.

Townsend, M. C. (2011). *Essentials in psychiatric mental health nursing* (5th ed.). Philadelphia, PA: F.A. Davis.

Varcarolis, E., & Halter, M. (2010). *Foundations of psychiatric mental health nursing: A clinical approach* (6th ed.). St. Louis, MO: Elsevier Saunders.

ANSWERS & RATIONALES

5

Anxiety Disorders

Chapter Outline

Overview/Theories
Etiology
Assessment

Nursing Diagnoses/Analysis
Planning and
    Implementation

Evaluation/Outcomes
Specific Disorders

 NCLEX-RN® Test Prep

Use the accompanying online resource, NursingReviewsandRationales, to test yourself with hundreds of NCLEX®-style practice questions.

Objectives

➤ Discuss at least three theories commonly cited to explain the origin of anxiety disorders.
➤ Explain six characteristics of anxiety disorders.
➤ Describe at least two physiological, behavioral, cognitive, and affective responses to anxiety disorders.
➤ Identify three specific treatment modalities used in the treatment of anxiety disorders.

Review at a Glance

acute stress disorder a *DSM-IV* diagnosis for the initial symptom of severe stress; a numbing and emotionally nonresponsive reaction to an extreme trauma

agoraphobia the fear of being incapacitated by being trapped in an unbearable situation with no escape; leads client to avoid places and situations that create anxiety

anxiety a state of apprehension, dread, uneasiness, or uncertainty generated by a real or perceived threat whose actual source is unidentifiable

burnout a state of mental and/or physical exhaustion

compulsion unwanted behavioral pattern or act

coping efforts to manage specific demands that are appraised as threatening

defense mechanism unconscious psychological response designed to diminish or delay anxiety and protect the person

fear a reaction to a specific danger

fight-or-flight reaction an automatic psychological state of high anxiety mediated by the sympathetic nervous system

general adaptation syndrome an automatic physical reaction to stress mediated by the sympathetic nervous system

obsession unwanted, persistent, intrusive thoughts, impulses, or images related to anxiety

panic attack a sudden episode of symptoms such as dizziness, dyspnea, tachycardia, palpitations, and feelings of impending doom and death

phobia an irrational fear of a specific activity, object, or condition that leads to a compelling desire to avoid the feared stimulus

stress a state of arousal when there is an imbalance between the demands placed on a person and the person's ability to deal with them; a normal state that may have a positive or negative reaction

stressor an internal or external event or situation that leads to feelings of anxiety

PRETEST

1 During client assessment, the nurse finds that the client is trembling and restless, blood pressure and pulse are elevated, and the client reports dry mouth, shortness of breath, inability to relax, loss of appetite, and an upset stomach. The nurse should conclude that this client is experiencing which level of anxiety?

1. Mild
2. Moderate
3. Severe
4. Panic

2 During an assessment interview the client tells the nurse, "I can't stop worrying about my makeup. I can't go anywhere nor do anything unless my makeup is fresh and perfect. I wash my face and put on fresh makeup at least once and sometimes twice an hour." The nurse's priority should be to adjust the client's plan of care so that which of the following will happen?

1. The client will be required to spend daytime hours out of own room.
2. The client will be given advance notice of approaching time for all group therapy sessions.
3. The client will be asked to keep a diary of feelings experienced if unable to groom self at will.
4. The client will be allowed to use own cosmetics and grooming products.

3 When assessing an apparently anxious client, the nurse ensures that questions related to the client's anxiety are which of the following?

1. Abstract and nonthreatening
2. Avoided until the anxiety disappears
3. Avoided until the client brings up the subject
4. Specific and direct

4 The nurse is working with a client who is anxious. Which nursing diagnosis has the highest priority at this time?

1. Defensive Coping
2. Ineffective Denial
3. Risk for Loneliness
4. Risk for Self-Directed Violence

5 The nurse has taught an anxious client a relaxation technique. The nurse would evaluate the effect of the instruction on which client goal? Select all that apply.

1. "The client will confront the source of the anxiety."
2. "The client will experience anxiety without feeling overwhelmed."
3. "The client will keep a journal of times anxiety is experienced."
4. "The client will suppress anxious feelings."
5. "The client will work through problems without being devastated."

6 The nurse has established the following long-term goal: "The client will learn new ways of coping with anxiety." For which level of anxiety is this goal most appropriate?

1. Mild
2. Moderate
3. Severe
4. Panic

7 Which of the following would be the best nursing action for a client who is having a panic attack?

1. Remain with the client.
2. Teach the client to recognize signs of a panic attack.
3. Instruct the client to remain alone until the symptoms subside.
4. Ask the client to describe what was happening before the anxiety began.

8 A client asks why a beta blocker medication has been prescribed for anxiety. When answering this question, the nurse should explain that this medication class is effective for treatment of which symptoms associated with anxiety? Select all that apply.

1. Confusion
2. Suicidal ideations
3. Insomnia
4. Palpitations
5. Rapid heart rate

9 A client who has refused to take the regular prescribed dose of clonazepam (Klonopin) reports irritability, insomnia, tremors, and sweating. The nurse concludes that the client is most likely experiencing symptoms associated with which of the following?

1. Anxiety
2. Manipulation
3. Overdose
4. Withdrawal

10 The nurse is caring for a client with posttraumatic stress disorder (PTSD). Which statement by the client would indicate the most improvement?

1. "I am responsible for what happened to me."
2. "I enjoy being back at work with my friends."
3. "I like to stay awake all night."
4. "I can't relax. I stay alert all the time."

➤ *See pages 114–116 for Answers and Rationales.*

I. OVERVIEW/THEORIES

A. *Anxiety*: a state of apprehension, dread, uneasiness, or uncertainty generated by a real or perceived threat whose actual source is unidentifiable
   1. Anxiety is an emotional, subjective response
      a. Anxiety is commonly experienced by all human beings
      b. Anxiety involves feelings of apprehension, worry, uneasiness, or dread
      c. Acute anxiety is also known as state anxiety
      d. Chronic anxiety is also known as trait anxiety
      e. Primary anxiety is related to psychological factors
      f. Secondary anxiety results as a reaction to a physical health problem
   2. **Fear:** a reaction to a specific danger
   3. **Stress:** a state of imbalance between demands placed on an individual and the individual's ability to deal with the demands
   4. **Stressor:** an internal or external event or situation that leads to feelings of anxiety
      a. Stressors are precipitating events that originate from the individual's internal or external environment
      b. Physical illness, hospitalizations, and medical treatment can be stressors
      c. It is not the stressor that causes anxiety; it is the person's perception of the stressor that leads to anxious feelings
      d. Individuals appraise stressors based on their past experiences, peer group practices, social circumstances, and current resources
   5. **Burnout:** a state of mental and/or physical exhaustion; may be caused by excessive, prolonged stress
B. Anxiety can be a healthy adaptive reaction when it alerts the person to impending threats
C. Anxiety is considered pathological when it is disproportionate to the risk, continues after the threat no longer exists, and/or interferes with functioning
D. Anxiety exists on a continuum
   1. Mild
      a. Associated with the tension of everyday life
      b. The person is alert, the perceptual field is increased, and learning is facilitated
      c. Physiological responses are within normal limits
      d. The affect is positive

2. Moderate
   a. Focus is on immediate concerns
   b. The perceptual field is narrowed
   c. Low-level sympathetic nervous system arousal occurs, such as increased pulse and respirations
   d. Tension and fear are experienced
3. Severe
   a. Focus is on specific details and behavior is directed toward relieving anxiety
   b. The perceptual field is significantly reduced, and learning cannot occur
   c. The sympathetic nervous system is aroused, possibly with somatic symptoms
   d. Severe emotional distress is experienced
4. Panic
   a. Associated with dread and terror
   b. Details are blown out of proportion, the personality is disorganized, and the person is unable to function
   c. Physiological arousal interferes with motor activities
   d. Overwhelming emotions cause regression to primitive or childish behaviors

E. *General adaptation syndrome*: an automatic physical reaction to stress mediated by the sympathetic nervous system; has two distinct stages—adaptive and maladaptive—that relate to an understanding of anxiety
   1. Stress is viewed as a nonspecific body response to any demand
   2. Stress is the initial response to a stressor
      a. As a result of hormonal activity, generalized physical arousal develops and physical and psychological defenses are mobilized
      b. The **fight-or-flight reaction**, an automatic psychological state of high anxiety mediated by the sympathetic nervous system, occurs
      c. Increased alertness is focused on the immediate task or threat
   3. The body mobilizes resources to combat stress
      a. The body stabilizes and adapts to stress, but functions below optimal level
      b. **Coping**, efforts to manage specific demands that are appraised as threatening, and **defense mechanisms**, unconscious psychological responses designed to diminish or delay anxiety and protect the person, are used
      c. Psychosomatic symptoms begin to develop
   4. Prolonged stress occurs when adaptational resources are depleted
      a. Results from inability to cope with overwhelming or long-lasting stress
      b. Thinking becomes disorganized and illogical
      c. The person may experience sensory misperceptions, delusions, hallucinations, and/or reduced orientation to reality
      d. Physical illness and even death can occur if the period of exhaustion is prolonged

F. Anxiety is related to how a person appraises stressors
   1. Events may be appraised as beneficial, benign, or stressful
   2. Primary appraisal is used to evaluate personal and environmental factors or events
   3. Secondary appraisal is used to determine how to cope with the anxiety generated by a stressful event

II. ETIOLOGY

A. **Several theories have been postulated** to account for a predisposition to anxiety
B. **One's theoretical viewpoint** affects the selection of treatment modalities
C. **Biological factors**
   1. Anxiety results from improper functioning of body systems involved in the normal stress response

2. Predisposition to the development of anxiety appears to be partially related to genetic factors
3. Hyperactivity of the autonomic nervous system is associated with anxiety
4. Several neurotransmitters have been associated with anxiety
   a. A low level of gamma-aminobutyric acid (GABA), a neurotransmitter that inhibits the reactivity of neurons, is associated with anxiety
   b. Norepinephrine is associated with the fight-or-flight reaction
   c. **Panic attacks**, sudden episodes of symptoms such as dizziness, dyspnea, tachycardia, palpitations, and feelings of impending doom and death, have been related to high levels of norepinephrine
   d. Obsessive-compulsive disorder is associated with dysregulation of serotonin
   e. Cholecystokinin, a neuropeptide that functions as a neurotransmitter, may be related to the etiology of panic disorders
5. Changes in the structure and function of the brain are associated with anxiety
   a. Anxiety appears to have its origin in the limbic system or the midline brainstem
   b. Heightened activity in the cortex has been associated with obsessive thinking
   c. PET scanning indicates that in some individuals anxiety leads to increased blood flow in the limbic system and certain areas of the midline brainstem

D. Psychodynamic factors

1. Anxiety is a warning of danger
   a. Primary anxiety begins in response to the stimulation and trauma of birth
   b. Subsequent anxiety represents a conflict between the instinctual drives (id) and the conscience (superego)
2. Anxiety and the personality are closely related
3. Symptoms of anxiety are a result of threatening unconscious mental content
4. Fear of punishment and pain may lead to anxiety
5. Unconscious repression of instinctual sexual drives may cause anxiety
6. Three types of anxiety have been identified
   a. Reality anxiety is a painful affective experience related to the perception of danger in the external environment
   b. Moral anxiety is related to feeling of guilt and/or shame
   c. Neurotic anxiety is related to threats to instincts

E. Interpersonal factors

1. All human behavior is directed toward the attainment of satisfaction and security; anxiety occurs when individuals' needs are not met
2. Anxiety is a response to external environmental factors arising out of contact with other human beings
   a. Anxiety is first conveyed from the mother to the infant
   b. Subsequent anxiety arises from fear of rejection, separation from significant others, and from feelings of inferiority
3. Symptoms of anxiety are a result of conflicts between individuals and their families, co-workers, and friends
4. Mild or moderate levels of anxiety may be expressed as anger
5. Severe anxiety produces confusion, forgetfulness, and decreased learning
6. Individuals with poor self-esteem are more susceptible to anxiety than are individuals with good self-esteem
   a. Individuals strive for security and relief from anxiety to protect the self
   b. The sense of self is based on how others evaluate the individual
   c. Individuals with low self-esteem have difficulty adapting to everyday events

F. Behavioral factors

1. Responses to stressors are often the result of learned or conditioned behavior
2. Anxiety may result from the inability to achieve desired goals

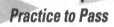

a. Experimental psychologists believe anxiety begins with the attachment of pain to a specific stimulus

b. Learning theorists believe individuals who have experienced intense fear early in life are likely to be anxious later in life

3. Anxiety may be generalized from specific stressors to similar objects and situations

4. When individuals experience too many life changes over a short period of time, they may be unable to adjust and may display dysfunctional or maladaptive behavior

G. **Other theories**

1. Social theorists emphasize the role of social condition, such as socioeconomic status and racial inequalities, in the development of anxiety

2. Intrapersonal theorists believe an external locus of control and fear of future dangers contribute to the development of anxiety

3. Cognitive theorists believe unrealistic ideas and thoughts lead to anxiety

4. Feminist theorists believe women are likely to develop anxiety because they are taught to be dependent, passive, and submissive

III. ASSESSMENT

A. **Stress affects each individual differently**, and leads to a variety of responses; the most common is anxiety

B. **Assessment should include data** to determine the level and stage of anxiety

C. **Several rating scales and diagnostic tools** are available to assess anxiety (e.g., Hamilton Anxiety Scale)

D. **Anxiety disorders are seen in all health settings**

1. Often individuals associate the symptoms of anxiety with physical disorders and seek treatment in medical-surgical health care settings

2. Shame and fear may prevent individuals from disclosing anxious feelings

3. All clients in all health care settings should be assessed for signs and symptoms of anxiety

a. Anxiety should be assessed using direct, specific questions

b. The person's cognitive ability, level of education, and language ability should be considered when formulating individualized assessment questions

4. Because anxiety can contribute to organic illness, and organic illness can lead to anxiety, physical assessment must be included in the assessment of anxious individuals

E. **Assessment should include internal and external stressors** and the individual's specific and objective reactions to the stressors

F. **Biological, psychological, and social factors** should be assessed

1. Biological assessment should include appearance, substance use, sleep patterns, nutrition, physical activity, sexual function, and menstrual cycle

2. Psychological assessment should include thought and behavioral patterns; mood and affect; self-esteem; coping patterns; defense mechanisms; orientation to time, place, and person; memory; insight; and suicide potential

3. Social assessment should include interpersonal relationships, support systems, diversional activities, ethnicity, and cultural factors

G. **Assessment should focus on the physical, affective, cognitive, social, and spiritual symptoms of stress**

1. The physical signs of anxiety include increased blood pressure, elevated respiration and heart rate, sweaty palms, diaphoresis, dilated pupils, dyspnea or hyperventilation, vertigo or light-headedness, blurred vision, urinary frequency, headache, sleep disturbance, muscle weakness or tension, anorexia, nausea, and vomiting

a. Physiologic symptoms of anxiety often mimic the symptoms of physical illness

  b. Abnormal laboratory findings, including elevated adrenocorticotropic hormones, cortisol, catecholamine levels, and hyperglycemia, may be evidence of anxiety
  c. Individuals may not associate the physical signs of anxiety with stress and may believe they have physical health problems

2. Affective symptoms include depression, irritability, apathy, crying, hypercriticism, and feelings of guilt, grief, anger, worthlessness, apprehension, and helplessness
3. Cognitive symptoms include an inability to concentrate, indecisiveness, inability to learn and reason, lack of interest, and forgetfulness
4. Social symptoms include changes in the quality and quantity of communications, fear of social interactions, and social withdrawal
5. Spiritual symptoms include feelings of hopelessness and despair, fear of death, and inability to find life meaningful

IV. NURSING DIAGNOSES/ANALYSIS

A. Several nursing diagnoses are appropriate for anxious clients
B. Anxiety (panic) related to situational and maturational crisis, real or perceived threat to self-concept or of death, unmet needs, and being exposed to a phobic stimulus
C. Fear related to phobic stimulus or phobia, being in place or situation from which escape might be difficult or implausible and causing embarrassment to self in front of others
D. Ineffective Individual Coping related to ritualistic behaviors, obsessive thoughts, inability to meet basic needs, inability to meet role expectations, and inability to problem solve effectively
E. Powerlessness related to lifestyle of helplessness, fear of disapproval from others, and unmet dependency needs
F. Social Isolation related to panic level of anxiety, past experience of difficulty in interactions with others, and repressed fears
G. A more detailed list is found in Box 5-1

V. PLANNING AND IMPLEMENTATION

A. Coping strategies
1. Coping is a process used by individuals to manage anxiety
2. The coping strategies selected by the individual are determined by the individual's intellectual ability, emotional state, physical health, beliefs, values, level of growth and development, and social status
3. Coping mechanisms may be effective or ineffective

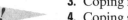

4. Coping strategies to prevent and alleviate anxiety include such specific actions as breathing exercises, guided imagery, meditation, listening to music, progressive muscle relaxation, recreational activities, crying, drinking, eating, exercising, laughing, sleeping, and swearing

Box 5-1		
Common Nursing Diagnoses for Anxious Clients	Ineffective Family Processes	Impaired Social Interaction
	Ineffective Role Performance	Ineffective Family Coping
	Decisional Conflict	Ineffective Individual Coping
	Disturbed Self-Esteem	Posttraumatic Stress Response
	Disturbed Sleep Pattern	Powerlessness
	Dysfunctional Grieving	Risk for Self-Harm
	Hopelessness	Social Isolation
	Impaired Adjustment	Spiritual Distress

Box 5-2		
Common Defense Mechanisms Used by Anxious Individuals	Conversion	Projection
	Compensation	Rationalization
	Denial	Reaction Formation
	Displacement	Regression
	Identification	Repression
	Idealization	Splitting
	Intellectualization	Sublimation
	Introjection	Suppression
	Isolation	Undoing

  5. General life management techniques related to diet, exercise, time management, and sleep can be used to prevent and alleviate stress
  6. "Problem-focused coping" is task-oriented and designed to eliminate or change the source of the anxiety or deal with the consequences of the stressor
  a. Cognitive processes are used to reduce anxiety, solve problems, and resolve conflicts

  b. Problem-focused coping utilizes the steps in the problem-solving process
   1) Assessment of the facts
   2) Development of goal
   3) Determination of alternatives for coping with the problem
   4) Identification of the risks and benefits of each possible coping alternative
   5) Selection of an alternative
   6) Implementation of the selected alternative
   7) Evaluation of the outcome
   8) Modification of actions based on evaluation
  7. "Emotional-focused coping" reinterprets the meaning of the situation
  a. Defense mechanisms are automatic unconscious emotionally focused coping strategies
  b. Defense mechanisms are often used to delay the onset of anxiety
  c. Common defense mechanisms used by anxious individuals are listed in Box 5-2

B. Psychopharmacology

  1. Anxiety disorders are treated with antidepressants (see Table 5-1)
  a. Selective serotonin reuptake inhibitors (SSRIs); these are a first line of treatment
  b. Tricyclic antidepressants (TCAs)
  c. Beta adrenergic blockers
  d. Antihistamines
  e. Anti-epileptics
  f. Buspirone (Buspar)
  2. SSRIs have a more rapid onset of action and fewer side effects
  a. Initially SSRIs may cause nausea, loose bowel movements, headaches, and insomnia
  b. A rare but serious adverse reaction is serotonin syndrome
  3. Benzodiazepines are also used for effective treatment of the symptoms of anxiety
  a. Prolonged use may lead to dependency and abuse
  b. Benzodiazepines appear to increase the effectiveness of GABA
  c. All benzodiazepines are readily absorbed in the gastrointestinal tract after oral administration

Table 5-1	Medications Commonly Used to Treat Anxiety	
Generic Name	**Trade Name**	**Clinical Use**
Selective Serotonin Reuptake Inhibitors (SSRIs)		
Citalopram	Celexa	Anti-anxiety
Escitalopram	Lexapro	Anti-anxiety
Fluoxetine	Prozac	Anti-anxiety
Paroxetine	Paxil	Anti-anxiety
Sertraline	Zoloft	Anti-anxiety
Benzodiazepines		
Alprazolam	Xanax	Anti-anxiety
Chlordiazepoxide	Librium	Anti-anxiety
Clonazepam	Klonopin	Anti-anxiety and anti-epileptic
Diazepam	Valium	Anti-anxiety
Lorazepam	Ativan	Anti-anxiety and hypnotic
Oxazepam	Serax	Anti-anxiety and hypnotic
Serotonin Partial Agonist		
Buspirone	Buspar	Anti-anxiety
Anti-epileptics		
Carbamazepine	Tegretol	Anti-anxiety and anti-epileptic
Gabapentin	Neurontin	Anti-anxiety and anti-epileptic
Valproic acid	Depakote	Anti-anxiety and anti-epileptic
Beta Blocker		
Propranolol	Inderal	Anti-anxiety
Antihistamine		
Diphenhydramine	Benadryl	Sedating antihistamine
Hydroxyzine hydrochloride	Atarax	Anti-anxiety
Tricyclics		
Amitriptylline	Elavil	Antidepressant and anti-anxiety
Clomipramine	Anafranil	Antidepressant and anti-anxiety
Imipramine	Tofranil	Antidepressant and anti-anxiety
Nortriptyline	Aventyl	Antidepressant and anti-anxiety

 d. The onset of action is very rapid and peak levels are often reached within an hour or less

 e. The doses of specific benzodiazepines vary

 f. Few drugs interact with benzodiazepines

 g. Common side effects include, ataxia, drowsiness, and impaired cognition, memory, and coordination

  1) Long-acting benzodiazepines tend to cause early-morning drowsiness

  2) Short-acting benzodiazepines may lose their effectiveness during the night, leading to nocturnal wakefulness and fatigue during the day

  3) Benzodiazepines reduce rapid-eye-movement (REM) sleep

h. Severe side effects are rare; however, sedation and death may occur when alcohol and benzodiazepines are used together

i. Benzodiazepines should be tapered to minimize symptoms of withdrawal and rebound

j. Withdrawal symptoms include difficulty concentrating, fatigue, irritability, insomnia, muscle aches, sweating, and tremors

4. Buspirone (Buspar) is a serotonin partial agonist used in the short-term treatment of anxiety

   a. Buspirone is well absorbed orally

   b. It generally takes two to three weeks for the anti-anxiety effects to become apparent and four to six weeks or longer for the drug to become fully effective

   c. Side effects of buspirone rarely occur

      1) Common side effects include dizziness, drowsiness, headache, nausea, nervousness, lightheadedness, and excitement

      2) Side effects generally decrease over time as the body adapts to the medication

   d. Buspirone is not habit forming and does not potentiate the depressant effects of alcohol, barbiturates, and other central nervous system (CNS) depressants

   e. Due to its short half-life, buspirone must be administered three times daily

   f. Because buspirone does not induce an immediate calming effect, it should not be used as a prn medication for anxiety

   g. Withdrawal symptoms do not occur when the drug is discontinued

   h. Because of its high cost and slow onset of action, buspirone is not widely prescribed

5. Beta blockers have a calming effect on the CNS

   a. Propranolol (Inderal) is a beta blocker sometimes used to treat anxiety

   b. Beta blockers are effective in treatment of physical symptoms of anxiety, such as tremors and tachycardia

6. The sedating antihistamines are used to treat lower levels of anxiety

   a. Are safe and nonaddictive and may be purchased without a prescription

   b. May be used to lower anxiety in clients with substance abuse problems

   c. Anticholinergic side effects, such as blurred vision and urinary hesitancy, may cause significant problems for elderly clients

C. **Individual and group therapy**

1. Most anxious individuals experience a marked decrease in their symptoms when they have the opportunity to discuss their feelings and problems with empathetic listeners

2. Individual and group therapy can be used to help anxious individuals develop insight into the reasons for their anxious feelings

   a. Insight therapy is most effective for highly motivated individuals who are not severely disabled by their symptoms

   b. Psychoanalysis is a form of insight therapy used by specially trained health care providers

3. Group therapy is an effective treatment modality for anxiety

   a. Group therapy provides multiple sources of feedback and an interpersonal testing ground for practicing new behaviors

   b. Group experiences increase security, satisfaction, self-esteem, and commitment

   c. Nurses can serve as group leaders and can facilitate group therapy by referring clients to groups, preparing clients for group meetings, and debriefing clients following group meetings

   d. There are several different types of groups

      1) Growth groups are designed to increase an individual's sensitivity and problem-solving ability

      2) Support groups assist individuals to deal with normal life changes and crises

Practice to Pass

An anxious client reports using over-the-counter Benadryl at bedtime to promote sleep and control "uncomfortable feelings." The client believes that because this medication is available without a prescription it is safe to use for an extended period of time. What information should you convey to the client?

                    3) Task groups use problem-solving strategies to achieve an outcome

                    4) Self-help groups are autonomous from mental health professionals and are designed to assist individuals who have common problems

                    5) Education groups are designed to provide information and teach new skills

    4. Guidelines for therapeutic nursing interventions to assist anxious clients are listed in Box 5-3

        a. An effective therapeutic relationship is based on trust

        b. The goal of nursing interventions is not to totally eliminate anxiety, but to assist the client to tolerate mild anxiety and use constructive coping mechanisms to deal with stressors and anxious feelings

        c. Client dependence on the nurse should be avoided

        d. The client should actively participate in planning goals and interventions and in evaluating outcomes

        e. When the client is hospitalized, the environment should be structured to protect the client and provide activities and therapeutic interactions to reduce anxiety

        f. Termination should occur when the client has gained optimal benefit

    5. Teaching is an important intervention for anxious clients

        a. Anxious clients should be taught to reduce their intake of caffeine, nicotine, and other stimulants

        b. Include information pertaining to diet, exercise, and general health maintenance in the teaching plan

        c. Teach relaxation techniques such as deep rhythmic breathing, progressive muscle relaxation, visualization, and meditation

        d. Social skill training and assertiveness training may also be useful

---

Box 5-3 **Guidelines for Therapeutic Nursing Interventions to Assist Anxious Individuals**	• Be aware of own level of anxiety. • Remain calm. • Establish a trusting relationship. • Protect and reassure the client. • Structure the environment to eliminate stressors. • Assess client's anxiety on an ongoing basis. • Assess the client's use of caffeine, nicotine, and other stimulants. • Assess the client for signs of depression and suicidal ideations. • Assist the client to identify stressors. • Encourage the client to express feelings and explore sources of feelings. • Help the client to examine cognitive processes and encourage positive self-talk. • Assist the client to maintain hope and find meaning in life. • Support the client's use of effective coping mechanisms. • Teach the client new coping behaviors. • Provide opportunities for the client to practice new coping behaviors. • Teach the client relaxation techniques. • Encourage appropriate grooming, sleep, diet, recreational activity, and exercise. • Facilitate the client's interactions with supportive significant others. • Use role-playing to assist the client to rehearse appropriate reactions to stressors. • Remain with clients who display high levels of anxiety; do not leave them alone. • Refer the client to community resources as needed.

D. Therapy for anxiety disorders

1. Cognitive therapy can assist individuals to identify errors in thinking and plan responses to stressors

    a. In cognitive restructuring, clients are encouraged to examine involuntary negative thoughts and to replace negative self-talk with more positive thoughts

    b. To discourage dependency, cognitive therapy is brief and time limited

    c. Cognitive therapy is structured and orderly

    d. Clients are encouraged to realistically appraise stressors

    e. Questions, rather than suggestions and advice, are used to encourage the clients to use and develop their own coping strategies

    f. "Homework" assignments are used to develop coping strategies

2. Behavioral therapy includes a variety of activities to decrease anxiety

    a. Response prevention is a form of behavior modification used to teach clients with obsessive-compulsive disorder how to prevent compulsive behaviors associated with obsessive thoughts

    b. Systematic desensitization is a form of behavior modification used to treat anxiety

        1) The client is first taught to relax

        2) While in a state of relaxation, the client is exposed to a progressive hierarchy of stress-provoking stimuli

        3) The client helps to develop the hierarchy used during the desensitization process

    c. Flooding, also known as implosion therapy, is a form of behavior modification used to treat anxiety

        1) Relaxation training is not used

        2) The client is exposed to imaginary or real-life stress provoking stimuli for an extended period of time

        3) The session is terminated when the client's anxiety decreases

    d. Thought stopping involves such techniques as instructing the client to shout "Stop!" or snap a rubber band placed on the wrist when unwelcome thoughts occur

    e. Other behavior modification techniques used to treat anxiety include modeling, shaping, token economy, role-playing, social skill training, aversion therapy, response prevention, and contingency contracting

Practice to Pass

An agoraphobic client verbalizes some interest in attending a support group designed to help people learn how to cope with stress. What strategies or actions can the nurse take to assist the client to connect with the group?

VI. EVALUATION/OUTCOMES

A. **The client's progress** toward the identified outcomes should be evaluated during each nurse–client interaction

B. **Complete remission of symptoms** and total avoidance of stress-producing stimuli is generally not an obtainable outcome

C. **Evaluation should focus on changes** in lifestyle, behavior, feelings, interpersonal relationships, level of anxiety, perception of stressors, ability to recognize signs and symptoms of anxiety, thought processes, coping skills, use of medications, utilization of community resources, client's understanding of the disorder, and view of the future

D. **Standardized rating scales** can be used to evaluate the client's level of anxiety

E. **Clients may be encouraged to keep logs of daily experiences**, which can be used to evaluate such factors as severity, frequency, and duration of panic attacks; ritualistic behaviors; feelings; and relaxation strategies

VII. SPECIFIC DISORDERS

A. **Phobic disorders**

1. Individuals with phobic disorders recognize that their **phobias** (fears of specific objects, activities, and situations) are irrational

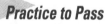

2. Contact with the feared stimuli, or mere thought of the stimuli, causes immediate, severe anxiety

 3. Individuals with phobic disorders attempt to manage their anxiety by avoiding the feared stimuli

4. Avoidance of the feared stimuli may drastically interfere with routine activities

5. There are three types of phobia

   a. **Agoraphobia** (the fear of being incapacitated by being forced into or trapped in an unbearable situation from which there is no escape) without panic attacks involves fear of places or situations such as crowds, standing in line, being on a bridge, and traveling in a plane, bus, train, or car

   b. Social phobia is excessive fear of embarrassment and humiliation in public settings

      1) A social phobia may be related to a specific situation or generalized to several similar situations

      2) Social phobias strain interpersonal relationships and the phobic individual may become more anxious when significant others attempt to provide support and assistance

      3) Treatment with alprazolam (benzodiazepine), propranol (beta blocker), SSRIs, and buspirone, and exposure therapy have been effective in reducing the anxiety associated with social phobias

   c. Specific phobia involves unrealistic fear of a particular object or situation

      1) The feared stimuli may be an object or a concern

      2) Panic level anxiety may be experienced

      3) Consider the ethnic or cultural background of the client during assessment

6. Cognitive therapy and graduated exposure or desensitization are generally used to treat phobias

7. Anti-anxiety medications may provide short-term relief of phobic anxiety

 8. Nursing care should include accepting but not supporting the phobia, exploring the client's perceptions of threats, discussing feelings that may contribute to irrational fears, and identifying strategies for change

B. Generalized anxiety disorder

1. Individuals with generalized anxiety disorder have a great deal of difficulty controlling unrealistic, excessive anxiety associated with common daily experiences

2. The continued high level of anxiety causes symptoms such as restlessness, irritability, fatigue, depression, difficulty concentrating, muscle tension, sleep disturbance, and feeling of helplessness

3. Symptoms interfere with normal daily activities

4. In an attempt to control the symptoms of generalized anxiety disorder, individuals sometimes become dependent on alcohol or other substances

5. Generalized anxiety disorder has been successfully treated by a combination of cognitive therapy and relaxation training

 6. Encourage clients with generalized anxiety disorder to rethink their perceptions of the stressor, recognize that some anxiety is a normal part of life, and learn new coping mechanisms

7. Selective serotonin reuptake inhibitors, tricyclic antidepressants, and buspirone are sometimes used to treat generalized anxiety disorders

C. Panic disorder

1. Individuals who have panic disorder have recurrent panic attacks

2. Between panic attacks, the individual may suffer from chronic worry about future panic attacks

3. The onset of a panic attack is sudden and the source of the anxiety may not be identifiable

---

Practice to Pass

A client being admitted to the hospital verbalizes fear of "shots and blood." The client reports, "My heart pounds and I can hardly breathe just thinking about shots and blood. I don't know how I am going to survive being in the hospital." How can you assist this client?

4. The symptoms of panic attacks include a desire to escape, chest pain, chills or hot flashes, choking sensations, depersonalization, dizziness, nausea, palpitations, shortness of breath, sweating, trembling, and fear of loss of control and mental illness
5. Individuals with panic attacks frequently associate their symptoms with physical illness and are concerned about death
6. Feelings of hopelessness, helplessness, and despair may lead to suicidal ideations
7. Agoraphobia may or may not be associated with panic disorder
8. During panic attacks the nurse should remain calm, stay with the client, offer reassurance, use short clear sentences, and reduce environmental stimuli
9. When the level of anxiety is mild or moderate, encourage the client to assume as much responsibility for self as possible, explore the possible causes of panic attacks, teach the signs and symptoms of escalating anxiety, reinforce appropriate coping, and teach new coping strategies
10. Benzodiazepines, selective serotonin reuptake inhibitors, and valproic acid are used to treat panic disorders; beta blockers may reduce autonomic symptoms associated with panic disorder

D. **Obsessive-compulsive disorder (OCD)**
1. Individuals with OCD recognize that their recurrent obsessive thoughts and uncontrollable compulsive behaviors are irrational
2. Control of self, others, and the environment is an important issue for obsessive-compulsive individuals
3. Common **obsessions** (unwanted, persistent, intrusive thoughts, impulses, or images related to anxiety) include thoughts about specific objects, contamination, questions, order, sex, aggressive feelings, and unacceptable impulses
4. Common **compulsions** (unwanted behavioral patterns or acts) include counting, praying, handwashing, repeating words, checking, and seeking assurance
5. In OCD, the obsessions and compulsions are either not realistically associated with preventing feared occurrences or are obviously excessive
6. Anxiety will increase if obsessive thoughts and compulsive behaviors are interrupted
7. Depression and/or substance abuse may occur as a complication of OCD
8. Behavioral techniques such as relaxation, flooding, and thought-stopping are used to treat OCD
9. Assist clients with OCD to identify situations that increase anxiety and lead to unwanted thoughts and ritualistic behaviors
   a. Assist the client to explore the meaning and purpose of thoughts and behavior
   b. Support client's attempts to decrease obsessions and compulsions
      1) Initially, time should be structured to allow the client to complete rituals
      2) Limits should gradually be applied to the time allowed for rituals
      3) The nurse and client should mutually agree on limitations of rituals
   c. Conduct teaching immediately following the completion of a ritual when the client's level of anxiety is at its lowest
10. Selective serotonin reuptake inhibitor (SSRI) antidepressant agents such as fluvoxamine (Luvox) and tricyclics such as clomipramine (Anafranil) are the most effective somatic treatments for OCD
11. Electroconvulsive therapy has been used to treat depressive symptoms associated with OCD

E. **Acute stress disorder**
1. Acute stress disorder is a *DSM-IV* diagnosis for the initial symptom of severe stress
2. Symptoms include feeling numb and emotionally nonresponsive, having a decreased awareness of one's environment, and possibly experiencing amnesia for part or all of the event; as with posttraumatic stress disorder, clients often experience recurrent images and flashbacks, which contribute to the avoidance of stimuli that remind

them of the trauma; symptoms usually begin within a month of the traumatic event, last at least two days, and go away within four weeks

F. Posttraumatic stress disorder (PTSD)
1. PTSD is associated with exposure to an extremely traumatic, menacing event such as military combat, rape, assault, kidnapping, torture, incarceration, disasters, and life-threatening illnesses
2. Symptoms of PTSD include blunted affect, inability to show affection, lack of trust, lack of responsiveness, social withdrawal, loss of interest in activities, hopelessness, restlessness, irritability, intrusive and unwanted memories of the traumatic event, amnesia for certain aspects of the trauma, depression, nightmares, flashbacks, and occasional outburst of anger and rage
3. Individuals with PTSD use denial, repression, and suppression to cope with anxious feelings
4. Nursing interventions include the following:
   a. Obtain an accurate account of the traumatic event
   b. Assess and acknowledge feelings of guilt, grief, and shame
   c. Provide a nonthreatening environment
   d. Encourage the client to discuss the traumatic event and feelings about the event
   e. Reinforce appropriate coping strategies
   f. Teach new coping strategies
   g. Assist the client to resume regular activities
5. Antidepressants (SSRIs and TCAs), carbamazepine (Tegretol), and beta-blockers seem to be somewhat effective in the treatment of PTSD

Case Study

An anxious client hospitalized on a psychiatric unit indicates her goal is to "feel more comfortable around other people." The client states, "I get so tense around other people my muscles hurt. I just don't know how to talk to other people. I am afraid I will do something wrong and offend someone. So I just stay home where it is safe. I don't have any friends here on the unit. I know I should go to the activities, but I just can't make myself do it. I wish I could relax more around others."

1. What would be the most important nursing diagnosis for this client?
2. What additional information would you need to obtain from this client?
3. How could you get this client involved in activities on the unit?
4. Which relaxation exercise would be best for you to teach this client?
5. How would you determine that the client had attained her goal?

For suggested responses, see page 297.

POSTTEST

1 Before a newly admitted anxious client begins treatment with benzodiazepines, it is most important for the nurse to assess which of the following?

1. Level of motivation for treatment
2. Situational and social support
3. Stressors and use of coping mechanisms
4. Recent use of alcohol or other depressants

2 A physician has just told a client that surgery will be required to treat a health problem. After the physician leaves, the client reports feeling angry, tense, and shaky. The nurse notes that the client's palms are sweaty and the pupils are dilated. The nurse interprets this to mean that the client is experiencing symptoms consistent with which level of the general adaptation syndrome (GAS)?

1. Alarm
2. Exhaustion
3. Generalized anxiety
4. Resistance

3 The nursing assessment indicates that a client is experiencing a panic attack. The client is unable to understand directions and is preoccupied with thoughts of danger. Which of the following would be the most appropriate nursing diagnosis?

1. Ineffective Health Maintenance
2. Impaired Thought Processes
3. Risk for Noncompliance
4. Impaired Communication

4 The nurse would formulate which goal as most appropriate for a client who has been diagnosed as having generalized anxiety disorder (GAD)?

1. The client will describe dissociative experiences.
2. The client will display the ability to cope with mild anxiety.
3. The client will relive the traumatic event.
4. The client will verbalize a sense of control over ritualistic behaviors.

5 A client who is receiving an anxiolytic medication is reluctant to participate in group therapy. The client states, "The pills I am taking will take care of my stress. I don't need to talk about my problems." In response to the client's statement which of the following should the nurse explain?

1. Many anxiolytics are habituating.
2. Medications relieve symptoms but do not change the source of the anxiety.
3. The client will need to attend group therapy only until the medication becomes effective.
4. The medications will not work unless the client participates in group therapy.

6 A client states, "I am always late for everything because I can't leave my room without checking every drawer and door to make sure they are locked. If I don't do that, I get so worried that I have to go back. I can't seem to stop my behavior." The nurse should take which action at this time?

1. Allow the client adequate time to carry out the ritual.
2. Explore childhood experiences that may have led to the behavior.
3. Encourage the client to remain in the room until the urge to recheck has decreased.
4. Remind the client that the staff will not allow others to enter the room.

7 The client is experiencing a panic attack. Which of the following actions by the nurse would be appropriate? Select all that apply.

1. Speak loudly and firmly.
2. Restrict the client's physical activity.
3. Use short simple sentences.
4. Remain calm and serene.
5. Teach cognitive restructuring skills.

8 A client has obsessive-compulsive disorder (OCD). Which of the following statements made by the client to the nurse would be the best indicator of improvement?

1. "I have more control over my thoughts and behaviors."
2. "I know that my thoughts and behaviors are not normal."
3. "I only do my ritual to reward myself when I have been good."
4. "My friends don't know about my disorder."

9 The client is taking triazolam (Halcion) to reduce anxiety related symptoms. Which statement indicates that the nurse should provide more teaching to the client? Select all that apply.

1. "The doctor wants me to take this drug at bedtime because it will help me sleep better."
2. "I should stop taking this medication abruptly."
3. "I might not be able to drive while I am taking this medication."
4. "I will probably have to take this medication for the rest of my life."
5. "I don't need to go to therapy since the medication is working."

10 A client with generalized anxiety disorder states, "I now know the best thing for me to do is just to try to forget my worries." How should the nurse evaluate this statement?

1. The client is developing insight.
2. The client's coping skills are improving.
3. The client needs to be encouraged to verbalize feelings.
4. The nurse–client relationship should be terminated.

➤ *See pages 116–118 for Answers and Rationales.*

ANSWERS & RATIONALES

Pretest

1 **Answer: 3 Rationale:** Severe is correct. The client's complaints indicate the fight-or-flight response that occurs at the severe level of anxiety. Mild anxiety is associated with the tension of everyday life; the person is alert, the perceptual field is increased, and learning is facilitated. In moderate anxiety, the perceptual field is narrowed, and low-level sympathetic arousal occurs. In panic anxiety, the perceptual field is narrowed, and low-level sympathetic arousal occurs. **Cognitive Level:** Analyzing **Client Need:** Psychosocial Integrity **Integrated Process:** Nursing Process: Assessment **Content Area:** Mental Health **Strategy:** Develop a mental picture of the client. Recall facts about behaviors associated with different levels of anxiety. Rule out two of the options immediately, as mild anxiety is normal and panic-level anxiety results in greatly disorganized and frightened behavior. **Reference:** Kneisl, C., Wilson, H., & Trigoboff, E. (2009). *Contemporary psychiatric–mental health nursing* (2nd ed.). Upper Saddle River, NJ: Prentice Hall, p. 144.

2 **Answer: 2 Rationale:** Giving the client advance notice for group therapy sessions is correct. Obsessive-compulsive (OC) behaviors represent attempts to relieve anxiety and decrease fear or guilt through controlling and ritualizing activities. People with obsessions and compulsions engage in a kind of magical thinking and believe that something terrible will happen if they do not act on their compulsion. If deprived of opportunity and adequate time to carry out a ritualistic compulsion, the person's anxiety will escalate significantly, resulting in an increased need to carry out the compulsive behavior. It is best to schedule a therapeutic activity just after the

client has completed a ritual. The client with OC symptoms is likely to have been socially isolated prior to admission and should be encouraged to participate in therapeutic and social activities on the unit. Instead of a diary connecting feelings experienced if unable to carry out the ritual, it would be more useful for the client to understand the relationship of feelings to the initiation of the ritual. The client should be allowed to use personal products, but this is not as important as allowing the client extra time to prepare for unit activities. **Cognitive Level:** Analyzing **Client Need:** Psychosocial Integrity **Integrated Process:** Nursing Process: Planning **Content Area:** Mental Health **Strategy:** Notice how much time the client's rituals are requiring. Recall that carrying out a ritual temporarily reduces anxiety. **Reference:** Kneisl, C., Wilson, H., & Trigoboff, E. (2009). *Contemporary psychiatric–mental health nursing* (2nd ed.). Upper Saddle River, NJ: Prentice Hall, p. 460.

3 **Answer: 4 Rationale:** Specific and direct is correct. Because of shame or difficulty organizing thoughts, clients may be reluctant to talk about anxiety. Questions should be specific, direct, and individualized to the client. Abstract and nonthreatening is incorrect because when a client is experiencing anxiety, abstract thinking is impaired. Both avoidance options are incorrect because the nurse should ask direct questions about the client's anxiety. **Cognitive Level:** Applying **Client Need:** Psychosocial Integrity **Integrated Process:** Caring **Content Area:** Mental Health **Strategy:** Recall behaviors associated with anxiety. Remember that an individual loses ability to process information as the level of anxiety escalates. **Reference:** Varcarolis, E., Carson, V., & Shoemaker, N. (2009). *Foundations of psychiatric mental health* *nursing: A clinical approach* (6th ed.). St. Louis, MO: Saunders Elsevier, pp. 227–229.

4 **Answer: 4** **Rationale:** Risk for Self-Directed Violence is correct. Safety needs have a higher priority than psychosocial needs, even when they are intense. The other options are applicable nursing diagnoses for anxious clients, but safety has the highest priority. **Cognitive Level:** Analyzing **Client Need:** Psychosocial Integrity **Integrated Process:** Nursing Process: Planning **Content Area:** Mental Health **Strategy:** Notice that three of the options indicate psychological needs. Recall Maslow's hierarchy to select the most basic need of the choices available. **Reference:** Varcarolis, E., Carson, V., & Shoemaker, N. (2010). *Foundations of psychiatric mental health nursing: A clinical approach* (6th ed.). St. Louis, MO: Saunders Elsevier, p. 229.

5 **Answer: 2, 5** **Rationale:** Two options are correct. The goal of teaching calming techniques such as relaxation therapy assists the client to learn to experience anxiety without feeling threatened and overwhelmed, and to work through problems without being devastated. Relaxation therapy does not assist a client to confront sources of anxiety, but rather to reduce the level of intensity of the anxiety. Keeping a journal is a self-monitoring technique but is not used to measure the outcome of relaxation. The goal is not to suppress anxious feelings but to make them more manageable. **Cognitive Level:** Applying **Client Need:** Psychosocial Integrity **Integrated Process:** Nursing Process: Planning **Content Area:** Mental Health **Strategy:** Think about times that you have used a relaxation technique. For what purpose did you decide to use it? **Reference:** Fontaine, K. (2009). *Mental health nursing* (6th ed.). Upper Saddle River, NJ: Prentice Hall, p. 251.

6 **Answer: 2** **Rationale:** Moderate is correct. Long-term goals for moderate anxiety should focus on assisting the client to understand the causes of anxiety and learn new coping strategies. Mild anxiety does not require nursing intervention. Clients at high (severe or panic) levels of anxiety have very narrowed attention and cannot focus on learning. **Cognitive Level:** Applying **Client Need:** Psychosocial Integrity **Integrated Process:** Nursing Process: Planning **Content Area:** Mental Health **Strategy:** Recall cognitive characteristics at different levels of anxiety. **Reference:** Fontaine, K. (2009). *Mental health nursing* (6th ed.). Upper Saddle River, NJ: Prentice Hall, p 251.

7 **Answer: 1** **Rationale:** Remaining with the client is correct. To promote safety, the nurse should stay with extremely anxious clients. It is important that the nurse remains calm and serene, use simple communication, and convey an attitude of calm authoritative competence. During a panic attack a client is unable to focus on learning how to recognize signs of a panic attack. The priority of the nurse is to provide safety, as clients at panic level anxiety are frantic and extremely disordered cognitively. Their judgment is impaired, they feel frantic, and they are therefore at high risk for injury if left alone until symptoms subside. Exploring possible sources of anxiety and what was happening before the anxiety began is appropriate when intervening in lower levels of anxiety. **Cognitive Level:** Analyzing **Client Need:** Psychosocial Integrity **Integrated Process:** Nursing Process: Implementation **Content Area:** Mental Health **Strategy:** Recall that at the panic level of anxiety, people are frantic and unable to make sound decisions. **Reference:** Kneisl, C., Wilson, H., & Trigoboff, E. (2009). *Contemporary psychiatric–mental health nursing* (2nd ed.). Upper Saddle River, NJ: Prentice Hall, p. 458.

8 **Answer: 4, 5** **Rationale:** Palpitations and rapid heart rate are correct. Beta blockers are effective in reducing cardiovascular symptoms (increased pulse and blood pressure, possible palpitations) associated with anxiety because they target the beta-adrenergic receptors in the sympathetic nervous system (fight-or-flight response). The other options are not cardiovascular symptoms and reflect symptoms that beta blockers will not relieve. **Cognitive Level:** Applying **Client Need:** Pharmacological and Parenteral Therapies **Integrated Process:** Teaching and Learning **Content Area:** Mental Health **Strategy:** Recall that beta blockers have their primary effects on cardiovascular functioning. Look for a cardiovascular-related answer in the options. **Reference:** Fontaine, K. (2009). *Mental health nursing* (6th ed.). Upper Saddle River, NJ: Prentice Hall, p. 241.

9 **Answer: 4** **Rationale:** Withdrawal is correct. Abrupt withdrawal from a benzodiazepine may lead to symptoms associated with hyperarousal. Benzodiazepine use can quickly lead to physical dependency. Although the client's symptoms could be related to anxiety, the nurse notes that these symptoms began after the client refused a benzodiazepine. Manipulation is a purposeful behavior aimed at getting one's needs met at the expense of someone else. No data is given to suggest manipulation on the part of the client. Signs of benzodiazepine overdose include severe drowsiness, ataxia, and impaired coordination. **Cognitive Level:** Analyzing **Client Need:** Psychosocial Integrity **Integrated Process:** Nursing Process: Assessment **Content Area:** Mental Health **Strategy:** Note the relationship of the onset of symptoms to the time of the client's having refused the medication. **Reference:** Varcarolis, E., Carson, V., & Shoemaker, N. (2009). *Foundations of psychiatric mental health nursing: A clinical approach* (6th ed.). St. Louis, MO: Saunders Elsevier, p. 410.

10 **Answer: 2** **Rationale:** "I enjoy being back at work with my friends" is correct. People with PTSD often avoid interactions and develop an isolated lifestyle that prevents them from working and socializing with others. Clients are likely to feel victimized by the traumatic event ("I am responsible for what happens to me"). The other options reflect symptoms of PTSD, indicating the client is not yet showing improvement. **Cognitive Level:** Analyzing **Client Need:** Psychosocial Integrity **Integrated Process:** Nursing Process: Evaluation **Content Area:** Mental Health **Strategy:** Recall behaviors common to persons experiencing PTSD. Notice that this question is asking for an indication of improvement. **Reference:** Varcarolis, E., Carson, V., & Shoemaker, N. (2009). *Foundations of psychiatric mental health nursing: A clinical approach* (6th ed.). St. Louis, MO: Saunders Elsevier, pp. 221–223.

Posttest

1 **Answer: 4** **Rationale:** Recent use of alcohol or other depressants is correct. Combined use of benzodiazepines and other central nervous system depressants can lead to death from respiratory failure. If the alcohol has been ingested shortly before admission (which is not at all uncommon for a client experiencing anxiety), giving a benzodiazepine could put the client at risk. Social support, coping mechanisms, and motivation for treatment (all the other options) are all important factors to document during the assessment. However, the client's immediate risk for safety is the priority at this point and must be assessed first. The other data can be compiled when the formal assessment is completed at a later time. **Cognitive Level:** Analyzing **Client Need:** Pharmacological and Parenteral Therapies **Integrated Process:** Nursing Process: Assessment **Content Area:** Mental Health **Strategy:** Recognize that benzodiazepines are central nervous system (CNS) depressants. Identify potential dangers that can be associated with them. **Reference:** Fontaine, K. (2009). *Mental health nursing* (6th ed.). Upper Saddle River, NJ: Prentice Hall, p. 209.

2 **Answer: 1** **Rationale:** Alarm is correct. The symptoms displayed by the client reflect an increased alertness and heightened level of arousal focused on an immediate concern or perceived threat. This is also referred to as fight-or-flight response and occurs during the alarm stage of the general adaptation syndrome. Exhaustion and resistance consist of more severe symptoms (both physical and psychological) experienced in the general adaptation syndrome. They occur in the second and third stages respectively of GAS. General anxiety is characterized by significant difficulty controlling unrealistic, excessive anxiety associated with common daily experiences. This type of anxiety is more generalized, or free floating, and does not necessarily have a specific focus. **Cognitive Level:** Analyzing **Client Need:** Physiological Adaptation **Integrated Process:** Nursing Process: Assessment **Content Area:** Mental Health **Strategy:** Recall theoretical information about the GAS. Look carefully at the client's presenting behaviors to guide your selection. **Reference:** Kneisl, C., Wilson, H., & Trigoboff, E. (2009). *Contemporary psychiatric–mental health nursing* (2nd ed.). Upper Saddle River, NJ: Prentice Hall, pp. 139–140.

3 **Answer: 2** **Rationale:** Impaired Thought Processes is correct. Impaired Thought Processes related to understanding directions and/or obsessive thoughts is an appropriate nursing diagnosis for clients with severe or panic-level anxiety. This is an important nursing diagnosis because the altered thought processes that occur at this level of anxiety are usually accompanied with overwhelming emotions and disorganization. These factors often result in a regression to more primitive behaviors putting the client at risk for injury. Ineffective Health Maintenance does not reflect the current cognitive state of the client. Risk for Noncompliance is an at-risk problem, and this client's current emotional state and risk for danger will take preference over any risk diagnosis. Impaired Communication does not reflect the current cognitive state of the client. **Cognitive Level:** Analyzing **Client Need:** Physiological Adaptation **Integrated Process:** Nursing Process: Diagnosis **Content Area:** Mental Health **Strategy:** Remember that safety is always a priority concern. Of the choices available, altered thought processes addresses impaired cognition that occurs with acute panic, creating risks for injury to self or others. **Reference:** Varcarolis, E., Carson, V., & Shoemaker, N. (2009). *Foundations of psychiatric mental health nursing: A clinical approach* (6th ed.). St. Louis, MO: Saunders Elsevier, pp. 226–227.

4 **Answer: 2** **Rationale:** Displaying the ability to cope with mild anxiety is correct. Clients with generalized anxiety disorder should be able to demonstrate effective coping with mild anxiety. Clients with generalized anxiety disorder do not generally have dissociative experiences or perform ritualistic behaviors. Dissociation and compulsive behaviors occur with more severe levels of anxiety. Neither of these symptoms is in the diagnostic criteria for GAD. Anxiety related to traumatic events is associated with posttraumatic stress disorder. **Cognitive Level:** Analyzing **Client Need:** Psychosocial Integrity **Integrated Process:** Nursing Process: Planning **Content Area:** Mental Health **Strategy:** Recall how GAD presents. Recognize that the behaviors in the other options are more dramatic than is generally true when a person has generalized anxiety disorder. **Reference:** Varcarolis, E., Carson, V., & Shoemaker, N. (2009). *Foundations of psychiatric mental health nursing: A clinical approach* (6th ed.). St. Louis, MO: Saunders Elsevier, pp. 220–222.

5 **Answer: 2** **Rationale:** Medications relieve symptoms but do not change the source of anxiety is correct. Anxiolytic medications alleviate or reduce symptoms of anxiety so the client can learn to identify stressors and develop effective coping mechanisms. Anxiolytics allow the client to benefit from individual and group therapy. Anxiolytics cannot change the source of the anxiety. While the statement that many anxiolytics are habituating is true, it does not provide the information that the client needs at this time. The statement about needing to attend group therapy only until the medication becomes effective is inaccurate. Anxiolytics are not curative. Persons with anxiety disorders need to change their coping behaviors. They cannot rely on drugs to address the underlying source of the anxiety. It is during group therapy that effective coping mechanisms can be introduced and practiced. The statement that the medications will not work without group therapy is inaccurate. The chemical effect of the anxiolytics can be realized whether the client is in group or not; however, the combination of anxiolytic and group therapy is considered to be more effective than either alone. **Cognitive Level:** Applying **Client Need:** Psychosocial Integrity **Integrated Process:** Teaching and Learning **Content Area:** Mental Health **Strategy:** Don't be misled by the statement that many anxiolytics are habituating; it contains an accurate statement but does not answer the question asked. **Reference:** Fontaine, K. (2009). *Mental health nursing* (6th ed.). Upper Saddle River, NJ: Prentice Hall, pp. 239–241.

6 **Answer: 1 Rationale:** Allowing the client time to carry out the ritual is correct. Ritualistic behaviors are related to heightened anxiety. The compulsive behaviors increase in intensity and/or frequency as the anxiety level escalates. The nurse should allow the client to complete the ritual in as reasonable and timely a manner as possible. Interrupting or stopping the ritual will increase anxiety, which in turn will increase the client's need to engage in the ritual. Exploring childhood experiences cannot be expected to bring about reductions in anxiety or ritualistic behavior. Clients who display compulsive behaviors need support and encouragement to manage their daily lives by modifying the environment and allowing time for the behaviors. Assigning solitude cannot be expected to decrease the client's need for the ritual. What causes the client to have a need to perform the ritual is not from the actual environment. Hence, remaining in the room will not necessarily decrease the urge to check and recheck compulsively. The nurse should recognize that the client's motivations for the rechecking arise from within the psyche and are not related to environmental events. While keeping others out of the room may spare the client from feelings of embarrassment, it will not necessarily decrease the compulsive behavior. **Cognitive Level:** Analyzing **Client Need:** Psychosocial Integrity **Integrated Process:** Nursing Process: Planning **Content Area:** Mental Health **Strategy:** Look beyond the rechecking behavior to what is thought to be underlying, or causing, it. **Reference:** Fontaine, K. (2009). *Mental health nursing* (6th ed.). Upper Saddle River, NJ: Prentice Hall, p. 230.

7 **Answer: 3, 4 Rationale:** Using short, simple sentences and remaining calm is correct. At panic-level anxiety, the individual will not be able to process complex ideas. Using short simple sentences will provide the best way to communicate information, directions, and support. Additionally, the nurse's highest priority is to reduce the client's anxiety to a more tolerable level. Speaking calmly and projecting an image of competence may have a calming effect on the client. The nurse should avoid communicating loudly and firmly. Speaking to the client in this manner would most likely further increase the client's fearfulness, anxiety, and agitation. The client in panic level of anxiety has an urgent need for physical

activity. Attempts to prevent or restrict the activity will result in increased agitation. The physical hyperactivity should be allowed, but in a protected and non-stimulating environment in which the nurse is physically present and attending to the client's safety needs. Clients in panic-level anxiety are not able to learn, because they cannot concentrate and have a very narrow self-focus. Learning best takes place when anxiety is at a mild or moderate level. Cognitive restructuring is appropriate for clients with chronic, lower level anxiety. **Cognitive Level:** Analyzing **Client Need:** Safety and Infection Control **Integrated Process:** Nursing Process: Implementation **Content Area:** Mental Health **Strategy:** Develop a mental picture of this client, who is feeling out of control and intensely anxious and fearful. Look for options that will address these feelings and reduce the anxiety while at the same time providing safety. **Reference:** Kneisl, C., Wilson, H., & Trigoboff, E. (2009). *Contemporary psychiatric–mental health nursing* (2nd ed.). Upper Saddle River, NJ: Prentice Hall, p. 458.

8 **Answer: 1 Rationale:** The statement about having more control is correct. Loss of control is a major concern for clients who have OCD. Goals related to control of unwanted thoughts and behaviors are appropriate for these clients. Clients with OCD are aware that their compulsive behaviors are not normal. Knowing this does not mediate or change their ability to manage or control the unwanted thoughts and behaviors. This statement only reflects the client's awareness of his or her disorder; it does not indicate control over the behaviors and thoughts. The compulsive behaviors are utilized to reduce anxiety, not to reward self for good behavior. The statement about friends not knowing about the disorder does not indicate control over behavior. **Cognitive Level:** Analyzing **Client Need:** Psychosocial Integrity **Integrated Process:** Nursing Process: Evaluation **Content Area:** Mental Health **Strategy:** Recall that clients with OCD report being unable to resist urges and stop unwanted thoughts. **Reference:** Fontaine, K. (2009). *Mental health nursing* (6th ed.). Upper Saddle River, NJ: Prentice Hall, p. 251.

9 **Answer: 2, 4, 5 Rationale:** Three options are correct. Hypnotic and anxiolytic agents should be taken for as short a period of time as possible. Physical dependence on these drugs can develop in a very short period of time. Additionally, anxious clients should be assisted to improve their coping mechanisms without relying on medication. Drugs should not be abruptly stopped; they need to be tapered off. Therapy is a healthy option to take to work through the anxiety. The statement about taking the drug at bedtime shows awareness of correct drug information. Triazolam (Halcion) has both anxiolytic and sedative effects. Its primary use is as a nighttime sedative. Since clients can become physically dependent on benzodiazepines in a very short period of time, abrupt discontinuation can precipitate a withdrawal response. The statement about not driving shows awareness of correct drug information: driving and operating heavy machinery are not recommended when clients take benzodiazepines or other drugs that have sedating effects. **Cognitive Level:** Analyzing **Client Need:** Pharmacological and Parenteral Therapies **Integrated Process:** Teaching and Learning **Content Area:** Mental Health **Strategy:** Apply what you know about benzodiazepines in general. Remember that these are one of the most popular "street drugs." **Reference:** Kneisl, C., Wilson, H., & Trigoboff, E. (2009). *Contemporary psychiatric–mental health nursing* (2nd ed.). Upper Saddle River, NJ: Prentice Hall, pp. 458–459.

10 Answer: 3 Rationale: The client needs encouragement to verbalize feelings is correct. Suppression of feelings requires energy and will lead to increased anxiety. Clients need to talk about their feelings. The client's statement does not suggest insight, which is the development of understanding of one's motivations. It

suggests that instead of addressing and managing worries, the client will use avoidant behaviors. Generalized anxiety is characterized by worrying. The client will not be able to independently reduce this behavior and improve coping. However, if the client is taught the technique of cognitive restructuring, this might help to reduce the worrying behaviors. The nurse–client relationship should be maintained because the client continues to require guidance and support. **Cognitive Level:** Analyzing **Client Need:** Psychosocial Integrity **Integrated Process:** Nursing Process: Evaluation **Content Area:** Mental Health **Strategy:** Compare and contrast symptoms of acute anxiety and generalized anxiety. **Reference:** Kneisl, C., Wilson, H., & Trigoboff, E. (2009). *Contemporary psychiatric–mental health nursing* (2nd ed.). Upper Saddle River, NJ: Prentice Hall, pp. 447–448.

References

American Psychiatric Association (2000). *Diagnostic and statistical manual of mental disorders, text revision* (4th ed.). Washington, DC: American Psychiatric Association.

Carpenito, L. J. (2011). *Nursing diagnosis: Application to clinical practice* (13th ed.). Philadelphia: Lippincott Williams & Wilkins.

Fontaine, K. L. (2009). *Mental health nursing.* (6th ed.). Upper Saddle River, NJ: Pearson Education, Inc.

Kneisl, C. R., Wilson, H. S., & Trigoboff, E. (2009). *Contemporary psychiatric–mental health nursing* (2nd ed.). Upper Saddle River, NJ: Pearson Education, Inc.

Stuart, G. W. & Laraia, M. T. (2009). *Principles and practice of psychiatric nursing* (9th ed.). St. Louis: Mosby.

Townsend, M. C. (2011). *Essentials of psychiatric/mental health nursing.* (5th ed.). Philadelphia: F.A. Davis.

Varcarolis, E. & Halter, M. (2010). *Foundations of psychiatric mental health nursing: A clinical approach* (6th ed.). St. Louis: Saunders Elsevier.

ANSWERS & RATIONALES

Somatoform Disorders

Chapter Outline

Overview
Etiology
Assessment

Nursing Diagnoses/
 Analysis
Planning and Implementation

Evaluation/Outcomes
Specific Disorders

Objectives

➤ Identify five characteristics associated with somatoform disorders.
➤ State examples of at least four nursing diagnoses frequently used in the management of clients experiencing somatoform disorders.
➤ Formulate three intervention strategies for clients with somatoform disorders.

NCLEX-RN® Test Prep

Use the accompanying online resource, NursingReviewsandRationales, to test yourself with hundreds of NCLEX®-style practice questions.

Review at a Glance

body dysmorphic disorder (BDD) a somatoform disorder characterized by preoccupation and/or fear due to an imagined or real defect in appearance

conversion disorder a somatoform disorder in which motor, sensory, or visceral function is impaired and indifferent whereby psychological factors versus biological factors are determined to be the etiology

hypochondriasis a somatoform disorder whereby bodily functions and/or bodily symptoms are misinterpreted as severe or life threatening; the obsession causes intense fear and worry

ideas of reference misinterpretation of external events as having a direct reference to oneself

la belle indifference an indifferent and unconcerned attitude toward

physical symptoms; persons with *la belle indifference* seek secondary gain

organic basis symptoms that are based upon pathophysiological, structural, and/or functional changes as supported by objective data such as a history and physical, laboratory, and/or diagnostic findings

pain disorder a somatoform disorder characterized by pain as the primary focus of the individual's need; psychological versus physiological factors are determined to be integral to the onset, severity, and exacerbations of the pain

primary gain symbolic resolution of unconscious conflict that decreases anxiety and wards off the psychological conflict from conscious awareness

pseudoneurological motor and sensory symptoms that have no

objective, laboratory, or diagnostic data to support an organic basis

secondary gain advantage person gains from being ill; the gain may be in the form of sympathy, empathy, disability benefits, and/or attention; persons with somatization disorders do not consciously/intentionally seek secondary gain

somatization disorder (formerly known as hysteria) a somatoform disorder characterized by numerous complaints in multiple body systems that include pain, sexual, gastrointestinal, and neurological symptoms; onset is prior to age 30 and lasts for years

somatoform disorder a psychiatric disorder whereby there is no organic basis for physical symptoms that are the primary individual's complaints

1 An older client diagnosed with chronic low back pain secondary to pain disorder receives cooking and cleaning help from her extended family. The mental health nurse anticipates that this client benefits from which of the following in this situation?

1. Primary gain
2. Secondary gain
3. Attention
4. Malingering

2 The spouse of a woman diagnosed with somatization disorder tells the nurse that he "is running out of patience with her" and feels that "she has all of those health problems on purpose." What is the best response by the nurse?

1. "Have you tried asking her? I think she'd tell you the truth."
2. "Your wife is trying to gain your attention."
3. "She doesn't have the problem on purpose; however, this is probably difficult for both of you."
4. "She has some significant emotional problems that she cannot admit."

3 The client has chronic pain to the back and is diagnosed with pain disorder. Which statement by the client indicates to the nurse that the plan of care has been successful?

1. "I realize that my pain can be influenced by stress."
2. "I should avoid most physical activity."
3. "Relaxation techniques only help when I am anxious about my pain."
4. "I should keep myself pain free by increasing my pain medication as I need it."

4 The client presents to an outpatient clinic with a history of conversion disorder reporting a new symptom of paralysis to the bilateral upper extremities. This is not the first time this has occurred. He states, "I cannot work anymore, and I've missed work for three weeks now." The nurse would infer which of the following about this client's condition? Select all that apply.

1. It causes significant distress in occupational, social, and or academic functioning.
2. It does sometimes manifest with paralysis.
3. It can sometimes cause psychosis; a mental status exam should be performed on the client.
4. It follows neurological pathways.
5. It may manifest with an affect of *la belle indifference*.

5 When completing the nursing history, what would the nurse expect the client who is diagnosed with somatization disorder to reveal?

1. Abrupt onset of physical symptoms at menopause
2. Episodes of personality dissociation
3. Ignoring physical symptoms until role performance was altered
4. Numerous physical symptoms in many organ systems

6 When caring for a client diagnosed with hypochondriasis, the nurse should take which of the following actions?

1. Explore the details and history of the client's early life and illnesses.
2. Encourage the client to seek second opinions about the symptoms experienced.
3. Assist the client to identify relationships between life events and physical symptoms.
4. Have the spouse encourage the client to talk more about the symptoms.

7 The nurse would anticipate that a health assessment of a client with a diagnosis of conversion disorder is likely to reveal which of the following?

1. Elevated serum calcium levels
2. Sensory loss along affected nerve tracks
3. No significant physical or laboratory findings
4. Motor loss to body parts along the nerve tracks

8 For a client diagnosed with a somatoform disorder, the nurse plans to write which nursing diagnoses in the client's plan of care? Select all that apply.

1. Ineffective Role Performance
2. Impaired Coping
3. Risk for Violence, Self-Directed
4. Impaired Oxygenation
5. Health-Seeking Behaviors

9 A hospitalized client diagnosed with a somatization disorder asks for as needed (prn) medication for complaints of abdominal pain. What is the nurse's best response?

1. Matter-of-factly assess the pain and administer prn medication.
2. Inform the client of negative gastroscopy findings.
3. Teach the client to take slow, deep breaths.
4. Delay fulfilling request for medication to see if the pain subsides first.

10 A client treated for a diagnosis of hypochondriasis would demonstrate understanding of the disorder by which statement to the nurse?

1. "I realize that tests and lab results cannot pick up on the seriousness of my illness."
2. "Once my family members realize how severely ill I am, they will be more understanding."
3. "I know that I don't have a serious illness, even though I still worry about the symptoms."
4. "I realize that exposure to toxins can cause significant organ damage."

➤ *See pages 134–136 for Answers and Rationales.*

I. OVERVIEW

   A. *Somatoform disorders* are a group of illnesses whereby there is no physical evidence to support the physical manifestations that the client presents

   B. **Physical symptoms**
      1. In persons with somatoform disorder symptoms are inorganic in nature; this means that the client's history and physical examination, as well as laboratory and/or diagnostic test results, show no evidence of structural or functional changes of the body

      2. Physical symptoms for which there is no **organic basis** allow clients to meet dependency needs without consciously understanding such dependency needs exist
   C. **Clients with somatoform disorders** may be admonished to be emotionally and psychologically "strong" and mentally intact; therefore, they do not confront and express any emotional needs
   D. **Requirements for a diagnosis of any somatoform disorder**
      1. The symptoms must cause significant distress and/or disruption in occupational, social, academic, and/or other areas of functioning
      2. Medical and/or substance abuse must be ruled out as the specific cause of the bodily manifestations

II. ETIOLOGY

   A. **Psychophysiological responses**
      1. Amplified awareness of somatic stimuli caused by impaired central nervous system inhibitory function
      2. Deficiency in communication between the right and left hemispheres of brain that impairs the ability of the individual to express emotions directly

B. Defense against anxiety

1. A person may express unconscious psychological conflict that results in uncomfortable feelings of anxiety that are manifested by physical/bodily symptoms
   a. Supported by the belief that physical illness versus psychological illness is more socially acceptable
   b. The physical symptoms facilitate the individual's dependency needs for nurturance, attention, and assistance
2. Allows for the individual to avoid acknowledgement of the psychological conflict
   a. It is less distressing for the client to seek relief from physical symptoms versus having to confront psychological conflicts
   b. Clients unconsciously do not want to resolve the physical symptoms because the bodily manifestation facilitates a decrease in anxiety levels

Practice to Pass

Explain how anxiety plays a role in the physical manifestations of somatoform disorders.

C. Family dynamics

1. Family rules and values may prevent direct expression of the psychological conflict
2. Family may view the physical illnesses as acceptable reasons (or rationalizations) for client not to have to meet expected age-related growth and development tasks
3. Family may perceive the physical illness as an acceptable means to allow the individual to avoid meeting various family and/or societal role expectations
4. Family may consciously, subconsciously, or unconsciously be largely contributing to or reinforcing to the client's secondary gain
5. The physical symptoms may be used by the client as a means to unconsciously control/manipulate other family members
6. The physical symptoms may be used by the client as an attempt to try to stabilize unhealthy family relationships

D. Culture influences physical expressions

1. Some cultures accept/expect distress when manifested in bodily symptoms, and deny and/or reject distress as psychological in nature
2. Somatization disorders in the *DSM-IV* are primarily from data collected specifically in the United States
3. Somatization symptoms are commonly culture-bound, and some symptoms appear exclusively in specific cultures; examples include the following:
   a. The feeling of "worms in the head" is seen in parts of Africa
   b. Male reproductive problems are reported as a syndrome in India due to the concern of semen loss

III. ASSESSMENT

A. History and physical is completed on the client and reveals the following:

1. The onset is variable, depending upon the specific somatoform disorder
2. The client often has sought care from multiple care providers without a history and physical, laboratory, and/or diagnostic criteria that supported a pathophysiological reason for the physical manifestations
3. The client often has sought care from multiple care providers, yet regardless of treatment continues to experience non-relief of physical symptoms
4. The client views the problem as physical in nature and denies any possibility of psychological/emotional influences on the physical symptoms
5. The client undermines (underreports) psychological, social problems, and/or current stressors that may be occurring in their life
6. **Primary gain**: the subjective data collected on the client may give clues that the illness allows for reprieve from various personal, family, and/or societal responsibilities
7. **Secondary gain**: sick role allows for dependency, attention, and nurturance needs to be met

Practice to Pass

Differentiate between primary and secondary gain.

8. As the psychosomatic illness progresses, the client is increasingly socially isolated, and physically less active or completely inactive
9. The family may have insisted that the client seek health care examination due to the client's altered role performance
10. Persons with somatoform disorder are often poor historians; it is important to assess for clues of an inconsistent history regarding diagnostic testing, hospitalizations, and treatments

B. Focused physical assessment

1. A physical assessment is imperative since physical symptomology is the primary manifestation of persons with somatic disorders
2. A thorough head-to-toe assessment of the client must be completed that includes both subjective and objective data; body systems that commonly manifest symptoms in persons with psychosomatic disorders include the following:
   a. Cardiovascular: fainting, hypertension, migraine headache, tachycardia, noncardiac chest pain
   b. Musculoskeletal: back pain, fatigue, tension headache, tremor
   c. Respiratory: bronchospasm, dyspnea, hyperventilation
   d. Gastrointestinal: bloating, nausea, constipation, difficulty swallowing, abdominal pain, vomiting
   e. Integumentary: pruritis
   f. Genitourinary: difficulties in micturation (voiding), menstrual disturbances, sexual dysfunction, pelvic pain
   g. Neurological (pseudoneurological): impaired coordination or balance, paralysis, paresthesias, dizziness, difficulty swallowing, urinary retention
   h. The five senses: blindness, double vision, deafness (somatization disorder), impairment in touch sensation

C. Mental status examination (MSE): in many cases persons with somatoform disorders do not seek psychiatric help, but if/when they do, a MSE is completed

1. **Appearance**: observe age, dress, posture, hygiene, gait, facial expressions, overall nutritional status, and overall health status; persons with body dysmorphic disorder are preoccupied with dissatisfaction with imagined or minor flaws (i.e., on the face, head, genitals, breasts, abdomen)
2. **Speech**: assess volume, rate, amount, and any other distinct features (i.e., slurred, stuttering)
3. **Motor activity**: examine level of activity, restless, agitation, appearance of pain; persons with somatoform disorders and pain disorder may manifest symptoms of pain
4. **Mood**: ask the client how he or she is feeling; in persons with psychosomatic illness the mood is often reported as indifferent, euthymic (normal), depressed, or anxious; persons with somatization disorder, hypochondriasis, pain disorder, and body dysmorphic disorder may display a depressed mood; persons with conversion disorder may have an 'indifferent' mood regarding the symptoms
5. **Affect**: objectively assess the client's expression of mood; observe both verbal and non-verbal cues; in persons with psychosomatic illness the affect may be normal (if they are indifferent), may be flat if depressed, may be labile, or may be anguished if in pain; persons with hypochondriasis may express anxiety over all the "worries" related to the overconcern of bodily manifestations; persons with body dysmorphic disorder may express extreme anxiety related to obsession with imagined or minor bodily flaws
6. **Perceptions**: observe for signs of auditory and/or visual hallucinations (ask the client if he or she is hearing voices or seeing anything/anybody); persons with somatization disorder and conversion disorder may experience hallucinations

7. **Thought content**: this reflects the thinking inside the client's head; ask the client about obsessions, compulsions, delusions, phobias; the thought content in persons with psychosomatic illness is usually preoccupation with physical symptoms; persons with body dysmorphic disorder may be obsessed, delusional, and/or have **ideas of reference** regarding an unimagined or minor physical defects

8. **Thought process**: this is expressed through the client's speech; these symptoms are not typically observed in persons with psychosomatic illness; persons with conversion disorder and somatization disorder may manifest dissociative symptoms

9. **Level of consciousness**: asses if the client is awake, alert, lethargic, stuporous; assess orientation to person, place, and time; persons with somatization disorder may manifest with symptoms of fainting, a loss of consciousness, amnesia, and/or seizures

10. **Memory**: assess short- and long-term memory (people with mood disorder may have impairment in both areas)

11. **Insight**: assess whether the client has insight into symptoms; persons with any somatoform disorder has poor insight into the psychological rationale for the physical manifestations/preoccupations

12. **Suicide assessment**: persons with body dysmorphic disorder are at an increased risk for suicidal ideation; suicidal attempts or completed suicide is commonly related to psychological impact of bodily obsessions

D. **Social assessment**
   1. Examines the individual's ability to interact and participate in life activities such as work, social interactions, and ongoing interpersonal relationships
   2. May include a client's inability to have an intimate relationship with another
   3. All persons with somatoform disorders have marked distress in social functioning; it is important to note that pain can lead to social isolation

E. **Physiological assessment**
   1. Is based on Maslow's hierarchy of needs theory; indicates priority needs for human survival
   2. Assess appetite (any increase or decrease): assess any weight loss in last several months, and whether it was purposeful; all persons with somatization disorders are at risk for depression; persons with a depressed mood may have recent weight loss or weight gain; persons with somatization disorder, hypochondriasis may have appetite changes due to perceived GI problems
   3. Assess hydration: assess skin turgor, mucus membranes, and specifically ask the client how much intake they have in a 24-hour period; inquire about urinary output; persons with somatization disorder, hypochondriasis may have hydration imbalances due to perceived gastrointestinal or other related problems
   4. Assess sleep patterns (amount, quality, duration): ask specifically how many hours of sleep they have per night (if any); when the last time they slept was; ask if they are taking any over-the-counter medicine, complementary medicine, alternative medicine, and/or prescribed sleep aides; persons with pain disorder are at particular risk for sleep disturbances, as pain interferes with sleep
   5. Assess bowel patterns: when was the last bowel movement? What was the size? Any constipation or diarrhea? Persons with depressed affect may have constipation secondary to slowed gastrointestinal system; persons with somatization and hypochondriasis may have problems with bowels (constipation, diarrhea) due to perceived GI problems
   6. Pain assessment: assess client's pain on a scale of 1–10, and location; assess level, onset, duration, what exacerbates it, what alleviates it; pain is the primary focus of persons with pain disorder and is also a criterion for diagnosis of somatization disorder

7. Sexual assessment: assess whether client is actively sexual; inquire if client has any pain during intercourse; persons with somatoform disorder may manifest pain in sexual and reproductive systems such as irregular menses, menorrhagia; men have reported erectile dysfunction or ejaculatory dysfunction

F. **Social assessment**
   1. Examines the individual's ability to interact and participate in life activities such as social interactions, ongoing interpersonal relationships, and work
   2. Inquire about the person's ability to have intimate relationships
   3. Social isolation increases in all psychosomatic illnesses as the disorder progresses

IV. NURSING DIAGNOSES/ANALYSIS

A. **Ineffective Coping** related to poor insight, unmet dependency needs, denial, moderate to severe levels of anxiety, low self-esteem, regression to earlier stage of development, inadequate coping skills, maladaptive coping mechanisms, poor support systems, and/or lack of resources

B. **Ineffective Family Processes** related to detachment, nonfamily acceptance of expression of emotionally related feelings, power struggles amongst family members, boundary issues, and/or stress of illness placed on family

C. **Ineffective Denial** related to threat to impaired sense of self (i.e., low self-esteem), having to confront psychological conflict

D. **Impaired Social Interaction** related to fear, anxiety, or panic to leave the home, physical manifestation of perceived illness, physical disability, pain, embarrassment, and shame

E. **Disturbed Body Image** related to low self-esteem, imagined or exaggerated physical defects, chronic physical manifestations, pain, pseudoneurological symptoms, sexual manifestations of the disorder

F. **Self-Care Deficit** related to paralysis of body part; sensory impairment (vision, hearing, speaking), physical manifestations, pain, or secondary gain

G. **Chronic Pain** related to moderate to severe levels of anxiety, and secondary gain received from the sick role

H. **Anxiety** related to excessive worry about illness, real or imaged physical deficits, pain

I. **Ineffective Role Performance** due to disability, clinical manifestations of physical illness, pain, social isolation, poor self-esteem

J. **Sleep Disturbances** related to medical manifestations of illness, pain, depressed mood

V. PLANNING AND IMPLEMENTATION

A. **Specific strategies**
   1. Establish trusting, therapeutic relationship
      a. Avoid describing the physical symptoms as "in the client's head"
      b. Note that the symptoms are not an attempt to get attention
      c. Recall that the client does not create symptoms consciously or on purpose
      d. Accept the reality of the symptoms as client presents them, avoiding dispute
   2. Client education
      a. Explain physiological symptoms, using understandable and acceptable language
      b. Present current knowledge of mind–body interaction, emphasizing how stress and anxiety affect physiological functioning
      c. Teach methods to reduce physiological arousal, including relaxation techniques, visual imagery, self-talk strategies, and physical exercise (see Box 6-1)
      d. Teach psychoeducation related to psychiatric disorder and any prescribed psychotropics

Box 6-1	1. Emphasize to the client the relationship between stress and physiological arousal/ symptoms.
Tips for Teaching Relaxation Training	2. Teach the client that relaxation techniques work by • Focusing attention to relaxation task, thus interrupting the preoccupation with symptoms. • Decreasing physiological arousal, which negates physical symptoms of anxiety. 3. Reinforce to the client that *he or she* effects the change (not the technique) by increasing a sense of control. 4. Help the client to maintain a physiological and psychological baseline that calms the mind and body. 5. Instruct the client that daily practice builds skill level; episodic use does not. 6. Suggest to the client to use additional relaxation techniques when anticipating a stressful situation, or when anxious. 7. Explain and teach a variety of relaxation to the client, the client can choose appropriate techniques as necessary.

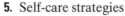

3. Encourage verbalization of thoughts and feelings, life events, and stressors
4. Assist in problem solving specific conflicts or situations
5. Self-care strategies
   a. Modify exercise/activity plan to individualize client's physical status, at a minimum of three times a week for 30 minutes at a time
   b. Employ nursing measures to promote sleep and rest, avoid taking naps if physically possible, avoid caffeine during the day, eliminate stimuli in bedroom (computers, televisions, radio), assess response to pharmacological or CAM sleep aides
   c. Promote healthy nutritional practices: three balanced meals a day, adequate amounts of fluids
   d. Teach day-to-day individualized client management of psychological and physical symptoms
   e. Teach stress management techniques, evidence indicates stress reduction can decrease symptomology
6. Encourage gradual assumption of expected work, family, and community roles, commensurate with physical capabilities

B. **Pharmacological treatment**
1. Hypochondriasis: SSRIs and SNRIs have been shown to be useful in the treatment of hypochondriasis
2. Somatization disorder: pharmacological treatment is not well understood in the treatment of somatization disorders
3. Conversion disorder: anxiolytics and antidepressants can be helpful in treating persons with conversion disorder during the rehabilitative phase; amobarbital (Amytal) (a mild sedative) may be administered per psychiatry to facilitate information regarding early or hidden conflicts
4. Body dysmorphic disorder: pharmacological treatment is still not well understood; SSRIs may be effective in treatment, but further studies are necessary
5. Pain disorder: antidepressants can decrease pain intensity in persons with pain disorder
6. Co-morbid problems such as anxiety and depression are treated symptomatically: anxiolytics for anxiety, and antidepressants for depression
7. Assess for symptoms of opium and benzodiazepine abuse in persons with pain disorder; approximately one fourth of persons prescribed opioids for chronic pain develop abuse or dependence

8. Medication for other physical symptoms
   a. Assess requests for medication and effectiveness of medication matter-of-factly
   b. Encourage client to express thoughts and feelings experienced at the time of discomfort
   c. Provide thorough client education on medications, emphasizing provider–client collaboration to reduce self-adjustment of dosages

C. Individual/group treatment

1. Cognitive-behavioral approaches
   a. Identify self-statements and assumptions about stress, anxiety, and sick role
   b. Challenge irrational beliefs and self-statements regarding seriousness of illness, inability to cope, and/or mind–body relationships
   c. Provide accurate data including psychoeducation to counter misinformation
   d. Encourage positive, self-coping statements
   e. Identify client strengths
   f. Teach client mindful meditation; can decrease pain in persons with pain disorder

2. Groups for clients and families
   a. Discussion of mind–body relationships
   b. Forum for discussion and encouragement to "talk" out problems as a deterrent to physical symptoms
   c. Correct misinformation about origin of somatoform disorders
   d. Support for families and/or clients as roles shift during recovery
   e. Refer client to National Alliance of the Mentally Ill (NAMI) for information on stigma reduction, family support, support groups, psychoeducation, and research

3. Supportive approaches
   a. Convey empathy: "This must be very trying for you"
   b. Convey respect: "I am impressed by how you have been able to do as much as you have, given how you feel"
   c. Explore with client ways to decrease isolation, improve role performance, and enhance self-esteem
   d. Focus on verbally expressing feelings and coping techniques rather than symptoms
   e. Keep discussion of symptoms brief and matter-of-fact, but without dismissal
   f. Reassure client by providing accurate information coupled with rehabilitation; this can be useful in some cases to decrease symptoms in clients with conversion disorder
   g. Consult with physical occupational therapy department as warranted, depending on presence of psychoneurological symptoms

4. Behavior modification
   a. In addition to cognitive behavioral approaches, engage client in self-modification to reward for engagement in treatment plan
   b. Teach family members to reinforce verbalization of stressors and life difficulties rather than symptoms

Practice to Pass

Describe what medications are used to treat the various somatoform disorders. What classifications of medications are used to treat anxiety and depression in persons with somatoform disorders?

Practice to Pass

Explain why a gradual assumption of responsibilities is indicated, especially since there is no organic basis for the disorder.

Practice to Pass

How might you teach family members to reinforce verbal expressions rather than symptoms?

VI. EVALUATION/OUTCOMES

A. Client identifies the interaction of mind and body and the effects of stress
B. Client increases ability to verbalize thoughts and feelings
C. Client identifies conflicts and/or problems in situations and relationships
D. Client seeks to actively solve problems through talking and concrete actions
E. Client assumes appropriate roles in work, family, and community

F. **Client employs self-help strategies**
1. Client challenges own irrational thoughts
2. Client corrects own misinformation
3. Client uses positive coping mechanisms
4. Client engages in physical activity on regular basis
5. Client employs relaxation techniques (i.e., visual imagery, mindfulness, breathing techniques)
6. Client consumes appropriate nutritional and hydration needs
7. Client obtains appropriate amounts of rest and sleep and demonstrates improved sleep hygiene practice

G. **Client manifests diminished or no somatic symptoms**

VII. SPECIFIC DISORDERS

A. *Somatization disorder*
1. Onset prior to age 30 with symptoms of several years' duration

2. The prevalence of somatization disorders ranges from 0.2% to 2% in women, and 0.2% in men

3. Multiple physical complaints in multiple body systems
    a. Must include four pain symptoms (i.e., back, head, abdomen, chest, pain during sexual intercourse)
    b. Must include two gastrointestinal symptoms not pain related (i.e., nausea, vomiting, intolerance of foods)
    c. Must include one sexual symptom (i.e., erectile or ejaculatory dysfunction, irregular menses)
    d. Must include one symptom suggesting a neurological disorder (i.e., paralysis, urinary retention)
    e. Many clients in addition to the above symptoms manifest chronic fatigue
4. Symptoms often arise or are exacerbated with increased psychological stressors that cause emotional distress
5. Is seen in 10–20% of female first-degree biological relatives
6. Lifestyle changes evoked by physical illness affect self-care, family, occupational, community relationships
    a. Client is often disabled, resulting in inability to work and economic hardship
    b. Constantly seeks treatment for physical symptoms (see Figure 6-1); may seek treatment from multiple providers; infrequently seeks care regarding psychological problems or impairment in social functioning
    c. Often a history of multiple hospitalizations, treatments, and surgeries
7. Special interventions
    a. Client requires long-term medical management, often in a medical setting
    b. Clients' physical symptoms should be treated in a conservative, matter-of-fact manner
    c. Antidepressants may be prescribed if depressive symptoms present
    d. Anxiolytics may be prescribed if anxiety symptoms do not respond to non-pharmacological approaches

B. *Conversion disorder*
1. Symptoms are associated with voluntary sensory or motor function so are called **pseudoneurological**
2. Pseudoneurological complaints are in two primary neurological regions:
    a. Motor symptoms (i.e., paralysis, difficulty swallowing, seizure) (Figure 6-2)
    b. Sensory symptoms (i.e., blindness, deafness, hallucinations)

Figure 6-1

Clients with somatization disorder seek relief for a multitude of symptoms

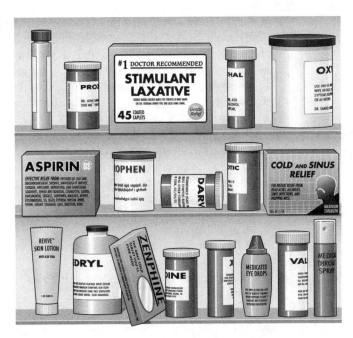

Figure 6-2

The client's symptoms reveal his or her needs

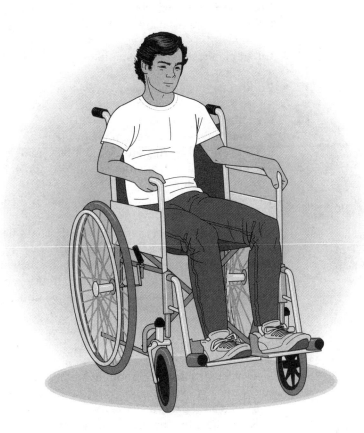

3. Research shows increased risk of conversion disorder in monozygotic twins
4. The less medically knowledgeable the client is, the more implausible the symptoms; the more medically knowledgeable the client, the more subtle the symptoms
    a. Symptoms correspond to the client's concept of the problem
    b. Symptoms do not follow neurological pathways
5. The identifiable psychological factors of stress and conflict are related to the onset or exacerbation of symptoms
6. The client's mood may be incongruent with the symptoms, displaying little or no affective concern (*la belle indifference*)
7. Symptoms are often symbolically related to primary gain
    a. Student may be unable to feel or move the hands prior to taking a comprehensive examination so that answers cannot be written and he or she does not have to graduate
    b. A man who is about to get married may manifest bilateral paralysis of lower extremities, so that he cannot "walk down the aisle" when uncertain of marital decision
8. The client may receive secondary gain from the conversion manifestations; but it is not intentional
9. Important nursing interventions
    a. Nurse must treat the symptom as "real," as the clients experience is subjective (real to them)
    b. Nurse must facilitate the client to apply problem-solving techniques to cope with conflicts and stressors

C. *Pain disorder*
    1. Characterized by pain as the dominant physical symptom
    2. Client seeks medical attention for severe, prolonged pain with no organic basis for the pain
    3. Client manifests a preoccupation with pain that is not insignificantly alleviated by analgesics
    4. Bodily manifestation vary (i.e., low back pain, headache, chronic pelvic pain)
    5. There is a historical relationship between stress and conflict prior to the onset and exacerbation of the pain
        a. Often follows physical trauma or injury
        b. Client usually refuses to consider psychological origin
    6. The diagnosis is difficult due to personal and cultural differences in definition of an expression of pain
    7. The diagnosis is commonly accompanied by a co-morbidity of major depressive disorder
        a. Symptoms of depression (i.e., hopelessness, helplessness, low self-esteem, changes in appetite, changes in sleep pattern)
        b. Behaviors such as anger and irritability may manifest
        c. Increased risk of suicide secondary to the depression
    8. There is an increased risk for substance abuse, particularly from anxiolytics and/or opioids
    9. There is an increase in sleep disturbances secondary to the pain
    10. Important nursing interventions
        a. Assess for suicidal threats, ideation; refer for immediate psychiatric evaluation; implement suicide precautions when indicated
        b. Teach client physiology of stress and increased muscle tension, which contributes to increased pain (the stress-tension-pain cycle)
        c. Refer client to acupuncture, biofeedback training, transcutaneous nerve stimulation

   d. Refer client to physical therapy and/or occupational therapy
   e. Teach client visualization and relaxation training
   f. Educate client regarding pain management techniques

D. *Hypochondriasis*
  1. Characterized whereby physical symptom(s) are interpreted as severe or life-threatening, resulting in exaggerated worry
  2. Physical symptoms may begin with sensitivity to vague physical sensations or mild physical symptoms that would go unnoticeable in most persons
  3. Exaggerated worry and preoccupation with physical symptoms and sensations occur
   a. Client interprets symptoms as severe or life-threatening when they are not
   b. Symptoms may be related to particular body function, such as constipation, or to organ system disease, such as coronary artery disease
   c. Client seeks information from clinicians
   d. Client seeks data from various sources (i.e., internet, textbooks) to substantiate concerns
  4. History of multiple visits to multiple practitioners
   a. May begin with physical illness in childhood
   b. May originate after severe medical problems as an adult
   c. Concern persists in spite of negative objective findings (i.e., labs, diagnostic tests), and clinician reassurances
  5. Often the disorder coexists with significant anxiety or depression
  6. Important nursing interventions
   a. Teach rational interpretation of bodily sensations
   b. Assist resolution of family conflict regarding the client's distress
   c. Assist resolution of family conflict regarding medical treatment
   d. Non-pharmacological treatment of anxiety (i.e., relaxation techniques)
   e. Pharmacological treatment of depression when indicated
   f. Referral to health care providers for treatment of coexisting anxiety and/or depression
   g. Set clear boundaries with client

E. *Body dysmorphic disorder (BDD)*
  1. Characterized by preoccupation with an imagined or exaggerated concern over a bodily defect or minor anomaly
   a. Causes significant distress or impairment in role function
   b. Common sites of complaints/concerns are areas of the head/face, wrinkles, scars, hair thinning, facial asymmetry)
   c. Any other body part may be the focus (i.e., genitals, breasts, buttocks, arms, spine)
  2. May frequently check defects, avoid reminders (removing mirrors), seek reassurances from others, or attempt to improve the defect (i.e., exercise, surgery, cosmetics)
  3. Often leads to social isolation
  4. Disorder is persistent; client has repeated surgeries, dental work, or dermatological treatment for defects
  5. Emotional distress may be severe for depression and/or suicidal ideation to coexist
  6. Important nursing interventions
   a. Respect preoccupation; avoid challenging the validity of client perceptions
   b. Focus on coping techniques
   c. Contract with client to increase social activities and relationships
   d. Conduct suicide assessment when applicable; refer to provider for treatment of suicidal threats/ideation when indicated

Case Study

A middle-aged man diagnosed with pain disorder has been unable to work for the past year. Usually affable and gregarious, the client has become increasingly irritable with friends and family and prefers to spend time alone. An infrequent drinker (several beers a month) in the past, he now easily finishes a six-pack of beer every evening. The client is now hospitalized on a psychiatric inpatient unit.

1. The client requests a prn pain medication that has been ordered. What principles would guide the nurse in handling his request?

2. In a meeting with the client and his wife, she asks why he is so irritable. How could the nurse explain his mood change?

3. The client questions going to group therapy: "I need my pain meds, not this jabbering about so-called problems." What is the best response?

4. One of the staff members comments that he just thinks the client is trying to get out of working. Explain what is known about the origin of somatoform disorders, and the roles of primary and secondary gain.

5. What are possible pain management strategies that could be included in a teaching plan for the client?

For suggested responses, see page 297.

POSTTEST

1. Which of the following is the most appropriate nursing diagnosis for a client with pain disorder who is homebound and unable to work in his previous profession for the past two years?

   1. Impaired Role Performance
   2. Anxiety
   3. High Risk for Injury
   4. Disturbed Sensory Perception

2. Which nursing intervention approaches would the nurse take that may be effective when caring for a client diagnosed with body dysmorphic disorder (BDD) who is preoccupied with a mole on her face? Select all that apply.

   1. Teach the client meditation and breathing relaxation techniques.
   2. Explain to the client that her perception of the mole is absolutely a misperception, and that it is all "in her head."
   3. Respect the client's preoccupation with the perceived physical defect.
   4. Encourage the client to participate in a self-help group.
   5. Focus on the client's positive relationships with family members.

3. The client who is diagnosed with body dysmorphic disorder says to the nurse, "I can't get rid of the idea that my ears are weird-looking." Which of the following is the most appropriate outcome criterion for this client?

   1. Consider plastic surgery to reshape the ears.
   2. List three benefits of having unusual ears.
   3. Understand how body image is affected by maturation.
   4. Explore possible explanations for dissatisfaction with body image.

4. A female client with an eight-year history of a diagnosis of somatization disorder is to be discharged from the first psychiatric hospitalization. Which client statement indicates that nursing care has been effective for the client?

   1. "I need to make sure that all of my medications are sent home with me."
   2. "I see now that when I get stressed, my 'body' speaks for me."
   3. "My family is so good to me when I am sick like this."
   4. "There are so many illnesses that you nurses simply do not know about."

5 A client treated for a diagnosis of hypochondriasis has an upsetting phone conversation with her husband and subsequently requests an analgesic. The client states, "My head is killing me, and I know there is a tumor in there somewhere, or it wouldn't hurt like this." Which of the following is the nurse's best response?

1. "You have no brain tumor. It is just your anger toward your husband."
2. "I'll get your vital signs and then call your doctor if they are abnormal."
3. "You must try not to rely on the pain pills so much since they are addictive."
4. "I'll get your medication and then let's talk about what just happened."

6 While taking the nursing history, a client with body dysmorphic disorder says, "After three surgeries, my jaw line still isn't right. Plus, it took five surgeries before my nose was finally fixed." Which of the following is the most appropriate nursing diagnosis?

1. Health-Seeking Behaviors
2. Disturbed Body Image
3. Disturbed Personal Identity
4. Risk for Self-Mutilation

7 Which of the following does the nurse expect to assess when taking the history of a client with a diagnosis of pain disorder?

1. Good responses to past pharmacological treatment
2. Indifference to the discomfort of pain
3. Pain does not respond well to medication
4. Insight into relationship between stress and pain

8 A nurse working on an inpatient psychiatric unit is orienting a new graduate nurse. The new graduate nurse asks what symptoms a person with a somatization disorder might manifest. The nurse replies by stating which of the following? Select all that apply.

1. Pain during intercourse
2. Menstrual irregularity
3. Shortness of breath
4. Nausea and vomiting
5. Urinary retention

9 A client says to the nurse, "I know you think this is in my head, but my pelvic pain is real. I have a serious malignancy and am going to die." The nurse is aware that the physician just informed the client that despite very extensive diagnostic testing, no abnormalities have been found. What is the nurse's best response?

1. "I guess it could be true. Sometimes doctors miss a diagnosis."
2. "I realize that you do have pain and hurt a lot."
3. "It must be hard for you to accept the testing results."
4. "How about resting now and asking your doctor more about it later?"

10 A client diagnosed with a somatization disorder has been attending group therapy on a regular basis. Which client statement suggests to the nurse that the therapy has been effective?

1. "I think I'd better get some pain pills. My back hurts from sitting in group."
2. "The other people in the group have mental problems!"
3. "I haven't said much, but I get a lot out of listening."
4. "I feel better physically just from getting a chance to talk."

➤ *See pages 136–138 for Answers and Rationales.*

ANSWERS & RATIONALES

Pretest

1 **Answer: 2** **Rationale:** Secondary gains are unintentionally sought benefits that result from an illness, such as support that otherwise might not be available. These benefits serve to reinforce illness behavior. The family's response (cooking and cleaning for the client) can be viewed as a secondary gain for the client. Primary gains are symbolic resolutions of unconscious conflict that decrease anxiety and keep the conflict from awareness. Attention-seeking behavior directly calls attention of others to the individual who has experienced lack of satisfaction of either conscious or unconscious needs. Attention-seeking behaviors are not indicated in the question. Malingering is used to achieve secondary gain, but in this question, the client has actual back pain. Malingering is motivated by deliberate conscious decisions of the individual. The individual offers a complaint, but has no actual dysfunction or symptom. **Cognitive Level:** Applying **Client Need:** Psychosocial Integrity **Integrated Process:** Nursing Process: Assessment **Content Area:** Mental Health **Strategy:** Consider how the responses of the family members might impact on the client's symptoms. Think also, "Would I be likely to work to give up a symptom if my family took over my cooking and cleaning?" **Reference:** Fontaine, K. (2009). *Mental health nursing* (6th ed.). Upper Saddle River, NJ: Prentice Hall, p. 277.

2 **Answer: 3** **Rationale:** "She doesn't have the problem on purpose; however, this is probably difficult for both of you" offers empathy and information about the spouse's illness. Family members must understand the mechanism of somatization disorder and have their own needs addressed. The chronic nature of the physical complaints is very frustrating and disruptive of family functioning. The nurse must be responsive to this. Suggesting that the spouse asks her about it suggests an approach that would be confrontational and therefore likely to increase relationship difficulties between the spouses. Suggesting that the woman is trying to gain the spouse's attention fails to offer empathy to the spouse. In fact, it could make the spouse feel defensive. In essence it says, "You aren't attentive enough." While the statement that she has some emotional problems that she cannot admit is perhaps factual, it does not offer empathy to the spouse. The nurse should be ever mindful that the chronic nature of the client's physical complaints is very frustrating and disruptive of family functioning. **Cognitive Level:** Analyzing **Client Need:** Psychosocial Integrity **Integrated Process:** Communication and Documentation **Content Area:** Mental Health **Strategy:** Notice that only one of the responses addresses the spouse's feelings in any

way. **Reference:** Varcarolis, E., Carson, V., & Shoemaker, N. (2010). *Foundations of psychiatric mental health nursing: A clinical approach* (6th ed.). St. Louis, MO: Saunders Elsevier, pp. 243, 260–261.

3 **Answer: 1** **Rationale:** The realization that the pain can be influenced by stress indicates beginning development of insight, which is a desired outcome for nursing intervention. Understanding the relationship between physical symptoms and stress helps the client to gain control of outcomes. Physical activity and limited use of pain medications are indicated when the client has pain disorder. The client tends to allow the pain to dominate all spheres of functioning. Relaxation techniques are most effective when practiced on a regular, not episodic basis, although they can be employed when pain levels are just beginning to rise. Clients with chronic pain disorders are at high risk for dependency on drugs, whether prescribed or non-prescribed. These clients should be taught non-pharmacologic methods of pain relief. **Cognitive Level:** Analyzing **Client Need:** Psychosocial Integrity **Integrated Process:** Nursing Process: Evaluation **Content Area:** Mental Health **Strategy:** Notice that the question is asking for an indication of progress on the spart of the client. Use this as a benchmark against which to evaluate each option. **Reference:** Kneisl, C., Wilson, H., & Trigoboff, E. (2009). *Contemporary psychiatric–mental health nursing* (2nd ed.). Upper Saddle River, NJ: Prentice Hall, p. 390.

4 **Answer: 1, 2, 3, 5** **Rationale:** Four options are correct. One of the criteria for conversion disorder in the *DSM-IV* is that the person, in addition to other problems, manifests significant distress in occupational, social, and/or academic functioning. A symptom of conversion disorder manifests with a motor and/or sensory function. The client is reporting paralysis. Sensory symptoms may involve hallucinations; therefore, a mental status exam should be performed. Persons with conversion disorder often have *la belle difference* as an affective feature—one that displays little or no concern for the problem. "It follows neurological pathways" is incorrect; for a diagnosis of conversion to occur, diagnostic testing must rule out existence of neurological pathways as an etiological factor for the paralysis. **Cognitive Level:** Analysis **Client Need:** Psychosocial **Integrated Process:** Nursing Process: Assessment **Content Area:** Mental Health **Strategy:** Examine the client's history; he reports a history of conversion disorder with paralysis. Also it is important to know *DSM-IV* criteria for conversion disorder in order to make inferences. His inability to work, history, and symptoms meet these criteria. **Reference:** Stuart, G. W. (2009). *Principles and practice of psychiatric nursing* (9th ed.). Mosby, Elsevier: St. Louis, p. 251.

5 **Answer: 4 Rationale:** Somatization disorder is characterized by chronic, multiple vague physical symptoms in multiple body systems that impair role performance. The disorder usually begins before age 30, and symptoms are a major source of concern throughout the client's life. The client reports significant distress and usually seeks out multiple providers for health care. Clients with somatization disorder do not generally have dissociative experiences or ignore their symptoms. Instead, they focus obsessively on their body. When one somatic complaint is managed, another emerges. **Cognitive Level:** Applying **Client Need:** Psychosocial Integrity **Integrated Process:** Nursing Process: Assessment **Content Area:** Mental Health **Strategy:** Remember that clients with somatization disorder are expressing psychologic distress through bodily symptoms and that the course of their illness is chronic and relapsing. **Reference:** Varcarolis, E., Carson, V., & Shoemaker, N. (2010). *Foundations of psychiatric mental health nursing: A clinical approach* (6th ed.). St. Louis, MO: Saunders Elsevier, p. 258.

6 **Answer: 3 Rationale:** Discharge criteria for clients with somatoform disorders, which are associated with anxiety, include understanding the relationships between symptoms and anxiety-provoking events. The nurse should focus on assisting the client to understand this relationship. When the client has hypochondriasis, it is important to avoid focusing on the client's past and associated physical conditions or complaints. These actions would likely increase the client's anxiety and increase the preoccupation with symptoms. The client with hypochondriasis usually has a number of care providers in succession, going from one to another in a search for a cure, so encouraging a second opinion may suggest the presence of a serious problem, thus increasing the client's anxiety and further intensifying symptoms. When the client has a somatoform disorder, family members must learn not to reinforce physical symptoms or illness behavior of the client. **Cognitive Level:** Applying **Client Need:** Psychosocial Integrity **Integrated Process:** Nursing Process: Planning **Content Area:** Mental Health **Strategy:** Recall principles of behavior therapy and remember that the attention of others can serve as a powerful social reinforcer. This will help eliminate some of the distracters in the question. **Reference:** Varcarolis, E., Carson, V., & Shoemaker, N. (2010). *Foundations of psychiatric mental health nursing: A clinical approach* (6th ed.). St. Louis, MO: Saunders Elsevier, p. 263.

7 **Answer: 3 Rationale:** Clients with a conversion disorder have no physiological basis for the symptoms. Three options have a physiological basis. Recall that conversion symptoms represent deficits in voluntary motor or sensory functioning for which there are no objective explanations or findings. **Cognitive Level:** Applying **Client Need:** Psychosocial Integrity **Integrated Process:** Nursing Process: Assessment **Content Area:** Mental Health **Strategy:** Notice that only one option does not relate to current

scientific understanding of the nervous system or functioning of the body. **Reference:** Varcarolis, E., Carson, V., & Shoemaker, N. (2010). *Foundations of psychiatric mental health nursing: A clinical approach* (6th ed.). St. Louis, MO: Saunders Elsevier, p. 259.

8 **Answer: 1, 2 Rationale:** Persons with somatoform disorders experience Ineffective Role Performance because the illness interferes with the usual responsibilities in life. These persons are controlled by their somatic symptoms and experiences, and significant others suffer greatly because of the preoccupations of the individual with somatoform disorder. Persons with somatoform disorders experience ineffective coping because they use their bodies to express emotional conflicts or needs (Impaired Coping), rather than expressing those needs more directly. Unless specific individual data is available that suggests Risk for Violence or Impaired Oxygenation, these NANDA problems are not an average part of somatoform disorder. Health-Seeking Behaviors is one of the nursing diagnoses that deals with healthy, adaptive efforts. The client with somatoform disorder cannot be expected to display behaviors that are consistent with this nursing diagnosis, because illness is a way of life with these clients. Their "doctor shopping" is not done in an effort to find wellness, but rather to confirm illness. **Cognitive Level:** Analyzing **Client Need:** Psychosocial Integrity **Integrated Process:** Nursing Process: Diagnosis **Content Area:** Mental Health **Strategy:** Recall that the client with somatoform disorder faces an ever-changing array of physical symptoms that suggest a physical disorder. Do you think that this person could fully meet role expectations, such as those of being a parent? **Reference:** Varcarolis, E., Carson, V., & Shoemaker, N. (2010). *Foundations of psychiatric mental health nursing: A clinical approach* (6th ed.). St. Louis, MO: Saunders Elsevier, p. 261.

9 **Answer: 1 Rationale:** The nurse should be aware that the client with somatization disorder is indeed experiencing pain, although physical diagnostic results may be negative. The client's pain should be relieved in a matter-of-fact manner. Prompt reduction of pain is the priority. Confronting the client with the negative physical findings will likely increase the client's anxiety level and therefore the level of pain. Once the client's pain is reduced, then the client can be taught relaxation techniques, like deep breathing. Teaching should not be attempted when the client is experiencing pain. The nurse should respond matter-of-factly to the client's request for medication and give the medication as ordered. Unnecessary delays will increase the client's anxiety and therefore the pain level. **Cognitive Level:** Analyzing **Client Need:** Psychosocial Integrity **Integrated Process:** Nursing Process: Implementation **Content Area:** Mental Health **Strategy:** Remember that the pain experience is real, even though an organic cause for the pain cannot be established. Avoid being critical and judgmental of the client. **Reference:** Varcarolis, E.,

Carson, V., & Shoemaker, N. (2010). *Foundations of psychiatric mental health nursing: A clinical approach* (6th ed.). St. Louis, MO: Saunders Elsevier, p. 263.

10 **Answer: 3** **Rationale:** The statement "I know that I don't have a serious illness, even though I still worry about the symptoms" indicates some basic level of understanding about the meaning of hypochondriacal concerns. Education for a client with hypochondriasis is effective if the client is aware that the symptoms present no real danger. Giving up the preoccupation with the serious nature of the symptoms is a gradual process of cognitive restructuring. The statement that tests and lab results cannot pick up on the seriousness of the illness suggests that the client believes that the illness is too serious to be identified. "Once my family members realize how severely ill I am they will be more understanding" indicates that the client feels ill and misunderstood by the family. The statement about exposure to toxins causing significant organ damage suggests that the client is searching for reasons to explain symptoms being experienced. **Cognitive Level:** Analyzing **Client Need:** Psychosocial Integrity **Integrated Process:** Nursing Process: Evaluation **Content Area:** Mental Health **Strategy:** Identify the most positive client behavior. Recall that successful cognitive restructuring occurs in gradual steps. **Reference:** Varcarolis, E., Carson, V., & Shoemaker, N. (2010). *Foundations of psychiatric mental health nursing: A clinical approach* (6th ed.). St. Louis, MO: Saunders Elsevier, pp. 258–259.

Posttest

1 **Answer: 1** **Rationale:** Impaired Role Performance is correct. Chronic pain interferes with social and occupational functioning, prompting further stress and anxiety. The diagnoses in the other options do not address the long-term homebound status and unemployment of the client. **Cognitive Level:** Analyzing **Client Need:** Management of Care **Integrated Process:** Nursing Process: Diagnosis **Content Area:** Mental Health **Strategy:** Note the duration of symptoms and the limitations imposed by them. **Reference:** Kneisl, C., Wilson, H., & Trigoboff, E. (2004). *Contemporary psychiatric–mental health nursing.* Upper Saddle River, NJ: Prentice Hall, p. 380.

2 **Answer: 1, 3, 4, 5** **Rationale:** Four options are correct. Meditation, breathing exercises, and other forms of relaxation are means to reduce anxiety; an underlying problem with persons with BDD is anxiety. Respect is a form of both establishing and maintaining a therapeutic relationship with the client, which is essential for trust and ongoing communication between the client and the nurse. Self-help groups are places where clients with BDD can feel safe and learn tools from peers to cope with their problems. Positive relationships provide assurance and support to clients with BDD. It is important not to confront the client and deny their perceptions. The disorder is a maladaptive coping mechanism.

Treatment is needed that involves long-term cognitive behavioral therapy. **Cognitive Level:** Analysis **Client Need:** Psychosocial **Integrated Process:** Nursing Process: Implementation **Content Area:** Mental Health **Strategy:** Nursing intervention approaches require an understanding of the psychological underpinnings of BDD. One problem is that of anxiety. Approaches must be therapeutic in nature and encourage support and resource usage. **Reference:** Stuart, G. W., & Laraia, M. T. (2009). *Principles and practice of psychiatric nursing* (9th ed.). St. Louis, MO: Elsevier Mosby, p. 252.

3 **Answer: 4** **Rationale:** Exploring possible explanations for dissatisfaction with body image is correct because it suggests that the client examine the interrelationship of personal emotion and body image. Additionally, it sets the stage for other interventions to deal with preoccupation with imagined physical defects. These include cognitive-behavioral approaches like (1) identifying and challenging distorted perceptions of the client and/or (2) interrupting self-critical thoughts. A crucial early intervention is to help the person to identify and express feelings. Considering plastic surgery, along with listing the benefits of having unusual ears, would support the client's preoccupation with appearance of the ears and would likely increase the client's level of anxiety and dissatisfaction. The client should examine the interrelationship of personal emotion and body image, not the relationship between body image and maturation. **Cognitive Level:** Applying **Client Need:** Psychosocial Integrity **Integrated Process:** Nursing Process: Planning **Content Area:** Mental Health **Strategy:** Notice that two options focus on the ears, with which the client is already preoccupied. Eliminate these choices very quickly and then decide between the remaining two options. **Reference:** Kneisl, C., Wilson, H., & Trigoboff, E. (2009). *Contemporary psychiatric–mental health nursing* (2nd ed.). Upper Saddle River, NJ: Prentice Hall, p. 392.

4 **Answer: 2** **Rationale:** Realizing that the body reacts to stress is correct because it indicates accurate awareness of mind–body interaction and shows that the client no longer persists in (1) identifying illness as physical in origin and (2) feeling that medication is necessary to control the symptoms. Both of these are characteristic of somatization disorder. Making sure all medications are sent home indicates that the client still sees symptoms as something to medicate. Commenting on how good the family is when the client is sick suggests that the client is receiving secondary gain from the family. A sign of progress would be a statement indicating recognition of secondary gain and its part in the chronicity of the symptoms. Stating that there are "so many illnesses that you nurses simply do not know about" indicates that the client is still focused on the idea of having an undiagnosed, untreatable problem. **Cognitive Level:** Analyzing **Client Need:** Psychosocial Integrity **Integrated Process:** Nursing Process: Evaluation **Content Area:** Mental

Health **Strategy:** Look for a positive change in behavior. Eliminate any options that indicate a static condition. **Reference:** Kneisl, C., Wilson, H., & Trigoboff, E. (2009). *Contemporary psychiatric–mental health nursing* (2nd ed.). Upper Saddle River, NJ: Prentice Hall, p. 392.

5 **Answer: 4** **Rationale:** "I'll get your medication and then let's talk about what just happened" is correct. The nurse should provide physical care for the client in a matter-of-fact manner and, at the same time, should help the client note how symptoms increase at the time of stress and can be a way of coping with stress. Denying the tumor and stating that the pain is due to anger is confrontational and interpretative and will likely cause the client to feel frustrated and angry, which can increase the intensity of the headache. Getting the client's vital signs and calling the doctor if they are abnormal would focus further attention on the physical aspects of the client's functioning without helping the client to move toward developing an awareness of the interrelationship between pain and emotions. It also suggests that the nurse requires physician guidance before intervening. The nurse should know that it is appropriate to provide physical care in a matter-of-fact manner, while at the same time helping the client to understand how symptoms increase in a time of stress and can be a way of coping with stress. Telling the client not to rely on pain pills due to the potential for addiction is a critical statement that will likely cause the client to feel frustrated and angry, which can increase the intensity of the headache. **Cognitive Level:** Analyzing **Client Need:** Psychosocial Integrity **Integrated Process:** Nursing Process: Implementation **Content Area:** Mental Health **Strategy:** Think about the nature of the pain and what underlies it. Ask yourself if symptomatic measures to relieve the pain will prevent future pain. **Reference:** Varcarolis, E., Carson, V., & Shoemaker, N. (2010). *Foundations of psychiatric mental health nursing: A clinical approach* (6th ed.). St. Louis, MO: Saunders Elsevier, p. 263.

6 **Answer: 2** **Rationale:** Disturbed Body Image is correct. This client is preoccupied with the appearance of the body, not the health of the body. Body dysmorphic disorder is characterized by preoccupation with imagined defects, usually on the face or head, that prompt the client to seek medical treatment. The client's behavior does not suggest Health-Seeking Behaviors, but rather relief from feelings that the body is defective. This client's history and statements show a preoccupation with the appearance of the body, not with personal identity. Although great dissatisfaction with the appearance of the body is expressed, there is nothing in the client's statement to suggest immediate threat for self-mutilation. **Cognitive Level:** Analyzing **Client Need:** Psychosocial Integrity **Integrated Process:** Nursing Process: Diagnosis **Content Area:** Mental Health **Strategy:** Look for the obvious. Don't try to make this question more difficult than it is.

Reference: Varcarolis, E., Carson, V., & Shoemaker, N. (2006). *Foundations of psychiatric mental health nursing: A clinical approach* (5th ed.). St. Louis, MO: Saunders Elsevier, p. 259.

7 **Answer: 3** **Rationale:** The correct option is that the pain does not respond well to medication because the pain of somatization disorder often begins after trauma or injury. The client with pain disorder continues to express discomfort even after medication is given, does not respond well to medication, and exhibits no insight into the role of stress on pain perception. Individuals with pain disorder generally do not show a good response to analgesics and are at high risk for substance abuse and dependency. In pain disorder, the client is not indifferent to the pain. Instead the client is consumed by the pain experience. Indifference to pain is most associated with pain of the conversion type. Clients with pain disorder see pain as something that is imposed on them (insight into relationship between stress and pain). **Cognitive Level:** Applying **Client Need:** Psychosocial Integrity **Integrated Process:** Nursing Process: Assessment **Content Area:** Mental Health **Strategy:** Recognize that this client's pain is not somatically caused. Consider possible psychological purposes of pain. **Reference:** Kneisl, C., Wilson, H., & Trigoboff, E. (2004). *Contemporary psychiatric–mental health nursing.* Upper Saddle River, NJ: Prentice Hall, p. 390.

8 **Answer: 1, 2, 4, 5** **Rationale:** Four options are correct. Criteria for a diagnosis of somatization disorder include pain symptoms (i.e., pain during intercourse), a sexual response (i.e., menstrual irregularities), gastrointestinal responses (i.e., nausea and vomiting), a pseudoneurological response (i.e., urinary retention). Shortness of breath is incorrect, shortness of breath is not a medical manifestation related to somatization disorder. **Cognitive Level:** Analyzing **Client Need:** Psychosocial Integrity **Integrated Process:** Nursing Process: Assessment **Content Area:** Mental Health **Strategy:** Nursing assessment of clients with a somatization disorder includes assessing for symptoms in the following categories: pain symptoms, gastrointestinal symptoms, sexual symptoms, and pseudoneurological symptoms. A history of physical complaints must be reported before 30 years of age before a diagnosis can be made. **Reference:** Kneisl, C. R., & Trigoboff, E. (2009). *Contemporary psychiatric–mental health nursing* (2nd ed.). pp. 479–480.

9 **Answer: 3** **Rationale:** Recognizing that it must be hard for the client to accept the test results is correct. It shows that when the nurse shows empathy by verbalizing the implied feeling of the client, an opportunity is created for the client. Specifically, the client can now express feelings and begin to connect these feelings to anxiety-producing situations and the symptoms being experienced. Stating that sometimes doctors miss a diagnosis leaves the client feeling that a misdiagnosis has occurred. It will not assist the client to verbalize feelings, nor will it assist the client to learn to express self in non-somatic ways. Recognizing the client's pain focuses totally on the physical aspect of the client's functioning and makes no effort to assist the client to recognize the interrelationship of emotions and the symptoms. Suggesting that the client rest now and ask the doctor about it later shows a lack of concern for the client and can lead to feelings of rejection, which can increase the client's anxiety and therefore the preoccupation with own physical health. **Cognitive Level:** Analyzing **Client Need:** Psychosocial Integrity **Integrated Process:** Communication and Documentation **Content Area:** Mental Health **Strategy:** Look for a response that could help the client connect anxiety with preoccupations about health. **Reference:** Kneisl, C., Wilson, H., & Trigoboff, E. (2009). *Contemporary psychiatric–mental health nursing* (2nd ed.). Upper Saddle River, NJ: Prentice Hall, p. 393.

10 Answer: 4 Rationale: Feeling better physically from getting a chance to talk is correct. This response shows that the client has profited from the opportunity to talk and gain support from others, both of which free up energy associated with unexpressed emotions. Unexpressed emotions and the energy associated with them play a significant role in the development of non-somatically caused pain. The statement about getting some pain pills for a painful back gives no indication that the group therapy has been effective. Instead, the client is still focused on the perceived pain. Stating that the other group members have mental problems suggests that the client does not recognize commonalities between other clients and self. Instead, the client is still focused on the perceived pain. The client's pointing out that he or she hasn't said much but benefits from listening suggests that the client has not participated fully in group therapy and cannot therefore be expected to have received full benefit from the therapy. **Cognitive Level:** Analyzing **Client Need:** Management of Care **Integrated Process:** Nursing Process: Evaluation **Content Area:** Mental Health **Strategy:** Look for the most insightful comment of the client. Eliminate any that show lack of change. **Reference:** Varcarolis, E., Carson, V., & Shoemaker, N. (2010). *Foundations of psychiatric mental health nursing: A clinical approach* (6th ed.). St. Louis, MO: Saunders Elsevier, p. 722.

References

American Psychiatric Association (2000). *Diagnostic and statistical manual of mental disorders, text revision* (4th ed.). Washington, DC: American Psychiatric Association pp. 485–511.

Carpenito, L. J. (2011). *Nursing diagnosis: Application to clinical practice* (13th ed.). Philadelphia, PA: Lippincott Williams & Wilkins.

Fontaine, K. (2009). *Mental health nursing* (6th ed.). Upper Saddle River, NJ: Pearson Education.

Kneisl, C. R., Wilson, H. S., & Trigoboff, E. (2009). *Contemporary psychiatric–mental health nursing* (2nd ed.). Upper Saddle River, NJ: Pearson Education, Inc.

National Alliance of the Mentally Ill (2011). *Inform yourself*. Retrieved on February 10, 2011, from www.nami.org/template.cfm?section=inform_yourself

Stuart, G. W., & Laraia, M. T. (2009). *Principles and practice of psychiatric nursing* (9th ed.). St. Louis, MO: Elsevier Mosby.

Townsend, M. C. (2011). *Essentials in psychiatric mental health nursing* (5th ed.). Philadelphia: F.A. Davis.

Varcarolis, E., & Halter, M. (2010). *Foundations of psychiatric mental health nursing: A clinical approach* (6th ed.). Philadelphia: Saunders.

Dissociative Disorders

7

Chapter Outline

Overview/Theories
Etiology
Assessment

Nursing Diagnoses/Analysis
Planning and
  Implementation

Evaluation/Outcomes
Specific Disorders

Objectives

➤ Identify five characteristic behaviors associated with dissociative disorders.
➤ State examples of at least four nursing diagnoses frequently used in the management of clients experiencing dissociative disorders.
➤ Formulate three intervention strategies for clients with dissociative disorders.

NCLEX-RN® Test Prep

Use the accompanying online resource, NursingReviewsandRationales, to test yourself with hundreds of NCLEX®-style practice questions.

Review at a Glance

alter personality state or identity that recurrently takes over the behavior of a person with dissociative identity disorder
continuous amnesia inability to recall successive events as they occur
depersonalization feeling of detachment or separation from one's self, as if in a dream-like state
derealization feeling that the external world is unreal or strange
dissociation defense mechanism in which experiences are blocked off from consciousness, so that affect, behavior, identity, memories, and/or thoughts are not integrated

dissociative amnesia dissociative disorder in which there is an inability to remember important personal information that cannot be accounted for by ordinary forgetfulness
dissociative fugue dissociative disorder characterized by suddenly wandering or taking a trip away from one's usual place, accompanied by amnesia for some or all of the past
dissociative identity disorder (DID) dissociative disorder characterized by two or more distinct personalities or identities (alters) in an individual person

generalized amnesia inability to recall entire life
host personality primary identity that holds the person's name
localized amnesia inability to recall events in a circumscribed time period
repression defense mechanism in which thoughts and feelings are kept from consciousness
selective amnesia inability to recall some events within a circumscribed time

PRETEST

1 The client, although oriented to person, place, and time, cannot remember being extracted from a burning automobile the day before. What term should the nurse use when documenting the client's inability to remember events surrounding the accident?

1. Suppression
2. Localized amnesia
3. Confabulation
4. Continuous amnesia

2 The nurse would select which of the following as appropriate nursing diagnoses for a client experiencing a fugue state? Select all that apply.

1. Anxiety
2. Disturbed Self-Esteem
3. Interrupted Family Processes
4. Relocation Stress Syndrome
5. Posttrauma Syndrome

3 The nurse assessing the client in a fugue state would look for which of the following? Select all that apply.

1. A history of childhood trauma
2. Coexisting depression
3. Exposure to a major stressor
4. Dissociative episodes
5. A recent history of being raped

4 A windstorm severely damaged a client's farm. The client recalls very little about the storm and repeatedly says, "I can't believe the farm is destroyed." When the nurse is providing care, which of the following client goals should take priority?

1. Report decreased depression by day two.
2. Express anger about his loss by day two.
3. Apply for job retraining by day two.
4. Attend a support group for disaster survivors by day two.

5 A nursing assistant (NA) asks for advice about talking with a client recently diagnosed with dissociative identity disorder (DID). When the NA asks, "Should I talk about her childhood abuse?" What is the best response?

1. "If she brings up the abuse, listen to her and be supportive."
2. "You will need to really push her to get it all out."
3. "Ask her to discuss this only with her therapist."
4. "Remind her that sometimes adults exaggerate their childhood experiences."

6 The client is experiencing dissociative amnesia. The nurse has taught the client about therapeutic methods for memory retrieval. The nurse determines that the teaching has been effective when the client makes which statement?

1. "Even if it does uncover hidden memories, I don't want to have electroconvulsive therapy."
2. "I'm a little uneasy about being hypnotized, but it does help release memories."
3. "If I use relaxation techniques properly, my memories will come back quickly."
4. "Anxiety causes this memory problem, and antianxiety agents will greatly reduce it."

7 The nurse determines that client education to manage dissociative episodes is effective if the client states to do which of the following if he starts to dissociate?

1. "Immediately take my anti-anxiety medication."
2. "Focus on what I can see and hear externally."
3. "Begin my relaxation technique."
4. "Focus on my internal feelings."

8 The client who has dissociative identity disorder (DID) is now 20 minutes late for cognitive therapy group. The client says, "I was never told to go to that group." What is the nurse's best response?

1. "You can't get out of group that easily."
2. "People with dissociative identity disorder forget quite a bit."
3. "Have you thought about just why you might be resisting treatment?"
4. "It is possible that you were not aware of group time."

9 The spouse of a client who is experiencing a fugue state asks the nurse if the spouse will be able to remember what happened during the time of the fugue. What is the nurse's best response?

1. "Your spouse will probably have no memory for events during the fugue."
2. "Your spouse will be able to tell you—if you can gently encourage talking."
3. "It is not possible to predict whether your spouse will remember the fugue state."
4. "Avoid mentioning it, or your spouse may start alternating old and new identities."

10 The client has dissociative identity disorder (DID). When the client is changing from one alter to another, which of the following would the nurse expect to observe?

1. Orthostatic hypotension
2. Blinking or rolling of the eyes
3. Dystonic reactions
4. Pallor

➤ *See pages 148–150 for Answers and Rationales.*

I. OVERVIEW/THEORIES

    A. In dissociative disorders, there is a sudden disruption in client's consciousness, identity, or memory; usually these are integrated functions

    B. Defense mechanisms used with dissociative disorders are dissociation and repression

        1. May experience considerable anxiety caused by expressed or fantasized forbidden wishes, often of sexual or aggressive nature

        2. May have considerable anxiety related to stressors or traumatic events

        3. Person does not consciously "decide" to dissociate

    C. Anatomical/physiological origins of "trance states" or dissociation

        1. Childhood trauma resulting in neurotransmitter and anatomical changes in the brain

        2. Genetic predisposition to dissociate is hypothesized

II. ETIOLOGY

      A. Traumatic experience (commonly accidents, natural disasters, assault)

        1. Strong emotional response

        2. Psychological conflict

        3. May be long-term, chronic stressors

    B. More easily induced if using psychoactive drugs (hallucinogens or cannabis)

      C. Severe childhood physical, sexual, or emotional abuse

        1. Implicated in dissociative identity disorder (DID)

        2. Child learns to detach or dissociate from intolerable situation (Figure 7-1)

        3. Continues to dissociate when experiencing stressful (even non-abusive) events as an adult, which interferes with normal functioning

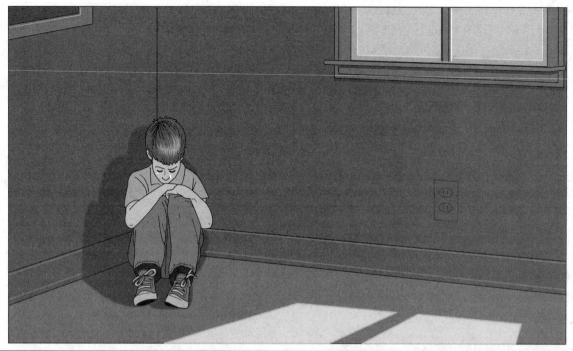

Figure 7-1

Children may learn to dissociate from intolerable situations such as severe abuse

III. ASSESSMENT

A. History
1. Recounts trauma and/or severe stress
   a. History of childhood abuse, but often does not recall trauma
   b. Symptoms appear in adulthood after stressful event(s)
   c. Symptoms appear immediately or may be delayed for years
2. Extent of dissociation or amnestic symptoms varies widely with different dissociative disorders
   a. **Dissociation** is a defense mechanism in which experiences are blocked off from consciousness, so that affect, behavior, identity, memories, and/or thoughts are not integrated
   b. **Repression** is a defense mechanism in which thoughts and feelings are kept from consciousness
3. May report symptoms of depression or anxiety

B. Physical symptoms
1. Headaches common with DID
2. Other dissociative disorders have no associated physical symptoms

C. Mental status examination
1. Appearance: facial expressions and mannerisms may vary widely within one session or appearance may vary widely from day to day (DID)
2. Mood: anxious, depressed; some clients have little mood change
3. Memory: amnesia for events (variable extent)
4. Perception: feelings of detachment from self or environment, feeling of physical change in body
5. Insight: impaired, unaware of memory impairment

Practice to Pass

How would you explain the stress–anxiety–dissociation relationship to a client who is dissociative and is puzzled about her behavior?

Practice to Pass

What questions could you routinely use in all assessments that might uncover a history of trauma?

VI. NURSING DIAGNOSES/ANALYSIS

A. **Anxiety** related to traumatic experience

B. **Ineffective Coping** related to childhood trauma, childhood abuse, low self-esteem, and inadequate coping skills

C. **Personal Identity Disturbance** related to threat to physical integrity, threat to self-concept, and underdeveloped ego

D. **Disturbed Sensory Perception** related to severe level of anxiety, repressed and decreased perceptual field

E. **Impaired Thought Processes** related to physical integrity and threat to self-concept

F. **Powerlessness** related to unmet dependency needs and fear of memory loss

G. **Risk for Self-Mutilation** related to response to increasing anxiety and inability to verbalize feelings

V. PLANNING AND IMPLEMENTATION

A. **Specific strategies**
  1. Create safe, calm environment
      a. Mutually develop plan of care
      b. Prevent stressors that could elicit dissociation; don't overwhelm client with data from the past
      c. Provide safety measures to prevent self-harm
  2. Teach stress management and coping techniques
      a. Progressive muscle relaxation
      b. Physical exercise
      c. "Grounding"—focus on external environment (what client can see and hear) rather than on internal feelings, thoughts, or sensations that can lead to "spacing out" (a lay term indicating lack of awareness of the immediate environment)
      d. Problem-solving strategies to resolve conflicts and stressors
      e. Provide a non-demanding simple routine
      f. Encourage journaling
  3. Discuss traumatic event and its meaning as client is able to recall event
  4. Reconstruct memories through client's account and those of others
  5. Educate about specific dissociative disorder
      a. Describe relationship between anxiety and dissociation
      b. Include family and significant others
  6. Assist staff and other clients to understand the disorder (especially DID)
  7. Plan for use of leisure time (anxiety often increases when alone without activities)

B. **Pharmacology**
  1. Drug-facilitated interviews using thiopental sodium (Pentothal) or sodium amytal to recovery memory
  2. Anti-anxiety agents for short-term symptomatic treatment
  3. Antidepressants for depression and antipsychotics for extreme agitation (if those symptoms are present)

C. **Individual/group**
  1. Hypnosis to recover memories
  2. Focus on emotional responses to trauma or stressors
  3. Work through unacceptable impulses or behavior verbally

Practice to Pass

A client who is dissociative remarks that he has tried using visual imagery to reduce stress, but finds it anxiety producing and "spacy." How could you explain this phenomenon and what alternatives could the client use to reduce stress?

Practice to Pass

Why are antianxiety agents recommended for short-term use?

Practice to Pass

How could you determine that the client's traumatic events are remembered with appropriate affect?

4. Refer to support groups
   a. Related to specific stressors such as parenting or occupational
   b. "Survivor" groups, particularly for natural disasters or abuse

D. Behavior modification
   1. Teach cognitive techniques to promote positive self-statements about coping ability
   2. Reinforce client's use of stress management and coping strategies rather than dissociation

VI. EVALUATION/OUTCOMES

A. **Client explains the relationship** between trauma/stress, anxiety, and dissociation
B. **Client can prevent dissociative states** by employing stress-management and positive coping behaviors
C. **Client can remember stressors** and traumatic events with congruent affect
D. **Client actively seeks to solve problems**
E. **Client assumes or resumes social and occupational roles**
F. **Client uses leisure time in constructive ways**

VII. SPECIFIC DISORDERS

A. *Dissociative amnesia*: a dissociative disorder in which the client cannot remember important personal information that cannot be accounted for by ordinary forgetfulness
   1. Suddenly unable to recall memories
      a. **Localized amnesia**: short time period (hours) after a disturbing event
      b. **Selective amnesia**: amnesia for some, but not all, events
      c. **Generalized amnesia**: amnesia for whole lifetime of experiences (very rare)
      d. **Continuous amnesia**: forgets successive events as they occur
   2. Not ordinary forgetfulness
   3. Able to recall other information, learn, and function coherently
   4. Most common during wars and natural disasters
   5. Primary gain: symbolic resolution of unconscious conflict that decreases anxiety and keeps the conflict from awareness
   6. Secondary gain: receipt of extra support and caring when experiencing an illness
   7. Usually terminates abruptly
   8. Special interventions
      a. Survivor support groups
      b. Gradual reconstruction of events through talking and listening/reading of others' accounts of the trauma

B. *Dissociative fugue*: a dissociative disorder characterized by suddenly wandering away or taking a trip away from one's usual place, accompanied by amnesia for some or all of the past (Figure 7-2)
   1. Travels from usual environment
   2. Unable to recall important aspects of identity and assumes new identity
      a. Old and new identities do not alternate
      b. Incomplete new identity
      c. Does not know information is forgotten
   3. Usually lasts from hours to days, rarely months; considerable confusion when returns to pre-fugue state
   4. Often is a response to psychological stressors (war, family, marital)
   5. Once the client has returned to pre-fugue state, he or she has no memory for events during the fugue
   6. Special interventions: hypnosis, drug-facilitated interviews, support groups

C. *Dissociative identity disorder (DID)*: a dissociative disorder characterized by two or more distinct personalities or identities (alters) in an individual person
   1. Client has two or more alters (separate, distinct identities or "personalities")
      a. An **alter** is a personality state or identity that recurrently takes over the behavior of a person with DID

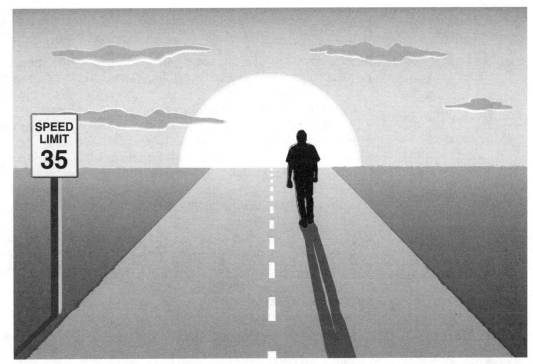

   b. Each alter has relatively enduring pattern of perceiving, relating to, and thinking about itself and the environment

   c. Formerly known as multiple personality disorder (MPD)

2. Personalities with different influences and power over one another

   a. May represent different ages, genders

   b. Alters each have different physiological responses and disorders (one alter may be myopic, while another is not)

   c. Communicate with one another through "executive" alter

   d. Some alters share "co-consciousness," aware of each other's experience and behavior, while others are only aware of own existence

   e. "Switching" occurs by dissociating from one alter to another

   f. Number of personalities range from 2 to over 100, with 50% of clients having more than 10 personalities

   g. **Host personality**: primary identity that holds the person's name

   h. The host personality is typically unaware of the alters (the anxiety-provoking aspects of personality), but the alters are typically aware of the host personality

 3. "Loses time" when alternate personality is present for a period of time

   a. Usually client is unable to give full account of childhood (few memories) because of dissociation

   b. May appear forgetful and is often accused of lying

 4. Mental status variations

   a. Marked variation in appearance from time to time

   b. Blinking, eye rolls, headaches, covering or hiding the face, and twitches may occur when "switching" from one alter to another

   c. Marked variation in speech for brief periods of time

   d. Impaired insight, usually unaware of alters

   e. May appear anxious or depressed

 5. Associated with severe physical or sexual abuse during childhood

   a. Many posttrauma symptoms (nightmares, flashbacks, hypervigilance)

   b. Self-mutilation, suicidal, or aggressive behavior

6. Special interventions
   a. No-harm contract and environmental safety if client is suicidal or is self-mutilating
   b. Meeting and recognizing alters and their unique experiences and needs
   c. "Mapping" personality system, noting characteristics of alters and co-consciousness
   d. Creation of emotionally safe environment for all alters
   e. Individual therapy with therapist skilled in working through trauma leading to integration (moving together of aspects of all identities)
   f. Development of new coping skills for integrated client and for clients who choose not to integrate so that dissociation is either not necessary or is under control
   g. Family therapy with partners and children to help client avoid dissociation, deal with hostile personalities, understand therapy process, and to confirm experience with client's behavior
   h. Hypnosis or drug-facilitated interviews; use is controversial because of the possibility of remembering "too much, too soon" and being overwhelmed with anxiety
   i. Issue: the therapist's "creating" memories and alters by his or her verbal and non-verbal behavior in suggestible client

D. **Depersonalization disorder**
   1. Experiences recurrent alterations in self-perception
      a. **Depersonalization**: feeling of detachment or separation from one's self, as if in a dreamlike state
      b. Client describes self as "detached from my body" or "being in a dream"
      c. Feels strange or unreal
      d. Able to function during the experience
   2. Client may report distress about experiences and become depressed and anxious
      a. Often fears being "crazy"
      b. May be accompanied by **derealization**, which is the feeling that the external world is unreal or strange
   3. Precipitated by stress and anxiety
   4. Most common in teenagers and young adults
   5. Special interventions
      a. Problem solving to reduce stress in general
      b. Stress-management techniques
      c. "Grounding" or focus on external environment

Case Study

A 35-year-old woman diagnosed with depression and dissociative identity disorder is hospitalized when outpatient therapy proved insufficient to manage her mood. You are part of the interdisciplinary team working with this client.

1. What are some of the safety issues you might anticipate?

2. You overhear one of the nursing assistants urging another to "go see the client and her eleven faces." How could you handle this situation?

3. What could you do to decrease confusion about which "personality" you are interacting with at a given point in time?

4. The client's husband is concerned about involving their two school-age children in family therapy. How might you explain how children might benefit from family therapy?

5. One of the evening nurses comments that the client does this "multiple business" just to get attention, even though she has a lovely family and a nice house. What is your best response?

For suggested responses, see page 298.

POSTTEST

1 The nurse is conducting a client teaching session about dissociative disorders. Which client statement indicates to the nurse that the client understands important concepts about the disorder?

1. "People with dissociative disorder usually have gradual loss of memory for names and phone numbers."
2. "Dissociative disorders serve as a means of avoiding adult responsibilities."
3. "Dissociative disorders are caused from past use of hallucinogens."
4. "People develop dissociative disorders to protect themselves from extreme anxiety."

2 The nurse determines that which of the following is a priority nursing intervention for a person recently admitted to an inpatient unit with a dissociative disorder?

1. Creation of a calm, safe environment
2. Increasing sensory stimulation
3. Working through past trauma
4. Promoting social skills

3 The nurse assessing a client with dissociative identity disorder (DID) is most likely to note which of the following? Select all that apply.

1. History of headaches
2. Elated mood
3. Intact memory for recent and remote events
4. Asthma
5. Irritable bowel syndrome

4 A client with dissociative identity disorder (DID) is admitted after an overdose of alcohol and benzodiazepines, claiming that another alter "did it." The nurse formulates which of the following as the priority nursing diagnosis?

1. Posttrauma Response
2. Risk for Self-Directed Violence
3. Disturbed Personal Identity
4. Anxiety

5 A client is brought to the emergency room after a brutal physical assault. Although oriented and coherent, the client cannot remember the assault or events surrounding it. The priority intervention by the nurse is to provide which of the following?

1. Frequent reality orientation
2. Physical comfort and safety
3. Thoughtful questioning for the police report
4. Referral to a community support group

6 A client with dissociative identity disorder (DID) suddenly begins to speak with a child's vocabulary and voice. The nurse should interpret this as which of the following?

1. An attempt to gain attention
2. A state of depersonalization
3. Changing to a child alter
4. Malingering

7 A client with dissociative identity disorder (DID) suddenly has a change in voice quality and sentence structure. What is the most therapeutic response by the nurse?

1. "You must be feeling very needy."
2. "I wonder why you're not acting your age."
3. "Can you tell me what is happening?"
4. "This behavior keeps you from working on your problems."

8 A client is diagnosed with depersonalization disorder. Which of the following is the nurse most likely to find in the assessment? Select all that apply.

1. Two or more personalities
2. Feelings like "being in a dream"
3. Indifference to the symptoms
4. Feeling like a robot
5. Amnesia about the event

9 The nurse formulates which priority nursing diagnosis for a client experiencing amnesia associated with high levels of anxiety?

1. Confusion
2. Powerlessness
3. Ineffective Coping
4. Disturbed Sensory Perception

10 A client reports episodic depersonalization experiences to the nurse. Which of the following is an appropriate goal of care?

1. The client will describe three stress management techniques by day two.
2. The client will report no suicidal thoughts by week one.
3. The client will create a chart of all personalities by week one.
4. The client will state five personal strengths by day two.

➤ *See pages 150–151 for Answers and Rationales.*

ANSWERS & RATIONALES

Pretest

1 **Answer: 2** **Rationale:** Localized amnesia is correct. The client's memory loss began a few hours after a disturbing event. Further, the client is unable to recall all memories of the event, and the memory loss is confined to this particular sphere of the individual's functioning. Suppression is a consciously motivated response of an individual to a stressful event. When suppression is used, the individual is fully aware of what is taking place and refuses to acknowledge it. This client does not evidence this type of awareness. Confabulation is the replacement of gaps in memory with imaginary information. This client is not showing this behavior. Continuous amnesia is that type of memory loss in which the individual forgets successive events as they occur. This type of amnesia includes loss of memory of present events and affects orientation. **Cognitive Level:** Applying **Client Need:** Psychosocial Integrity **Integrated Process:** Communication and Documentation **Content Area:** Mental Health **Strategy:** Notice that this client has just experienced an intensely stressful event. Doesn't it make sense that the psyche would try to protect the individual by blocking out memory of the event? **Reference:** Fontaine, K. (2009). *Mental health nursing* (6th ed.). Upper Saddle River, NJ: Prentice Hall, p. 234.

2 **Answer: 1, 5** **Rationale:** Anxiety and posttrauma syndrome are correct. A fugue state is a result of dissociation, a defense against overwhelming anxiety. It is often precipitated by sub-acute chronic stress and/or a major stressful event. This condition is rare and can last for varying periods of time. During the fugue state the person often behaves in ways that are inconsistent with normal personality and values. Without further data, it is impossible to determine that the stress and anxiety are related either to family difficulties, self-esteem, or relocation. **Cognitive Level:** Applying **Client Need:** Psychosocial Integrity **Integrated Process:** Nursing Process: Diagnosis **Content Area:** Mental Health **Strategy:** Consider the concept of unconscious motivators of behavior. Notice also that no information is given about the client's family, living circumstances, or self-esteem. **Reference:** Fontaine, K. (2009). *Mental health nursing* (6th ed.). Upper Saddle River, NJ: Prentice-Hall, p. 251.

3 **Answer: 3, 5** **Rationale:** Exposure to a major stressor and a recent history of being raped are correct. Fugue states usually begin abruptly after a major stressor such as war or natural disaster, and end abruptly. The client experiencing a fugue state may or may not have a history of childhood trauma or depression. During the fugue state the person either appears totally normal to others or appears dazed and confused. Depression, if it occurs, is likely to precede or follow the fugue state. If the stressor is severe enough, the client can enter a fugue state without ever having had other dissociative responses. **Cognitive Level:** Applying **Client Need:** Psychosocial Integrity **Integrated**

Process: Nursing Process: Assessment **Content Area:** Mental Health **Strategy:** Recall various types of dissociative responses. Identify the common underlying factor in each of them. Apply that knowledge to this situation. **Reference:** Fontaine, K. (2009). *Mental health nursing* (6th ed.). Upper Saddle River, NJ: Prentice Hall, p. 234.

4 **Answer: 4** **Rationale:** Attend a support group is correct. At this time the client needs an opportunity to work through the disaster event, acknowledge its reality, and reduce anxiety. This will best occur in a disaster survivor support group in which other survivors of disaster and the client will talk about the reality of the loss. If this does not happen, the client is at risk for experiencing a crisis response. Feelings of depression and anger, while a part of coping with loss, may occur later than two days after an event and will take more than a few days to resolve. It is too early to consider whether job retraining is necessary or whether funds are available for rebuilding. **Cognitive Level:** Analyzing **Client Need:** Psychosocial Integrity **Integrated Process:** Nursing Process: Planning **Content Area:** Mental Health **Strategy:** Apply theoretical information about crisis responses and balancing factors. **Reference:** Fontaine, K. (2009). *Mental health nursing* (6th ed.). Upper Saddle River, NJ: Prentice Hall, p. 251.

5 **Answer: 1** **Rationale:** Listening and being supportive if the client mentions the abuse is correct. Trust is the basis of a therapeutic relationship, and the client should proceed at a self-determined rate, particularly if the subject is painful. Self-pacing avoids flooding the client with severe anxiety. This self-disclosure should be accepted nonjudgmentally by all persons with whom the client has contact. Pushing the client to get it all out would result in flooding the client with anxiety, which is not recommended. Additionally, the nurse should recognize that a nursing assistant is not properly prepared for this sort of intervention. Asking the client to discuss it only with her therapist could interfere with trust and the client's readiness to disclose. Reminding the client that sometimes adults exaggerate their childhood experiences is non-accepting and demeaning to the client. **Cognitive Level:** Applying **Client Need:** Psychosocial Integrity **Integrated Process:** Caring **Content Area:** Mental Health **Strategy:** Notice to whom the nurse is responding. Consider the level of complexity necessary for intervening in dissociative states. **Reference:** Varcarolis, E., Carson, V., & Shoemaker, N. (2009). *Foundations of psychiatric mental health nursing: A clinical approach* (6th ed.). St. Louis, MO: Saunders Elsevier, pp. 521–523.

6 **Answer: 2** **Rationale:** Recognizing that hypnosis helps release memories is correct. Hypnosis may be effective to access memories and, if present, other personalities that result from dissociation. The statement about electroconvulsive therapy is incorrect because ECT does not enhance the recovery of memories. Instead, it can interfere with recall and memory, particularly of recent events. While overwhelming anxiety is associated with dissociative identity disorders, normal relaxation techniques do not enhance memory retrieval. While overwhelming anxiety is associated with dissociative identity disorders, anti-anxiety medications are symptomatic measures to reduce anxiety and are not directly associated with retrieval of memories. **Cognitive Level:** Analyzing **Client Need:** Psychosocial Integrity **Integrated Process:** Nursing Process: Evaluation **Content Area:** Mental Health **Strategy:** Consider that dissociative states result from the unconscious mental activities designed to reduce anxiety. Look for the treatment that is most expected to access the unconscious mind. **Reference:** Kneisl, C., Wilson, H., & Trigoboff, E. (2009). *Contemporary psychiatric–mental health nursing* (2nd ed.). Upper Saddle River, NJ: Prentice Hall, p. 469.

7 **Answer: 2** **Rationale:** Focusing on what can be seen and heard externally is correct. Objects or surroundings can be used to reorient the client by promoting concentration and an external focus. Internal focusing only augments dissociation. Taking an anti-anxiety medication at the time of dissociation will not be an effective deterrent, since the dissociation has already begun. It is also unlikely that the person can actually take the medicine, because dissociation will already be interrupting integrated functioning. Beginning a relaxation technique at the time of dissociation will not be an effective deterrent, since the dissociation has already begun. It is also unlikely that the person can focus on the relaxation technique because integrated functioning has already been interrupted by the dissociation. **Cognitive Level:** Analyzing **Client Need:** Psychosocial Integrity **Integrated Process:** Nursing Process: Evaluation **Content Area:** Mental Health **Strategy:** Think about the psychological purposes served by dissociation. Look for an option that would promote a more realistic coping response. **Reference:** Varcarolis, E., Carson, V., & Shoemaker, N. (2009). *Foundations of psychiatric mental health nursing: A clinical approach* (6th ed.). St. Louis, MO: Saunders Elsevier, pp. 521–523.

8 **Answer: 4** **Rationale:** Recognizing the possibility that the client was not aware of group time is correct. This is a supportive response. Many clients with DID have lack of awareness of events because another personality was present when these events were discussed. Thus, the host personality has no knowledge of them. Although the client eventually must be accountable for all actions of the personalities to the greatest extent possible, this may not initially be under the client's control. The statement that people with dissociative identity disorder forget often could be construed as somewhat condescending. The information is true, but there is no attempt to be supportive of this individual client. The nurse should not look upon the client's lateness as resistance. Many other causative possibilities exist, including presence of an alter personality that emerged and controlled the individual's behavior. Also, this response is somewhat accusatory. **Cognitive Level:** Analyzing **Client Need:** Psychosocial Integrity **Integrated Process:** Caring **Content Area:** Mental Health **Strategy:** Think about the most basic thing you know about DID: multiple personalities exist in the same person. Use this information to evaluate each option. **Reference:** Kneisl, C., Wilson, H., & Trigoboff, E. (2009). *Contemporary psychiatric–mental health nursing* (2nd ed.). Upper Saddle River, NJ: Prentice Hall, p. 467.

9 Answer: 1 Rationale: Stating that the client will probably have no memory of events during the fugue is correct. The client who has experienced a fugue is generally unable to remember events occurring during the fugue state, despite encouragement. During fugue states, clients are generally reclusive and quiet, so their behavior rarely attracts attention. Amnesia for the events occurring during the fugue state can be predicted. The client does not have the ability to alternate personal identity with the partial identity assumed during the fugue state. **Cognitive Level:** Applying **Client Need:** Health Promotion and Maintenance **Integrated Process:** Caring **Content Area:** Mental Health **Strategy:** Recall basic facts about fugue states and the unconscious purposes that they serve. **Reference:** Kneisl, C., Wilson, H., & Trigoboff, E. (2009). *Contemporary psychiatric–mental health nursing* (2nd ed.). Upper Saddle River, NJ: Prentice Hall, p. 467.

10 Answer: 2 Rationale: Blinking or rolling the eyes is correct. Changing from one alter to another is manifested in a variety of ways including blinking, facial changes, and changes in voice and train of thought. Orthostatic hypotension, dystonic reactions, or pallor are not usually associated with changing from one alter to another. **Cognitive Level:** Applying **Client Need:** Psychosocial Integrity **Integrated Process:** Nursing Process: Assessment **Content Area:** Mental Health **Strategy:** Consider that among multiple personalities, the common means of communicating with the external world is through both verbal and non-verbal means. Choose blinking/rolling the eyes over dystonic reactions as a non-verbal behavior because dystonic reactions can occur as an adverse effect of some medications. **Reference:** Varcarolis, E., Carson, V., & Shoemaker, N. (2009). *Foundations of psychiatric mental health Nursing: A clinical approach* (6th ed.). St. Louis, MO: Saunders Elsevier, pp. 519–520.

Posttest

1 Answer: 4 Rationale: "People develop dissociative disorders to protect themselves from extreme anxiety" is correct. Dissociative disorders result from using the defense mechanism of dissociation. This dissociation prevents anxiety about traumatic events or stressors from entering conscious awareness. Dissociation is not consciously employed and does not involve a gradual loss of memory. The process of changing alters generally occurs very quickly. Regressive behaviors are common in dissociative states, but dissociation is intended to

reduce anxiety, not avoid adult responsibilities. Use of hallucinogens can result in dissociation in persons who are prone to "trance states" or spacing out, but when this occurs, current use of the drug is most likely to have occurred. **Cognitive Level:** Analyzing **Client Need:** Psychosocial Integrity **Integrated Process:** Teaching and Learning **Content Area:** Mental Health **Strategy:** Look for an accurate and simply stated option. **Reference:** Fontaine, K. (2009). *Mental health nursing* (6th ed.). Upper Saddle River, NJ: Prentice Hall, p. 232.

2 Answer: 1 Rationale: Creation of a calm, safe environment is correct. Dissociation occurs when anxiety is high; thus, a calm, safe, and supportive environment is essential to decrease emotional arousal. Increasing sensory stimulation will increase psychological arousal and can lead to increased dissociation. Working through past trauma is not an immediate priority. Even if a history of trauma is a causative factor, anxiety must be reduced to a level compatible with verbal exploration. Social skills may or may not be problematic when the client is dissociating. This is dependent on the alter that emerges and its "function" within the group of personalities. **Cognitive Level:** Analyzing **Client Need:** Psychosocial Integrity **Integrated Process:** Nursing Process: Planning **Content Area:** Mental Health **Strategy:** Remember that dissociation occurs because of—and in—states of high emotional arousal and anxiety. Look for an option that would be likely to decrease anxiety. **Reference:** Varcarolis, E., Carson, V., & Shoemaker, N. (2009). *Foundations of psychiatric mental health nursing: A clinical approach* (6th ed.). St. Louis, MO: Saunders Elsevier, pp. 521–523.

3 Answer: 1, 4, 5 Rationale: Three options are correct. Clients with DID often have particular physical problems including headache, irritable bowel syndrome, and asthma. Elated mood could be a co-morbid condition associated with one more of the alters. However, it is not a universal symptom of dissociative identity disorder (DID). Memory is discontinuous in states of DID. Each personality has a memory of its own. **Cognitive Level:** Applying **Client Need:** Psychosocial Integrity **Integrated Process:** Nursing Process: Assessment **Content Area:** Mental Health **Strategy:** Look for an answer that will be true in the vast majority of persons with DID. **Reference:** Kneisl, C., Wilson, H., & Trigoboff, E. (2009). *Contemporary psychiatric–mental health nursing* (2nd ed.). Upper Saddle River, NJ: Prentice Hall, p. 465.

4 Answer: 2 Rationale: Risk for Self-Directed Violence is correct. The overdose of alcohol and benzodiazepines is particularly lethal, which demonstrates that the client is potentially harmful to self. The presenting personality may not be depressed or may not have enough power to prevent the alter that is self-destructive from acting out again, so substantial risk remains. Physical safety is a priority over all other options, including psychological needs, even when they are intense. **Cognitive Level:** Analyzing **Client Need:** Safety and Infection Control **Integrated Process:** Nursing Process: Diagnosis **Content Area:** Mental

Health **Strategy:** Notice that only one diagnosis is not a psychological one and remember that safety and physical needs always take precedence over psychological or sociologic needs. **Reference:** Varcarolis, E., Carson, V., & Shoemaker, N. (2009). *Foundations of psychiatric mental health nursing: A clinical approach* (6th ed.). St. Louis, MO: Saunders Elsevier, pp. 521–523.

5 **Answer: 2** **Rationale:** Physical comfort and safety is correct. The client needs to have critical physical needs met, including physical comfort, as the first priority. Creating a sense of safety after an assault is essential as anxiety may fluctuate. The nursing interventions in the other options are relevant, but not a priority and can be deferred to a later time. **Cognitive Level:** Analyzing **Client Need:** Psychosocial Integrity **Integrated Process:** Nursing Process: Diagnosis **Content Area:** Mental Health **Strategy:** Consider the nature of what has happened to this client. Recognize that unexpressed terror is probably present. **Reference:** Varcarolis, E., Carson, V., & Shoemaker, N. (2009). *Foundations of psychiatric mental health nursing: A clinical approach* (6th ed.). St. Louis, MO: Saunders Elsevier, pp. 516–518.

6 **Answer: 3** **Rationale:** Changing to a child alter is correct. The change in the client's voice indicates a change to a child alter. Reasons for this change include regression, resistance, needing sustenance, wanting to be understood, or other possibilities that are connected to severe underlying anxiety. Persons with DID do not dissociate in order to gain attention. Dissociation is an unconscious mechanism used to reduce overwhelming anxiety. Depersonalization involves a person's feeling disengaged and removed from one's surroundings, as if viewing things in a dream state. The person remains aware of personal identity during the time of depersonalization. Dissociation is not shown in this situation. Malingering is a consciously motivated behavior in which the individual behaves as if ill or feigns an emotion. Malingering is not shown in this situation. **Cognitive Level:** Analyzing **Client Need:** Psychosocial Integrity **Integrated Process:** Nursing Process: Assessment **Content Area:** Mental Health **Strategy:** Remember that states of dissociation develop as a protective response to reduce awareness of anxiety and stressors causing it. **Reference:** Varcarolis, E., Carson, V., & Shoemaker, N. (2009). *Foundations of psychiatric mental health nursing: A clinical approach* (6th ed.). St. Louis, MO: Saunders Elsevier, pp. 517, 519–520.

7 **Answer: 3** **Rationale:** Asking what is happening is correct. Changing alters often occurs with increases in anxiety. Asking the client to explain more will help the nurse understand what is happening on a system level, and why the child alter was emergent. Stating that the client must be very needy would increase the client's anxiety level. Asking why the client is not acting his or her age would not help the client become aware of feelings that preceded the dissociation. It is somewhat critical and represents a sort of private musing of the nurse that should not be verbalized to the child alter. Stating that

this behavior is preventing the client from working on his or her problems would also increase the client's anxiety level. **Cognitive Level:** Analyzing **Client Need:** Psychosocial Integrity **Integrated Process:** Caring **Content Area:** Mental Health **Strategy:** Identify the option that is most likely to keep the client focused on the reality of the present situation. **Reference:** Kneisl, C., Wilson, H., & Trigoboff, E. (2009). *Contemporary psychiatric–mental health nursing* (2nd ed.). Upper Saddle River, NJ: Prentice Hall, p. 469.

8 **Answer: 2, 4** **Rationale:** Feeling like "being in a dream" and feeling like a robot are correct. Feeling detached and/or being an outside observer of their body are characteristic of clients with depersonalization disorder. Multiple personalities or alters are not part of depersonalization disorder. Indifference to the symptoms (*la belle indifference*) and amnesia are usually related to conversion disorder. In depersonalization, the client remembers the event and usually is distressed by the experience. **Cognitive Level:** Analyzing **Client Need:** Psychosocial Integrity **Integrated Process:** Nursing Process: Diagnosis **Content Area:** Mental Health **Strategy:** Compare and contrast primary presenting symptoms of the different dissociative responses. **Reference:** Fontaine, K. (2009). *Mental health nursing* (6th ed.). Upper Saddle River, NJ: Prentice Hall, p. 234.

9 **Answer: 3** **Rationale:** Ineffective Coping is correct. Amnesia is a result of being unable to cope with high levels of anxiety. While heightened anxiety can be associated with this diagnosis, there is no indication that the diagnoses in the other options are present at this time. However, it is universally true that when amnesia results from increased anxiety, the individual is coping ineffectively. **Cognitive Level:** Analyzing **Client Need:** Psychosocial Integrity **Integrated Process:** Nursing Process: Diagnosis **Content Area:** Mental Health **Strategy:** Look for an option that will be universally true. Remember that amnesia and other dissociative responses result from unhealthy or ineffective attempts at coping. **Reference:** Varcarolis, E., Carson, V., & Shoemaker, N. (2009). *Foundations of psychiatric mental health nursing: A clinical approach* (6th ed.). St. Louis, MO: Saunders Elsevier, pp. 516–519.

10 **Answer: 1** **Rationale:** Describing three stress management techniques by day two is correct. Reducing anxiety through the use of stress management techniques will prevent depersonalization that is a reaction to high levels of anxiety. There is no data to support suicidal thoughts or multiple identities. Imsproving self-concept is helpful, but is not a priority when anxiety leads to dissociation. **Cognitive Level:** Applying **Client Need:** Psychosocial Integrity **Integrated Process:** Nursing Process: Planning **Content Area:** Mental Health **Strategy:** Remember that depersonalization is considered to be an anxiety disorder. **Reference:** Kneisl, C., Wilson, H., & Trigoboff, E. (2009). *Contemporary psychiatric–mental health nursing* (2nd ed.). Upper Saddle River, NJ: Prentice Hall, p. 468.

ANSWERS & RATIONALES

References

American Psychiatric Association (2000). *Diagnostic and statistical manual of mental disorders text revision* (4th ed.). Washington, DC: American Psychiatric Association, pp. 257, 527.

Carpenito, L. J. (2011). *Nursing diagnosis: Application to clinical practice* (13th ed.). Philadelphia, PA: Lippincott Williams & Wilkins.

Fontaine, K. (2009). *Mental health nursing* (6th ed.). Upper Saddle River, NJ: Pearson Education.

Kniesl, C., Wilson, H., & Trigoboff, E. (2009). *Contemporary psychiatric–mental health nursing* (2nd ed.). Upper Saddle River, NJ: Pearson Education.

Stuart, G. (2009). *Principles and practice of psychiatric nursing* (9th ed.). St. Louis: Elsevier Science.

Townsend, M. (2011). *Essentials of psychiatric–mental health nursing* (5th ed.). Philadelphia, PA: F. A. Davis.

Varcarolis, E., & Halter, M. (2010). *Foundations of psychiatric mental health nursing: A clinical approach* (6th ed.). Philadelphia: Saunders.

Personality Disorders 8

Objectives

➤ Identify four predisposing factors that contribute to personality disorders.
➤ Describe five characteristics associated with each personality disorder.
➤ State examples of at least four nursing diagnoses frequently used for clients experiencing personality disorders.
➤ Formulate four intervention strategies for clients with personality disorders.

NCLEX-RN® Test Prep

Use the accompanying online resource, NursingReviewsandRationales, to test yourself with hundreds of NCLEX®-style practice questions.

Review at a Glance

antisocial personality disorder a disorder characterized by a pattern of disregard for, and violation of the rights of others, and the inability to experience guilt in relation to untoward behaviors, exploits others to achieve goals

avoidant personality disorder a disorder characterized by a pattern of feelings of inadequacy, social inhibition, and hypersensitivity to negative feedback/evaluation

axis I disorders psychiatric problems such as mood disorders, psychotic disorders, eating disorders, somatoform disorders are coded per the *DSM-IV* as axis I

axis II disorders personality disorders and mental retardation are coded per the *DSM-IV* as axis II

borderline personality disorder (BPD) a disorder characterized by a pattern of instability in self image, interpersonal relationships, and marked impulsivity; carries a high risk for suicide and self-mutilation

Cluster A personality disorder descriptive characteristics include eccentric and odd; paranoid, schizoid, and schiotypal personality disorders are classified in this category

Cluster B personality disorder descriptive characteristics include emotional, dramatic, and erratic; antisocial, borderline, narcissistic, and histrionic personality disorders are classified in this category

Cluster C personality disorder descriptive characteristics are anxious and fearful; obsessive-compulsive, dependent, and avoidant personality disorders are classified in this category

dependent personality disorder a disorder characterized by a pattern of submissive and clinging behavior, with an excessive need for others to make decisions for, care for, and/or support them

dichotomous thinking also known as black and white thinking: where one can see no grey area; linked to splitting behavior in persons with BPD

egodystonic describes when patterns of personal behavior are perceived as uncomfortable, unnatural, or foreign to the self; life problems are perceived as internal causes; associated with a willingness to try to change behavior

egosyntonic describes when patterns of personal behavior are perceived as comfortable, natural, and a part of the self; life problems are perceived as external causes; associated with an unwillingness to try to change behavior

histrionic personality disorder a disorder characterized by a pattern of excessive emotionality, attention seeking, and suggestible behaviors

impulsivity human behavior done without thought; unplanned and rapid reactions to stimuli without regard for the potential untoward consequences of these reactions

manipulation a behavior whereby people treat other persons as objects; controlling others to meet one's own needs is of central concern

narcissistic personality disorder a disorder characterized by a pattern of grandiosity, need for admiration, and lack of empathy; exploits others to achieve personal goals

obsessive-compulsive personality disorder a disorder characterized by a pattern of preoccupation with orderliness, perfectionism, and control; includes focus on detail and difficulty with decision making, which is related to a fear of making a mistake and/or losing control

paranoid personality disorder a disorder characterized by a pattern of distrustful and suspicious behavior such that others' motives are interpreted as malevolent

personality disorder (PD) a disorder characterized by personality patterns or traits that are inflexible, enduring, pervasive, maladaptive, and cause subjective distress and impairment in social, occupational, and/or interpersonal functioning

personality traits enduring patterns of relating to, perceiving, and thinking about the self and the environment; these patterns are manifested in a wide range of personal and social contexts

projection a defense mechanism where a person unconsciously denies his or her own thoughts, attributes, and emotions, and ascribes them to the outside world

schizoid personality disorder a disorder characterized by a pattern of detachment from social relationships and whereby the person experiences a restricted range of emotions; the person is not influenced by praise nor criticism

schizotypal personality disorder a disorder characterized by a pattern of acute discomfort in close relationships, cognitive or perceptual distortions, and eccentricities of behavior

splitting the thought/behavior of switching from idealizing someone to hating them

PRETEST

1 The nurse is responsible for providing care to a group of clients with various personality disorders. The nurse should anticipate that a characteristic common to each client will be which of the following?

1. An ability to charm and manipulate people
2. A desire for interpersonal relationships
3. A diminished need for approval
4. A disruption in some aspect of his or her life

2 A client has been diagnosed with borderline personality disorder. The client is impulsive, shows labile affect, displays frequent angry outbursts, and has difficulty tolerating angry feelings without self-injury. The nurse selects which of the following as the priority nursing diagnosis for this client?

1. Anxiety
2. Risk for Self-Mutilation
3. Risk for Violence toward others
4. Ineffective Coping

3 The client is diagnosed with borderline personality disorder and engages in dichotomous thinking. When considering possible etiologies for this type of thinking, the nurse should give particular attention to a client history of which of the following?

1. Gender stereotyping
2. Family enmeshment
3. Perfectionistic standards
4. Physiological underarousal

4 A client recently released from prison for embezzlement has a history of becoming defensive and angry when criticized and blaming others for personal problems. The client has expressed no remorse or emotion about the actions that resulted in the prison term, but instead says that the embezzlement was justifiable because the employer "did not treat me fairly." The nurse concludes these behaviors are consistent with which of the following mental health problems?

1. Narcissistic personality disorder
2. Histrionic personality disorder
3. Antisocial personality disorder
4. Borderline personality disorder

5 The mental health nurse is reviewing a 35-year-old client's history before conducting an interview. The client's history indicates fear of criticism and rejection from others, having few friends, and withholding information about thoughts and feelings in anticipation of rejection by others. Based on the data, the nurse suspects that the client may have which personality disorder?

1. Schizotypal
2. Paranoid
3. Avoidant
4. Schizoid

6 The nurse caring for a client diagnosed with antisocial personality disorder would place highest priority on which nursing diagnosis?

1. Disturbed Personal Identity
2. Fear
3. Risk for Violence directed at others
4. Social Isolation

7 The nurse is preparing to orient a new graduate to the psychiatric unit. When teaching the new nurse about general principles related to psychopharmacology and personality disorders, the nurse includes which information about pharmacologic treatment? Select all that apply.

1. It is aimed at treating various psychiatric target symptoms in persons with personality disorders.
2. Carbamazepine (Tegretol) may be a prescribed treatment for mood stabilization in Cluster B disorders.
3. They have no role in treating any of the Cluster A, Cluster B, or Cluster C personality disorders.
4. Quetiapine (Seroquel) may be used to treat symptoms manifested in Cluster A personality disorders.
5. Benztropine (Cogentin) is useful in treating avoidant symptoms in Cluster C personality disorders.

8 The client diagnosed with narcissistic personality disorder arrives late to group therapy. Without apologizing, the client interrupts another client and says, "Well, I'm here. The group can start now." The nurse interprets this behavior as which of the following?

1. Splitting
2. Hypersensitivity
3. Suspiciousness
4. Entitlement

9 Which intervention strategy should the nurse routinely include in the nursing care plan for a client diagnosed with antisocial personality disorder?

1. Establish clear and enforceable limits.
2. Vary unit rules based on client demands.
3. Vary unit rules based on staff needs.
4. Let the client have a voice in when unit rules should apply.

10 Which nursing interventions would be appropriate for the nurse to implement when caring for the client diagnosed obsessive-compulsive personality disorder? Select all that apply.

1. Assertiveness training
2. Decision-making skills
3. Anxiety management
4. A 12-step program
5. Distraction techniques

➤ *See pages 169–170 for Answers and Rationales.*

I. OVERVIEW

A. *Personality*

1. Composed of enduring patterns or traits that determine how individuals perceive, relate to, and think about the self and the environment
2. Develops as individuals adjust to their physical, emotional, interpersonal, social, and spiritual experiences
3. **Personality traits** enduring patterns of relating to, perceiving, and thinking about the self and the environment; these patterns are manifested in a wide range of personal social context

B. Personality disorders

1. **Personality disorders (PDs)** are diagnosed when personality patterns or traits are inflexible, enduring, pervasive, maladaptive, and cause significant functional impairment or subjective distress
2. Reflect patterns of inner experience and behavior that differ from cultural, ethnic, and/or social expectations
3. Result in impairment and distress in everyday life rather than a manifestation of clinical symptoms
4. Clients perceive and experience their personality patterns as natural or comfortable (**egosyntonic**) rather than painful or uncomfortable (**egodystonic**)
5. If personality patterns are experienced as egosyntonic, clients rarely seek treatment as they tend to externalize the cause of any functional impairment or subjective distress
6. If personality patterns are experienced as egodystonic, clients are more likely to seek treatment to ease their distress
7. Are coded under **axis II disorders** (personality disorders or mental retardation) using the American Psychiatric Association's *Diagnostic and Statistical Manual of Mental Disorders, fourth edition text revision* (*DSM-IV-TR*) diagnostic criteria
8. Frequently overlap: individuals may exhibit patterns or traits associated with more than one personality disorder
9. Develop before or during adolescence and persist throughout life; symptoms may become less obvious by middle or old age
10. Diagnosis of a personality disorder is made at the age of 18 unless traits are evident for at least one year
11. A diagnosis of antisocial personality disorder cannot be made until the age of 18
12. Prevalence of PD in the United States is 9.1%
13. Symptoms/behaviors of PD may be exacerbated by a significant loss (i.e., job, family, home)
14. May coexist with clinical disorders coded as **axis I disorders** (i.e., mood disorder, psychotic disorder, eating disorder)
15. Are organized into three diagnostic clusters
    a. **Cluster A disorders**: individuals with these disorders manifest as odd and eccentric
    b. **Cluster B disorders**: individuals with these disorders manifest as dramatic and erratic
    c. **Cluster C disorders**: individuals with these disorders manifest as anxious and fearful
16. Characteristics of personality disorders are manifested in four areas
    a. Behavioral: a common problem is impulse control
    b. Affective: varies dependent on the disorder, may be flat, restricted, labile, or incongruent
    c. Cognitive: misinterpreted reflection of self, others, or events (i.e., narcissism, paranoia)

Practice to Pass

What untoward qualities must personality patterns reflect for an individual to be diagnosed with a personality disorder?

      d. Interpersonal/social: provokes, has enduring ways of provoking negative responses from people

II. ETIOLOGY

A. Neurobiological/anatomical theories
1. Limbic system dysregulation and central nervous system (CNS) irritability may result in decreased impulse control
2. Decreased levels of serotonin (5-HT) have been associated with a tendency to self-mutilate, experience intense rage, and behave aggressively toward others
3. Elevated levels of norepinephrine (NE) have been associated with hypersensitivity to the environment
4. Abnormal levels of dopamine (DA) may explain the brief psychotic episodes associated with borderline, schizoid, and schizotypal personality disorders
5. Physiological underarousal to stimulation may contribute to the risk taking associated with some disorders
6. Studies reveal decreased volume of prefrontal grey matter in persons with antisocial personality disorder

B. Genetic/familial
1. In individuals with certain personality disorders, there is an increased prevalence of the disorder in first degree biological relatives
2. A familial relationship exists between certain personality disorders and some axis I disorders
3. Research indicates that persons with PD have higher than normal rate of first degree biological relatives with a substance abuse problem
4. Specific personality disorders are diagnosed more frequently in certain genders

C. Intrapersonal theories
1. Hostility toward the self may be projected onto others resulting in fear, mistrust, and defensive withdrawal to avoid being hurt or avoid taking responsibility for behavior
2. Individuals may try to live up to perfectionistic standards imposed on them by their parents or caregivers during childhood development
3. An underdeveloped superego may result in a failure to both internalize authority and morals that results in the inability to feel guilt or remorse; this explains their disregard for others, exploitation, and violation of rules
4. Inadequate parenting that results in unmet and/or unsatisfied needs may lead to hostility toward significant others, fear of abandonment, anger, and rage; this explains their fear of intimacy, acting out of rage (to self or others) and/or guilt

D. Social theories
1. Social oppression may have a negative effect on the development of self-esteem and a healthy identity
2. Changes in societal values from a focus on group needs versus personal needs may be reflected in narcissistic behaviors associated with Cluster B PDs

E. Family theories
1. The inconsistent parenting inadequate supervision, inappropriate discipline, and poor parental role modeling may affect personality development
 2. Growing up in an enmeshed family (poor boundaries) that disallows for development of self may be associated with dichotomous thinking and/or splitting manifested in BPD
3. A chaotic, neglectful, and/or abusive environment is associated with the development of BPD in some persons

F. Feminist theory: the diagnosis of a PD is reflected by the influence of rigid gender-role stereotyping versus that of genetic factors

III. ASSESSMENT

A. **Many persons with PDs do not access or seek care** unless symptomatic for anxiety, depression, and/or suicidal ideation, suicide threats, or self-mutilation behaviors

B. **Mental status examination**

1. Appearance: observe age, dress, posture, hygiene, gait, facial expressions, overall nutritional status, an overall health status; persons with schizotypal, paranoid, or schizoid may have an appearance of being odd or eccentric; persons with antisocial PD may be cocky and charming as observed in facial expression; persons with narcissistic PD may show haughty, arrogant expressions

2. Speech: assess volume, rate, amount, and any other distinct features (i.e., slurred, stuttering); persons with schizotypal may manifest odd speech (circumstantial, stereotyped, vague); persons with borderline PD may have verbal outbursts

3. Motor activity: examine level of activity, restless, agitation, grimaces, tics, tremors, psychomotor retardation, compulsions; persons with antisocial PD may be aggressive and irritable; persons with paranoid PD may be guarded; persons with obsessive-compulsive disorder may demonstrate compulsions (i.e., repeated handwashing, rechecking)

4. Mood: ask the client how he or she is feeling; persons with schizotypal may have social anxiety; persons with antisocial PD and borderline PD may have depressed mood, boredom, dysphoria

5. Affect: objectively assess the client's expression of mood; observe both verbal and non-verbal cues; persons with schizoid, schizotypal, or paranoid PD may have a flat or restricted affect; persons with antisocial PD may have depressed affect and exhibit "superficial charm"; persons with borderline PD may have intense anger, panic, despair; persons with narcissism may have intense disdain/rage

6. Perceptions: observe for signs of auditory and/or visual hallucinations (ask the client if he or she is hearing voices/seeing anything/anybody); persons with schizotypal, schizoid, or borderline PD may exhibit brief psychotic episodes; persons with schizotypal PD may have bodily illusions: they may sense another person is present or hear a murmur; persons with borderline PD may hallucinate

7. Thought content: reflects thinking inside client's head; ask client about obsessions, compulsions, delusions, phobias; persons with schizotypal PD may have magical thinking, may experience brief psychotic episodes, and/or may have paranoid ideation; persons with antisocial PD or narcissistic PD may have grandiose ideas about self

8. Thought process: this is observed through the client's speech; examples of distortions in thought process include tangentiality, circumstantiality, word salad, thought blocking, perseveration, neologisms, loose associations, and flight of ideas; persons with schizotypal or borderline PD may have ideas of reference; persons with antisocial, narcissistic, borderline, or histrionic PD have problems with impulse control

9. Level of consciousness: is the client awake, alert, lethargic, stuporous; ask the client if he or she is oriented to person, place, and time

10. Memory: assess short- and long-term memory (persons with mood disorder may have impairment in both areas)

11. Insight: assess whether the client has insight into symptoms; persons with PDs have poor insight into their illness

12. Self-mutilation/suicide: persons with BPD may have thoughts of self-mutilation and/or suicidal threats or suicidal ideation due to a fear of abandonment; complete a suicide assessment as indicated; when suicidal these clients are at high risk for completed suicide

C. Social assessment
1. Examines individual's ability to interact and participate in life activities such as work, social interactions, and ongoing interpersonal relationships, and also includes client's ability to have an intimate relationship with another
2. Clients with schizoid PD may be socially isolated, have a lack of desire for intimacy and sexual experience
3. Clients with paranoid or schizotypal PD may prefer to be alone
4. Persons with borderline PD have a pattern of unstable relationships
5. Persons with narcissistic PD may become socially isolated when feeling rejected
6. Persons with avoidant PD may be lonely and/or socially isolated due to severe low self-esteem

IV. NURSING DIAGNOSES/ANALYSIS

A. Cluster A disorders (paranoid personality, schizoid personality, and schizotypal personality)
1. Ineffective Coping related to inability to trust others
2. Fear related to perceived threats from others or the environment; paranoia ideation
3. Social Isolation related to craving of solitude
4. Spiritual Distress related to lack of connectedness to others
5. Disturbed Thought Process related to (varies depending on medical diagnosis)
6. Defensive Coping related to related to anxiety, lack of insight
7. Risk for Loneliness related to social withdrawal, fear of refection, low self-esteem

B. Cluster B disorders (antisocial personality, borderline personality, histrionic personality, and narcissistic personality)
1. Impaired Social Interaction related to **manipulation** of others, unstable mood, poor impulse control, extreme emotional reactions, **splitting**, self-centeredness, and/or seductive behavior
2. Risk for Violence Self-Directed (suicide) related to intense emotional pain including rage and a sense of emptiness, and poor impulse control
3. Risk for Self-Mutilation related to fear of rejection, abandonment, need to punish self, anxiety
4. Risk for Violence directed at others or objects related to intense rage, poor impulse control, **projection**
5. Disturbed Personal Identity related to lack of a sense of self, changes in perceptions of body image, dissociation
6. Fear related to feelings of abandonment, rejection, poor self-esteem

C. Cluster C disorders (avoidant personality, dependent personality, and obsessive-compulsive personality)
1. Ineffective Coping related to high dependency needs, rigid thoughts and behavior, fear of rejection, high need for approval from others, or inability to make independent decisions
2. Fear related to feelings of abandonment, disapproval, or losing control
3. Impaired Social Interaction related to rigid behavior, fear of rejection, low self-esteem
4. Powerlessness related to extreme need for dependency on others, fear of losing control, inability to make decisions

V. PLANNING AND IMPLEMENTATION

A. Basic principles of nursing intervention

1. Establish at best a trusting nurse–client relationship
2. Recognize that clients have the right to change or not to change; if patterns of behavior are egosyntonic, clients may lack the motivation required to effect change
3. Facilitate clients to see how behavior affects specific aspects of their lives to motivate them to develop a more adaptive lifestyle
4. Recall that personality traits are ingrained; interventions should be based on short-term goals and should focus on small steps designed to improve role functioning and decrease distress
5. Instill hope for each client's improved quality of life; all clients have the potential for change
6. Identify your own emotional responses; intense feelings may be aroused when caring for persons with PD
7. Clients may split staff and power struggles may arise between staff members that creates staff divisiveness and a chaotic milieu

B. Specific strategies: cluster-specific nursing interventions can be individualized for each client

1. Cluster A disorders (paranoid personality, schizoid personality, and schizotypal personality)
   a. Approach client in a gentle, interested, nonintrusive manner
   b. Respect client's needs for distance and privacy
   c. Be cognizant of own non-verbal cues, as a client may perceive others as threatening
   d. Gradually encourage interaction with others, if and when appropriate

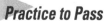

2. Cluster B disorders (antisocial personality, borderline personality, histrionic personality, and narcissistic personality)
   a. Remain patient in response to emotional, erratic, aggressive behavior
   b. Provide a consistent and structured milieu to avoid manipulation and power struggles
   c. Protect clients from suicide and self-mutilation until they can protect themselves
   d. Implement suicide precautions when necessary; implement one-on-one care to persons at risk for self-injury

   e. If client self-mutilates, treat wounds in a matter-of-fact manner
   f. Set limits to help clients maintain impulse control in order to protect self and others from injury
   g. Engage in frequent staff conferences to counteract client's ability to play one staff member against another (splitting)
   h. Encourage clients to recognize and discuss fear of abandonment
   i. Facilitate clients to recognize the presence of **dichotomous thinking** (the perception that self and/or others are perceived as all good or all bad)
   j. Encourage direct communication to minimize attention seeking through the use of dramatic, seductive behavior
   k. Redirect clients who display a sense of entitlement so as to help them acknowledge the needs of others
   l. Nurse will role-model healthy behaviors and effective communication

3. Cluster C disorders (avoidant personality, dependent personality, and obsessive-compulsive personality)
   a. Address avoidance behaviors related to losses and any secondary gain

---

Practice to Pass

Identify three specific PDs that may manifest with brief psychotic episodes. What is the psychopharmacologic treatment for psychosis in PDs?

Practice to Pass

Explain the rationale for the importance of nursing interventions related to limit setting in managing persons with antisocial personality disorder.

      b. Provide problem solving and assertiveness training to increase self-confidence and independence

      c. Encourage expression of feelings to decrease rigidity and need for control

      d. Facilitate clients to recognize any impairment or distress related to the need for perfection and control

      e. Encourage clients to acknowledge and discuss a sense of inadequacy and/or fear of rejection

C. Psychopharmacology: symptomatic treatment is the standard for persons with PD

    1. Psychosis: low dose atypical and typical antipsychotic agents may be prescribed on a short-term basis to alleviate brief psychotic symptoms associated with schizotypal, paranoid, schizoid, and borderline personality disorders

    2. Depression: antidepressants may be prescribed to treat a comorbidity of major depression in persons with PD

    3. Benzodiazepines and buspirone (Buspar) may be prescribed to alleviate anxiety symptoms in persons with PD

    4. Impulse control: mood stabilizers such as lithium, carbamazepine (Tegretol), valproates, and gabapentin (Neurontin) may be used to reduce suicidal tendencies, angry outbursts, and anxiety, as seen in persons with antisocial personality disorder and borderline personality disorder

    5. Mood dyregulation: mood stabilizers such as lithium, some antiepileptics (i.e., lamotrigine, carbamazepine, gabapentin), and certain antipsychotics (haloperidol, quetiapine [Seroquel], and olanzapine [Zyprexa]) can assist with mood stabilization

    6. Asocial behavior: some of the causes of asocial behavior may be related to depression; in this case SSRIs or MAOIs may help; in some cases, emotional/social detachment can be alleviated by atypical antipsychotics such as risperidone (Risperdal), quetiapine (Seroquel), and olanzapine (Zyprexa) as seen in persons with Cluster A PD and Cluster C PD (avoidant PD)

    7. Obsessions/compulsions: some of these symptoms can be alleviated by the use of SSRIs

D. Individual and group therapy

    1. Due to poor insight, ineffective coping mechanisms, and problems with interpersonal relationships, resistance to change is an issue with individual and group therapy for persons with PD

    2. Frequent sessions (once a week) are necessary to establish trust and work on contracts for behavioral changes

    3. A decision to participate in individual or group therapy is based on client's willingness to participate, on the a client's level of function, and specific psychosocial needs

    4. Self-help groups provide a safe and trusting environment where clients can receive feedback from peers and facilitator(s), share effective coping skills amongst the group, and increase self-awareness

E. Cognitive behavioral therapy (CBT)

    1. CBT is an action-oriented form of therapy; evidence supports successful treatment for BPD, relapse for prevention of depression, and behaviors such as anger issues, suicidal attempts, social anxiety, and obsessive-compulsive behaviors; therefore, techniques are useful in treating various behaviors associated with PDs

    2. Impulse-control training is designed to support client safety by decreasing the risk of suicide or self-mutilation through the use of anti-harm contracts, staff and client (self) monitoring, and identifying triggers and patterns related to self-destructive behavior; it also includes identifying alternative coping strategies

Practice to Pass

Explain the rationale for the importance of nursing interventions that diminish dichotomous thinking/splitting in persons with borderline personality disorder.

3. Limit setting is designed to discourage the tendency to test and manipulate others
   a. Involves establishing a structured environment with clear ground rules
   b. Limit setting reflects three principles: limits must be clearly stated, setting must be necessary, and must be enforceable
   c. Clearly stating limits and seeking clarification from clients of their understanding of the limit setting decreases attempts at manipulation as there is no excuse for "not understanding what is expected"
   d. Limit setting lays the foundation that staff members are professional authority figures rather than individuals who are perceived as harsh, judgmental, or punitive; this foundation diminishes a client's tendency to attempt to engage in a power struggle
   e. Limits must be enforceable or they encourage/reinforce rather than discourage the manipulative behaviors
   f. Staff must be consistent in enforcing limits and teamwork, and interdisciplinary conferences are essential to success

Practice to Pass

Why is impulse-control training crucial to the effective nursing management of some individuals diagnosed with a personality disorder?

4. Cognitive and behavioral measures

   a. For clients who are helpless and dependent, the goal is to increase coping skills and independent functioning
      1) Acknowledge client's feelings of helplessness and fear of gaining independence
      2) Explore client's dichotomous thinking (the tendency to see the self as totally dependent or totally independent)
      3) Help client to identify perceived gains and losses of becoming less helpless
      4) Engage client in problem-solving exercises to increase self-confidence
      5) Provide assertiveness training, referral as necessary
      6) Maintain healthy nurse–client relationship: do not take the role as "rescuer"

   b. For clients who are socially isolated secondary to a fear of rejection, abandonment, and/or low self-esteem, the goal is to increase the client's self-confidence
      1) Help client to acknowledge the fear of criticism and rejection; assist the client to identify both the perceived losses and gains, risking being criticized or rejected
      2) Encourage clients to identify the interpersonal effects of social isolation and associated emotional feelings (impact)
      3) Engage clients in problem-solving exercises to increase self-confidence
      4) Provide assertiveness training; make a referral as indicated

   c. For clients who are socially isolated related to suspiciousness and mistrust of others, do the following:
      1) Respect the client's need to be socially isolative; gradually encourage interaction with others
      2) When appropriate, facilitate the client to identify the interpersonal effects of social isolation and associated emotional feelings (impact)

   d. For clients who seek out relationships through attention-seeking behaviors (i.e., dramatic, seductive, hypersexual), do the following:
      1) Help the client to interact interpersonally in a more direct matter-of-fact manner
      2) Assist the client to identify both the perceived losses and gains if he or she were to communicate in a direct and non-superficial manner

   e. For clients whose relationships are based on manipulation, do the following:
      1) Confront the client's attempts at manipulation
      2) Assist the client to identify means to interact that are collaborative and less power and control-based
      3) Help the client to identify both the perceived losses and gains if manipulative behaviors were reduced

    5. Dialectical behavior: insight-oriented

        a. Evidence-based treatment for BPD

        b. Based on behavioral and cognitive therapy

        c. Includes both individual and/or group therapy

        d. Includes identifying and labeling emotions, examining obstacles to change, increasing mindfulness of current emotions, using distress tolerance techniques

F. Psychological comfort promotion and anxiety reduction

    1. For clients who avoid making decisions in an effort to decrease the anxiety of failure, do the following:

        a. Encourage the client to make decisions individually; this will promote a sense of competence and development of an internal locus of control

        b. Teach the client that making an imperfect decision may be better than making no decision at all; teach the client that decision making is a process, and can be reevaluated

    2. For clients who manifest perfectionistic behaviors to guard against anxiety, low self-esteem, and/or feelings of inferiority, facilitate the client to explore specific reasons for fear from the evaluation of others

    3. For clients whose anxiety prevents them from asking for help due to fear of rejection, assist the client to identify both the perceived losses and gains if they were to seek or ask for help

VI. EVALUATION/OUTCOMES

    A. Based on assessment of behavioral, affective, cognitive, and sociocultural manifestations; identify realistic, specific, and measurable short-term goals for each nursing diagnosis

    B. Goals must be realistic, by reflecting small steps that decrease subjective distress and improve overall function; personality traits are too ingrained to expect immediate, radical, and long-term change

    C. Evaluate the effectiveness of the nursing interventions in relationship to stated outcomes (goals)

VII. SPECIFIC DISORDERS

    A. Cluster A disorders (using *DSM-IV-TR* diagnostic criteria)

        1. Paranoid personality disorder: pattern of distrust and suspiciousness such that others' motives are interpreted as malevolent (APA, 2000)

            a. Behavioral manifestations

                1) Secretive due to unwarranted fear that others are out to get them

                2) Hyperalert to danger due to paranoid ideation

                3) Argumentative to maintain a safe distance between self and others

            b. Affective manifestations

                1) Avoids expression of feelings unless brief expression (i.e., anger)

                2) Fear of losing own power or control to others

            c. Cognitive manifestations

                1) Pervasive distrust and suspicion without justification

                2) Suspects/expects to be used, exploited, or harassed by others

                3) Looks for hidden, demeaning, or threatening meanings behind people's behavior

                4) May experience brief psychotic episodes

            d. Sociocultural manifestations

                1) Interacts in a cold and aloof manner to avoid intimacy

                2) Expects to be harmed or exploited by others and questions the loyalty or trustworthiness of family and friends

                3) Often pathologically jealous of a significant other

2. **Schizoid personality disorder**: pattern of detachment from social relationships that manifests in restricted range of emotions (APA, 2000)
   a. Behavioral manifestations
      1) Neither desires nor enjoys relationships with others
      2) Has little interest in activities or sexual relationships
   b. Affective manifestations
      1) Mood stable but restricted range of expression of emotions
      2) May become anxious if forced into a close interaction
      3) Affect is bland, blunted, or flat
      4) Emotion is expressed in a cold manner
   c. Cognitive manifestations
      1) Appears to have poverty of thought
      2) Thoughts are expressed vaguely
      3) Indifferent to the attitudes and feeling of others
      4) Not influenced by praise or criticism
      5) May experience brief psychotic episodes
   d. Sociocultural manifestations
      1) Interacts with others in a cold, aloof manner
      2) Desires no close friends
      3) Chooses activities that are solitary
3. **Schizotypal personality disorder**: pattern of acute discomfort in close relationships, cognitive or perceptual distortions, and eccentricities of behavior (APA, 2000)
   a. Behavioral manifestations
      1) Exhibits odd and eccentric behaviors
      2) Speech is coherent but tangential, vague, or overelaborated
   b. Affective manifestations
      1) Emotionally constricted affect
      2) Inappropriate affect
   c. Cognitive manifestations
      1) Paranoid ideation may be present
      2) Ideas of reference may be present
      3) Illusions may be present
      4) Magical thinking may be present
      5) May have brief psychotic episodes
   d. Sociocultural manifestations
      1) Discomfort with intimate relationships
      2) Avoids relationships with others (has no friends except first-degree relatives)
      3) Manifests social anxiety

B. **Cluster B disorders**
   1. **Antisocial personality disorder**: pattern of disregard for and violation of the rights of others (APA, 2000); the disorder cannot be diagnosed until age 18
      a. Behavioral manifestations may first appear in childhood and/or adolescence (i.e., lying, stealing, truancy, vandalism, fighting, and running away from home)
      b. Behavioral manifestations in adults: failing to conform to social norms (i.e., pathological lying, conning others for personal gain or profit, failing to meet financial obligations, failing to comply with work behaviors, reckless disregard for own safety and that of others, malingering, **impulsivity**, manipulation)
      c. Affective manifestations: superficial expression of emotion (i.e., charm, glib, cocky, self-assured); lack of guilt or remorse; is irritable and/or aggressive

  d. Cognitive manifestations: egocentric and grandiose; perceives self as more clever than others

  e. Sociocultural manifestations: consistently violates the rights of others as well as societal values, unable to sustain interpersonal relationships; may be abusive

2. **Borderline personality disorder**: pattern of instability in interpersonal relationships, self-image, and affect, and has marked **impulsivity** (APA, 2000)

  a. Behavioral manifestations

    1) Unpredictable, impulsive, manipulative

    2) Fear of real or imagined abandonment

    3) Engages in self-destructive behaviors such as reckless driving, substance abuse, and binge-eating

    4) High risk for suicide and self-mutilation secondary to feelings of emptiness, feelings of anger/rage, and/or fear of rejection

    5) Behavior may labile (vary from one moment to the next)

  b. Affective manifestations

    1) Mood is intense dysphoria, instability, anxiety, irritability

    2) Difficulty in moderating anger, can escalate rapidly

  c. Cognitive manifestations

    1) Identity disturbance related to feelings of chronic emptiness and a lack of or unstable sense of self

    2) Splitting or dichotomous thinking: tend to see self and others as all good (idealization) or all bad (devaluation)

    3) Paranoid ideation or dissociation may be present

  d. Sociocultural manifestations: intense, unstable interpersonal relationships alternating between extremes of idealization and devaluation of others

3. **Histrionic personality disorder**: pattern of excessive emotionality and attention seeking (APA, 2000)

  a. Behavioral manifestations

    1) Uncomfortable unless the center of attention

    2) Displays inappropriate seductive or provocative behavior

    3) Conversation is superficial

    4) Uses physical appearance to gain attention

  b. Affective manifestations

    1) Overly dramatic, theatrical

    2) Rapidly shifting

    3) Shallow expression of emotion

  c. Cognitive manifestations: tends to be guided by feelings rather than logic; is suggestible

  d. Sociocultural manifestations

    1) Assume role of victim or prince/princess in relationships

    2) Consider relationships to be more intimate than they are

4. **Narcissistic personality disorder**: pattern of grandiosity, need for admiration, and lack of empathy (APA, 2000)

  a. Behavioral manifestations

    1) Preoccupied with fantasies of power, success, beauty, brilliance

    2) Grandiose sense of self-importance

    3) Exploits others to achieve personal goals

    4) Seeks constant admiration from others

    5) Maintains a sense of entitlement; sees self as favorable

          b. Affective manifestations: labile moods varying from anger to anxiety

          c. Cognitive manifestations

            1) Arrogant, egotistical, sees self as more important/special than others

            2) Lack of empathy; refuses to recognize others needs or feelings

            3) Believes others are envious, or may be envious of others

          d. Sociocultural manifestations

            1) Disturbed relationships secondary to using others to meet own goals

            2) Own needs are perceived as more important than the needs of others

    C. Cluster C disorders

        1. Avoidant personality disorder: pattern of social inhibition, feelings of inadequacy, and hypersensitivity to negative evaluation (APA, 2000)

          a. Behavioral manifestations

            1) Avoids interpersonal contact and new situations related to concern of disapproval from others, embarrassment, and/or criticism

            2) Lacks self-confidence; is extremely sensitive to rejection

            3) Goes out of way to obtain nurturance, even if volunteering for an activity may be uncomfortable

          b. Affective manifestations: fearful, shy, hurt by criticism

          c. Cognitive manifestations

            1) Views self as inadequate and inferior

            2) Remains fearful of shame, criticism, and ridicule

          d. Sociocultural manifestations

            1) Desires relationships but reluctant to enter without a guarantee of unconditional acceptance

            2) Few close friends due to avoidant behaviors

        2. Dependent personality disorder: pattern of submissive and clinging behavior related to a need to be taken care of (APA, 2000)

          a. Behavioral manifestations

            1) Desires help with everyday decisions

            2) Expects others to take care of them

            3) Difficulty in disagreeing with others related to fear of rejection and abandonment

          b. Affective manifestations: anxious when left alone secondary to fear of being unable to do things independently

          c. Cognitive manifestations

            1) Lacks self-confidence, poor self-esteem

            2) Preoccupied with fear of being abandoned

          d. Sociocultural manifestations

            1) Constantly strives to obtain support from others

            2) Uncomfortable unless involved in a supportive relationship

        3. Obsessive-compulsive personality disorder: pattern of preoccupation with orderliness, perfectionism, and control (APA, 2000)

          a. Behavioral manifestations

            1) Excessive need for routine, rules, order, schedules, details

            2) Decreased ability to focus on the major goal of activity due to overinvolvement in details

            3) Difficulty with task completion related to a need for perfection

            4) Inflexibility related to values, morals, and ethics

            5) Unable to discard worthless or worn-out objects

            6) Resists delegation of tasks for fear that others will not meet expectations

            7) Hoards money to be used later

      b. Affective manifestations: rigid, stubborn, and emotionally constricted

      c. Cognitive manifestations

          1) Believes in a correct solution for every problem

          2) Procrastinates related to fear of making mistakes

      d. Sociocultural manifestations

          1) Impaired interpersonal relationships due to overdevotion to productivity/work

          2) Absence of leisure activities due to excessive devotion to productivity and work

D. Concomitant disorders: there is a correlation between certain personality disorders and several axis I disorders such as substance abuse, mood disorders, anxiety disorders, and psychotic disorders

Case Study

A client admitted to the psychiatric unit with a diagnosis of borderline personality disorder describes dissatisfaction with her boyfriend, stating, "My boyfriend seemed so kind, and wonderful at first. But then he let me down, he sometimes ignores my phone calls; I think I hate him now." When asked how she responds to this disappointment, she states, "Sometimes I'm filled with a sense of overwhelming rage, but most of the time I don't care, I am just plain bored..." When asked to describe how she copes with these feelings, she states, "I try not to think about it, but sometimes I cut or burn myself. I know I shouldn't but I can't always stop myself." She then shows you burn marks on her anterior left forearm that appear to be infected. She states two days ago she used a car cigarette lighter to inflict the wounds.

1. Identify two to three priority nursing diagnoses for this client.

2. What personal input do you expect from the client in terms of development of the goals for these nursing diagnoses?

3. Identify two to three nursing interventions that you will implement based on each goal.

For suggested responses, see page 298.

4. What comments might you make or not make to the client while performing wound care to the burn sites?

5. On what basis will you evaluate the effectiveness of your interventions?

POSTTEST

❶ The client diagnosed with a personality disorder says, "There is no need for me to be treated. I've always acted this way. It's normal for me." What term should the nurse use when describing this statement in documentation?

1. Narcissistic
2. Egosyntonic
3. Schizotypal
4. Avoidant

❷ A client is admitted to the unit with a diagnosis of a personality disorder (PD). The client is withdrawn and refuses to go to group. In addition the client acts very fearful when approached by staff. The nurse considers that this behavior is consistent with which type of PD? Select all that apply.

1. Antisocial PD
2. Avoidant PD
3. Histrionic PD
4. Dependent PD
5. Obsessive compulsive PD

3 The client diagnosed with antisocial personality disorder persists in asking for the address and other personal information about the nurse. The client states, "I just want to get to know you better. You're the only one I can really talk to." What is the most effective response by the nurse?

1. "You're getting too involved with me. Maybe another nurse would be more appropriate for you."
2. "Let's talk about my purpose in working with you and your feelings about it."
3. "Why are you focusing on me all the time?"
4. "Are you trying to avoid talking about yourself and your problems?"

4 A client arrives for her mental health appointment wearing a cocktail dress and theatrical makeup. She announces loudly, dramatically, and in a flirtatious manner that she needs to be seen immediately because she is experiencing overwhelming psychological distress. The nurse should recognize behaviors suggestive of which axis II diagnosis?

1. Borderline personality disorder
2. Narcissistic personality disorder
3. Histrionic personality disorder
4. Antisocial personality disorder

5 A client diagnosed with antisocial personality disorder tells Nurse A, "You're a much better nurse than Nurse B said you were." The client then tells Nurse B, "Nurse A is upset with you for some reason." To Nurse C, the client states, "I think you're great, but Nurse A said she saw you make three mistakes this morning." The nurse should conclude that these behaviors are intended to have which effect?

1. Gain acceptance
2. Gain attention
3. Create guilt in the staff
4. Manipulate the staff

6 The client with a diagnosis of antisocial personality disorder has reportedly physically abused his spouse. During a nurse–client interview, the client makes all of the following comments listed. The nurse concludes that which of the comments are likely to be insincere? Select all that apply.

1. "I've done a stupid thing, but I've learned my lesson."
2. "I'm feeling awful about the way I've hurt my wife."
3. "I have a quick temper, but I can usually keep it under control."
4. "I hit her because she nags at me."
5. "If I was a little too forceful, I do apologize."

7 The client diagnosed with borderline personality tells the nurse, "You are so much smarter than the other nurses. You're an ideal nurse." The nurse should interpret this behavior as an example of which of the following?

1. Secondary gain
2. Acting out
3. Passive aggression
4. Dichotomous thinking

8 The client's behavior is characterized by repeated attempts at manipulation of staff members and other clients. Which of the following is the most important short-term client goal for the nurse to establish?

1. Spend more time alone.
2. Sustain lasting relationships.
3. Explore childhood experiences.
4. Acknowledge own behavior.

9 When the nurse is evaluating the progress of the client whose interpersonal relationships are based on manipulation, which statement by the client indicates that progress has been made?

1. "I plan to stop taking advantage of other people."
2. "I've promised myself that I will be kind to others."
3. "I did not try to take advantage of anyone today."
4. "I can be more kind if I make an effort to do so."

POSTTEST

10 The axis II diagnosis of a client is schizoid personality disorder. Which approach should the nurse plan to use when interacting with this client?

1. Helpful and nurturing
2. Matter-of-fact and calm
3. Light and playful
4. Warm and friendly

➤ *See pages 170–172 for Answers and Rationales.*

ANSWERS & RATIONALES

Pretest

1 **Answer: 4 Rationale:** To meet *DSM-IV-TR* diagnostic criteria for a personality disorder, behavioral patterns must be pervasive and maladaptive, resulting in functional impairment or subjective distress. The other behavioral patterns are associated with some but not all personality disorders. **Cognitive Level:** Applying **Client Need:** Psychosocial Integrity **Integrated Process:** Nursing Process: Assessment **Content Area:** Mental Health **Strategy:** Look for the answer that is most comprehensive. It must be true of persons with personality disorders in general. **Reference:** Varcarolis, E., Carson, V., & Shoemaker, N. (2010). *Foundations of psychiatric–mental health nursing: A clinical approach* (6th ed.). St. Louis, MO: Saunders Elsevier, p. 276.

2 **Answer: 2 Rationale:** The priority of care is always client safety. Intervening to minimize a client's risk of self-harm maintains a safe environment. The nursing diagnoses of Anxiety and Ineffective Coping are of secondary importance to the maintenance of the client's safety. Although the client is impulsive and exhibits angry outbursts, more assessment data would be needed to determine if the client is at risk for violence directed toward others. **Cognitive Level:** Analyzing **Client Need:** Psychosocial Integrity **Integrated Process:** Nursing Process: Diagnosis **Content Area:** Mental Health **Strategy:** Consider Maslow's hierarchy of needs or any other system of prioritization with which you are familiar. Recognize that basic physiologic and safety needs take precedence over all other needs. **Reference:** Varcarolis, E., Carson, V., & Shoemaker, N. (2006). *Foundations of psychiatric–mental health nursing: A clinical approach* (5th ed.). St. Louis, MO: Saunders Elsevier, pp. 282–283, 291.

3 **Answer: 2 Rationale:** Growing up in a multigenerational enmeshed family system and failure to separate/individuate the self are associated with the development of borderline personality disorder. Conflict in the area of separation/individuation can result in splitting or dichotomous thinking—perceiving the self and others as all good or all bad. Although each of the other etiologic factors in the other options is associated with the development of personality disorders in general, none of them is associated with the development of dichotomous thinking. **Cognitive Level:** Applying **Client Need:** Psychosocial Integrity **Integrated Process:** Nursing Process:

Assessment **Content Area:** Mental Health **Strategy:** Look for the answer that applies specifically to the person with borderline personality disorder, not to persons with other personality disorders. Some questions may require the opposite type of thinking. **Reference:** Fontaine, K. (2009). *Mental health nursing* (6th ed.). Upper Saddle River, NJ: Prentice Hall, p. 492.

4 **Answer: 3 Rationale:** All four options indicate Cluster B disorders, as defined in *DSM-IV-TR* diagnostic criteria. However, the disregard for others, lack of guilt and remorse, and involvement in illegal actions are specific behaviors associated with antisocial personality disorder. The client's behaviors do not indicate narcissism because there is no indication of grandiosity or need for admiration. Histrionic qualities are absent because there is a lack of emotion rather than heightened emotionality. There is no indication of borderline personality because the client is not showing a pattern of instability in interpersonal relationships, self-image, and affect. **Cognitive Level:** Analyzing **Client Need:** Psychosocial Integrity **Integrated Process:** Nursing Process: Assessment **Content Area:** Mental Health **Strategy:** Recall the principal characteristics of each of the Cluster B disorders in *DSM-IV-TR*. Focus on the client's absence of remorse and guilt. **Reference:** Fontaine, K. (2009). *Mental health nursing* (6th ed.). Upper Saddle River, NJ: Prentice Hall, pp. 481–482.

5 **Answer: 3 Rationale:** According to *DSM-IV-TR* criteria for avoidant personality disorder, the individual will show a pattern of social inhibition, feelings of inadequacy, and avoidance of interpersonal contact and new situations related to fear of rejection and embarrassment. Avoidant personality disorder is a Cluster B disorder, while schizotypal, paranoid, and schizoid personality disorders are Cluster A disorders in *DSM-IV-TR*. **Cognitive Level:** Analyzing **Client Need:** Psychosocial Integrity **Integrated Process:** Nursing Process: Assessment **Content Area:** Mental Health **Strategy:** The wording of the question indicates that you should not look for generalities. Look instead for something specific about each of the different personality disorders. **Reference:** Fontaine, K. (2009). *Mental health nursing* (6th ed.). Upper Saddle River, NJ: Prentice Hall, p. 485.

6 **Answer: 3 Rationale:** Individuals diagnosed with antisocial personality disorder display decreased impulse control, can be irritable and aggressive, and lack remorse for their actions. Recognizing the potential risk for violence and maintaining client safety is the first priority of nursing care. Clients with antisocial personality disorder do not have personal identity disturbance, which is an anxiety disorder. Clients with antisocial personality disorder do not show excessive fearfulness, which is a characteristic of Cluster C disorders in *DSM-IV-TR*. Instead of being socially isolated, the client with antisocial personality disorder often has a wide range of social contacts and activities, although they occur at a superficial level without regard for the feelings of the other persons. **Cognitive Level:** Analyzing **Client Need:** Psychosocial Integrity **Integrated Process:** Nursing Process: Diagnosis **Content Area:** Mental Health **Strategy:** Recall characteristic behaviors of persons with antisocial personality disorder. Remember that they feel no concern or regard for others. **Reference:** Fontaine, K. (2009). *Mental health nursing* (6th ed.). Upper Saddle River, NJ: Prentice Hall, p. 482.

7 **Answer: 1, 2, 4** **Rationale:** Three options are correct. There are no pharmacological agents to treat personality disorders, rather medication is used to treat various psychiatric symptoms. Persons with Cluster B personality disorder may manifest with mood swings; Tegretol is a mood stabilizer and can be effective in treating these mood swings. Some persons with Cluster A personality disorder manifest with psychotic features. Antipsychotics can be used to alleviate these symptoms. (Two options are incorrect.) Cogentin is used to treat extrapyramidal symptoms. **Cognitive Level:** Analyzing **Client Need:** Psychosocial Integrity **Integrated Process:** Nursing Process: Implementation **Content Area:** Mental Health **Strategy:** The role of psychopharmacology in the treatment of personality disorders is limited. Medications are used to alleviate symptoms such as mood swings, aggression, impulsivity, anxiety, and depression. **Reference:** Stuart, G. W. (2009). *Principles and practice of psychiatric nursing* (9th ed.). Mosby, Elsevier: St. Louis, p. 384.

8 **Answer: 4** **Rationale:** A sense of entitlement, or believing that one is so special that others should defer to his or her needs, is included in the *DSM-IV-TR* diagnostic criteria for narcissistic personality disorder. Additionally, these clients lack empathy and have very disturbed interpersonal relationships due to their arrogance and focus on self. Splitting, or dichotomous thinking, is associated with borderline personality disorders and involves seeing the world, the self, and others in extremes: all good or all bad; totally perfect or totally awful; etc. Hypersensitivity, especially when combined with suspiciousness, is more associated with paranoid personality disorder. **Cognitive Level:** Analyzing **Client Need:** Psychosocial Integrity **Integrated Process:** Nursing Process: Assessment **Content Area:** Mental Health **Strategy:** Look carefully at the client's behavior. Notice the self-centeredness of the client and the lack of apology to others. **Reference:** Fontaine, K. (2009). *Mental health nursing* (6th ed.). Upper Saddle River, NJ: Prentice Hall, p. 484.

9 **Answer: 1** **Rationale:** Because the behavioral patterns of individuals diagnosed with antisocial personality reflect a tendency to test and manipulate others, it is important to establish the parameters of acceptable behavior upon admission through limit setting. The interventions in the other options result in an unstructured environment with no consistent limits on behavior. This would increase rather than decrease an individual's tendency to test and try to manipulate others in the environment. **Cognitive Level:** Applying **Client Need:** Psychosocial Integrity **Integrated Process:** Nursing Process: Planning **Content Area:** Mental Health **Strategy:** Recall the major characteristics of persons with antisocial personality disorder, particularly the fact that they easily manipulate and take advantage of others with no hesitation or remorse. **Reference:** Kneisl, C., Wilson, H., & Trigoboff, E. (2009). *Contemporary psychiatric–mental health nursing* (2nd ed.). Upper Saddle River, NJ: Prentice Hall, p. 503.

10 **Answer: 1, 2, 3** **Rationale:** Individuals with obsessive-compulsive personality disorder tend to become aggressive and argumentative when someone is stressing the importance of routine, rules, and regulations. Assertiveness training would be useful for these individuals. Obsessions and compulsions are attempts to control anxiety; therefore anxiety management would be useful. Because persons with obsessive-compulsive personalities need perfection and control, they usually have trouble making decisions, which can negatively affect their occupational functioning. Learning that decisions do not always have to be perfect and that they can be changed may be a first small step toward improvement (decision-making skills). 12-step programs are appropriate for treating individuals with addictive disorders. Distraction techniques are not likely to be effective with persons with obsessive-compulsive symptoms. Their attention is riveted to the obsessions and accompanying compulsions. **Cognitive Level:** Analyzing **Client Need:** Psychosocial Integrity **Integrated Process:** Nursing Process: Implementation **Content Area:** Mental Health **Strategy:** Consider how restricted and anxious the world of the obsessive-compulsive person is. Look for approaches that will help them to function better in their interactions with others. **Reference:** Fontaine, K. (2009). *Mental health nursing* (6th ed.). Upper Saddle River, NJ: Prentice Hall, pp. 486–487.

Posttest

1 **Answer: 2** **Rationale:** Clients diagnosed with personality disorders view their personality patterns as natural, or egosyntonic. They think their behavior is normal, and it is neither painful nor uncomfortable to them. For this reason, they rarely seek treatment. This view is directly opposite that of egodystonia, in which the individual is greatly distressed by behaviors and symptoms. Narcissistic responses involve a grandiose sense of entitlement and focus on the self. Schizotypal individuals demonstrate eccentricities in behavior and avoidant responses.

Avoidant behaviors involve social inhibition and feelings of inadequacy. **Cognitive Level:** Applying **Client Need:** Psychosocial Integrity **Integrated Process:** Communication and Documentation **Content Area:** Mental Health **Strategy:** Remember that personality disorders are fixed, lifelong patterns of behavior. **Reference:** Varcarolis, E., Carson, V., & Shoemaker, N. (2010). *Foundations of psychiatric mental health nursing: A clinical approach* (6th ed.). St. Louis, MO: Saunders Elsevier, p. 789.

2 **Answer: 2, 4, 5** **Rationale:** Three options are correct. Avoidant PD, Dependent PD, and Obsessive compulsive PD are all categorized under the Cluster C PDs. The predominant features of Cluster C PDs are anxiety and fearfulness. The client in this case is manifesting both of these symptoms. (Two options are incorrect.) Antisocial PD and histrionic PD are categorized under Cluster B PDs; these PDs' predominant features include dramatic, erratic, overemotional, and impulsive behaviors. **Cognitive Level:** Analyzing **Client Need:** Psychosocial Integrity **Integrated Process:** Nursing Process: Assessment **Content Area:** Mental Health **Strategy:** Pay careful attention to client behaviors. The client manifests fearful and withdrawn behaviors. Persons with Cluster C, due to their fear, withdraw from occupational and social situations. As a nurse it is important to distinguish predominant features in each of the three (A, B, C) categories of PD. **Reference:** Stuart, G., W., (2009). *Principles and practice of psychiatric nursing* (9th ed.). Mosby, Elsevier: St. Louis, p. 372.

3 **Answer: 2** **Rationale:** In returning the focus of the conversation to the client, the nurse intervenes in the attempts at manipulation. The manner in which the nurse does this is professional and businesslike without appearing uncomfortable. Asking why the client is focusing on the nurse and asking if the client is trying to avoid talking about him- or herself makes the nurse seem uncomfortable. Sensing this, the client will feel in control of the interaction and use even more manipulative behaviors. Stating that the client is getting too involved and suggesting finding another nurse is defensive and shows the client that the manipulative attempt has "gotten under your skin." This will encourage the client to continue with other manipulative efforts. **Cognitive Level:** Analyzing **Client Need:** Psychosocial Integrity **Integrated Process:** Communication and Documentation **Content Area:** Mental Health **Strategy:** Remember that attempts at manipulation are aimed at allowing the manipulating individual to remain in control of the situation. **Reference:** Kneisl, C., Wilson, H., & Trigoboff, E. (2009). *Contemporary psychiatric–mental health nursing* (2nd ed.). Upper Saddle River, NJ: Prentice Hall, p. 499.

4 **Answer: 3** **Rationale:** The client's pattern of attention-seeking behavior reflects *DSM-IV-TR* diagnostic criteria for histrionic personality disorder. Dramatic attention-seeking behaviors are not as common in borderline personality disorders as are those in which the individual is unstable and impulsive because of fears of abandonment.

Dramatic and theatrical attention-seeking behaviors are not characteristic of narcissistic personality disorders. Narcissistic individuals show a sense of entitlement and lack of empathy for others. Dramatic attention-seeking is not a common behavior associated with antisocial personality disorders. Instead, even though they may be superficially charming and sociable, they have utter disregard and consideration for the rights of others and often violate the rights of others if it is to their own personal advantage. **Cognitive Level:** Applying **Client Need:** Psychosocial Integrity **Integrated Process:** Nursing Process: Assessment **Content Area:** Mental Health **Strategy:** Recall which type of personality disorder is most likely to be referred to by others as a "drama queen." **Reference:** Kneisl, C., Wilson, H., & Trigoboff, E. (2009). *Contemporary psychiatric–mental health nursing* (2nd ed.). Upper Saddle River, NJ: Prentice Hall, pp. 492–494.

5 **Answer: 4** **Rationale:** Individuals diagnosed with antisocial personality disorder frequently attempt to play one staff member against another. This behavior is referred to as splitting. Their goal in doing this is to manipulate others or control their environment. Individuals diagnosed with antisocial personality disorder have no regard for others and lack the capacity to empathize. Their behavior is not driven by attempts to gain acceptance or attention or to create guilt. Rather, it is to gain control by manipulation. **Cognitive Level:** Applying **Client Need:** Psychosocial Integrity **Integrated Process:** Nursing Process: Evaluation **Content Area:** Mental Health **Strategy:** Recall that persons with antisocial personality disorder lack positive regard or empathy. **Reference:** Kneisl, C., Wilson, H., & Trigoboff, E. (2009). *Contemporary psychiatric–mental health nursing* (2nd ed.). Upper Saddle River, NJ: Prentice Hall, p. 495.

6 **Answer: 1, 2, 3, 5** **Rationale:** Individuals diagnosed with antisocial personality disorder rarely take responsibility for their behavior. Statements of this nature are likely to be insincere. They feel their behavior is justified and typically blame others in an irritable fashion for their socially unacceptable actions. In addition, they feel that their physical aggression toward another is not only justifiable but even deserved by the other person. They are not remorseful, and it would be very unlikely that they would apologize. They characteristically assign blame to others. **Cognitive Level:** Analyzing **Client Need:** Psychosocial Integrity **Integrated Process:** Nursing Process: Assessment **Content Area:** Mental Health **Strategy:** Remember that the person with antisocial personality disorder does not experience guilt, shame, or remorse. Note the word *insincere* in the question. **Reference:** Fontaine, K. (2009). *Mental health nursing* (6th ed.). Upper Saddle River, NJ: Prentice Hall, pp. 481–482.

7 **Answer: 4** **Rationale:** Individuals diagnosed with borderline personality disorder frequently display a tendency to engage in dichotomous thinking or splitting. They perceive the self and others as all good or all bad. The client may be seeking secondary gain from the nurse, but the manipulative behavior itself is not a manifestation of secondary gain. Acting-out behavior involves displacing anxiety from one situation to another in the form of some observable response like crying or being violent. Passive aggression involves behaviors that appear passive on the surface but are actually motivated by unconscious anger. Examples are being obtuse, arriving late, and making "mistakes." **Cognitive Level:** Applying **Client Need:** Psychosocial Integrity **Integrated Process:** Nursing Process: Assessment **Content Area:** Mental Health **Strategy:** Recognize that clients with borderline personality disorders have an intense fear of abandonment. **Reference:** Varcarolis, E., Carson, V., & Shoemaker, N. (2010). *Foundations of psychiatric mental health nursing: A clinical approach* (6th ed.). St. Louis, MO: Saunders Elsevier, pp. 282, 289, 784, 792.

8 **Answer: 4** **Rationale:** Being encouraged to acknowledge attempts at manipulation is a small, but important step in recognizing maladaptive communication patterns and their effect on relationships. Spending more time alone cannot be expected to lead to a decrease in manipulative behavior. The manipulative person should be taught ways to have social interactions without manipulating and taking advantage of others. The manipulative person will have a great deal of difficulty sustaining lasting relationships. Working toward a change in this area would be a long-term goal. Exploring childhood experiences is not a short-term goal. **Cognitive Level:** Analyzing **Client Need:** Psychosocial Integrity **Integrated Process:** Nursing Process: Planning **Content Area:** Mental Health **Strategy:** Recall relevant steps in change theory and apply to this situation. **Reference:** Kneisl, C., Wilson, H., & Trigoboff, E. (2009).

Contemporary psychiatric–mental health nursing (2nd ed.). Upper Saddle River, NJ: Prentice Hall, p. 499.

9 **Answer: 3** **Rationale:** Change is reflected in action and behavior. Even if stated clearly and with apparent conviction, plans, promises, and words do not reflect actual behavioral change. Statements of plans and promises (three options) indicate intentions. In order to evaluate actual change, behavior must be observed. **Cognitive Level:** Analyzing **Client Need:** Psychosocial Integrity **Integrated Process:** Nursing Process: Evaluation **Content Area:** Mental Health **Strategy:** Look for an indication of actual change in behavior. **Reference:** Varcarolis, E., Carson, V., & Shoemaker, N. (2010). *Foundations of psychiatric mental health nursing: A clinical approach* (6th ed.). St. Louis, MO: Saunders Elsevier, p. 289.

10 **Answer: 2** **Rationale:** *DSM-IV-TR* criteria for schizoid personality disorders indicate that such individuals are aloof and remote when interacting with others, as they have no desire for close relationships. The nurse should accept this behavior pattern with calmness. To the schizoid client, helpful and nurturing, light and playful, and warm and friendly approaches might seem like the nurse is attempting to be interpersonally close. This feeling would make the client uncomfortable and could be experienced as overwhelming. **Cognitive Level:** Analyzing **Client Need:** Psychosocial Integrity **Integrated Process:** Caring **Content Area:** Mental Health **Strategy:** Place yourself in the framework of the client's thinking. Imagine how you would respond to each approach. **Reference:** Varcarolis, E., Carson, V., & Shoemaker, N. (2010). *Foundations of psychiatric mental health nursing: A clinical approach* (6th ed.). St. Louis, MO: Saunders Elsevier, p. 288.

References

American Psychiatric Association (2000). *Diagnostic and statistical manual of mental disorders* (4th ed. text revision). Washington, DC: American Psychiatric Association.

Beck Institute of Cognitive Behavioral Therapy and Research (2011). *What research shows?* Retrieved January 3, 2011, from www.beckinstitute.org/

Carpenito, L. J. (2011). *Nursing diagnosis: Application to clinical practice* (13th ed.). Philadelphia, PA: Lippincott Williams & Wilkins.

Fontaine, K. (2009). *Mental health nursing* (6th ed.). Upper Saddle River, NJ: Pearson Education.

Kniesl, C., Wilson, H., & Trigoboff, E. (2009). *Contemporary psychiatric–mental health nursing* (2nd ed.). Upper Saddle River, NJ: Pearson Education.

National Institute of Mental Health (2011). *Any anxiety disorder among children.* Retrieved on February 1, 2011, from www.nimh.nih.gov/statistics/1ANYANX_child.shtml

Stuart, G. (2009). *Principles and practice of psychiatric nursing* (9th ed.). St. Louis: Elsevier Science.

Townsend, M. (2011). *Essentials of psychiatric–mental health nursing* (5th ed.). Philadelphia, PA: F.A. Davis.

Varcarolis, E., & Halter, M. (2010). *Foundations of psychiatric mental health nursing: A clinical approach* (6th ed.). Philadelphia: Saunders.

Schizophrenia and Other Psychotic Disorders

9

Chapter Outline

Overview/Classification
Etiology
Assessment for
    Symptomatology
    (Subjective/Objective)

Nursing Diagnoses/Analysis
Planning and Implementation
    of Specific Treatment
    Modalities

Evaluation/Outcomes
Specific Disorders

Objectives

➤ Describe at least three factors regarding the development
   of schizophrenia.
➤ Differentiate between positive and negative symptoms
   of schizophrenia.
➤ Describe four treatment modalities for clients with schizophrenia.
➤ Differentiate between schizophrenia and other psychotic disorders.

NCLEX-RN® Test Prep

Use the accompanying online resource,
NursingReviewsandRationales, to test
yourself with hundreds of NCLEX®-style
practice questions.

Review at a Glance

catatonic position of the body in a fixed, waxlike state

clang association rhyming of words in a sentence that make no sense

delusional ideation a false belief brought about without appropriate external stimulation and inconsistent with the individual's own knowledge and experience

echolalia an involuntary parrotlike repetition of words spoken by others

echopraxia a meaningless imitation of motions made by others

hallucination a false sensory perception that may involve any of the five senses (auditory, visual, tactile, olfactory, and gustatory)

ideas of reference a cognitive distortion in which a person believes that what is in the environment is related to him or her, even when no obvious relationship exists; also called personalization

illusion an inaccurate perception or misinterpretation of sensory impressions

milieu therapy a method of psychotherapy that controls the environment of the client to provide interpersonal contacts in order to develop trust, assurance, and personal autonomy

neologisms new words that are invented by and have meaning to only one person

psychosis a disorderly mental state in which a client has difficulty distinguishing reality from his or her own internal perceptions

thought broadcasting the delusional belief that others can hear one's thoughts

thought control the delusional belief that others can control a person's thoughts against one's will

thought insertion the delusional belief that others have the ability to put thoughts in a person's mind against one's will

word salad the combining of words in a sentence that have no connection and make no sense

PRETEST

1 A client diagnosed with schizophrenia, paranoid type, is admitted to an acute-care psychiatric hospital unit. Which nursing diagnosis should be given highest priority in the initial nursing care plan?

1. Interrupted Thought Processes
2. Social Isolation
3. Impaired Verbal Communication
4. Risk for Violence Directed at Self or at Others

2 The client diagnosed with schizophrenia says, "Everyone here is part of the secret police and wants to torture me," and refuses to be weighed by a member of the nursing staff. What is the most appropriate response by the nurse?

1. "That is a strange idea. We aren't secret police persons."
2. "That must be a frightening thought. We are nurses who work at this hospital."
3. "Being suspicious isn't easy, is it? You won't be tortured here."
4. "There is no need to be frightened. We will keep you safe from torture."

3 A male client is taking a second-generation antipsychotic drug. The client's spouse tells the nurse that she read that the drug is effective to treat negative symptoms of schizophrenia and asks the nurse to explain what these are. What should the nurse include in a response to the spouse? Select all that apply.

1. Abnormal thoughts
2. Diminished pleasure
3. Blunted affect
4. Hallucinations
5. Difficulty making decisions

4 The nurse is assessing a client who recently began taking a typical antipsychotic medication. The client says, "All of a sudden I can't breathe right." The nurse observes generalized body rigidity and diaphoresis. The body temperature is 103°F, or 39°C, and the pulse is 130. What should the nurse do next?

1. Administer the ordered prn anticholinergic medication.
2. Assess the client for indications of orthostatic hypotension.
3. Begin preparing the client for immediate transfer to an emergency department.
4. Arrange for an additional physician's visit later in the day.

5 While the nurse is meeting with the family of a client with schizophrenia, a family member asks the nurse to explain what causes this disorder. What is the nurse's best response?

1. "Research indicates that schizophrenia is caused by a genetic predisposition."
2. "The exact cause of schizophrenia is unclear at this time."
3. "It is likely that poor parenting skills cause schizophrenia to occur."
4. "It is clear that early-age psychological traumas cause schizophrenia."

6 The nurse is working with a severely withdrawn client. Which of the following should the nurse formulate as an appropriate short-term client goal?

1. Attend one group meeting accompanied by a staff member within three days.
2. Voluntarily lead the unit community meeting by the time of discharge from the hospital.
3. Be more comfortable in group situations by three days.
4. Enjoy participating in group therapy by the time of discharge.

7 The client has catatonic schizophrenia and demonstrates rigidity, waxy flexibility, and extreme psychomotor retardation. The nurse anticipates that this client is at risk for which of the following? Select all that apply.

1. Aggressive outbursts
2. Constipation
3. Ineffective coping
4. Nutritional deficiency
5. Memory deficit

8 A client diagnosed with schizophrenia says, "I want to go home to tome in a dome." When documenting, the nurse will refer to this as which of the following?

1. Echopraxia
2. Echolalia
3. Clang associations
4. Associative looseness

9 The client is to begin taking olanzepine (Zyprexa). The nurse makes it a priority to assess which of the following before administering the first dose?

1. Usual sleep pattern
2. Food and fluid preferences
3. Body weight
4. History of indigestion

10 A client diagnosed with schizophrenia tells the nurse that another client is "creating negative thoughts in me against my will." The nurse documents that the client is exhibiting which of the following features of schizophrenia?

1. Thought broadcasting
2. Thought blocking
3. Thought insertion
4. Thought control

➤ *See pages 185–187 for Answers and Rationales.*

I. OVERVIEW/CLASSIFICATION

A. **Schizophrenia is one of a cluster** of related psychotic brain disorders of unknown etiology

B. **Schizophrenia is a combination** of disordered thinking, perceptual disturbances, behavioral abnormalities, affective disruptions, and impaired social competency

C. **Symptoms of schizophrenia typically include the following**

1. **Delusional ideation**: a false belief brought about without appropriate external stimulation and inconsistent with the individual's own knowledge and experience

2. **Hallucinations**: false sensory perceptions that may involve any of the five senses (auditory, visual, tactile, olfactory, and gustatory)

3. Disorganized speech patterns

4. Disorganized or catatonic behaviors

5. Negative symptoms (lack of or reduced behaviors usually seen as "normal")

D. **At least two of these symptoms** must be present for a significant portion of the time during a one-month period

E. **Other manifestations** include social impairment and cognitive impairment: the subtypes of schizophrenia have similar features, but differ in their clinical presentations

F. **Critical essential features of each subtype of schizophrenia**

1. Paranoid type

   a. Auditory hallucinations

   b. Preoccupation with one or more delusions usually of a persecutory nature

   c. May appear hostile or angry

   d. None of the following are present: flat or inappropriate affect, disorganized speech or behavior, or **catatonic** behavior; in catatonic behavior the body remains in a fixed position, waxlike state

    2. Catatonic type

      a. Stupor (state of daze or unconsciousness); motor immobility or restricted movement, or extreme motor agitation

      b. Excessive negativism or inability to speak

      c. Inappropriate or bizarre body postures

      d. Echolalia (an involuntary parrotlike repetition of words spoken by others) or **echopraxia** (a meaningless imitation of motions made by others)

    3. Residual type

      a. Absence of prominent psychotic symptoms

      b. Social withdrawal and inappropriate affect

      c. Eccentric behavior

      d. Lack of interest, initiative, or energy

      e. Past history of at least one episode of schizophrenia

    4. Disorganized type

      a. Disorganized speech

      b. Disorganized behavior

      c. Inappropriate or flat affect

      d. Oddities of behavior (i.e., grimacing)

    5. Undifferentiated type

      a. Disorganized behaviors

      b. Psychotic symptoms (including delusions and hallucinations)

II. ETIOLOGY

    A. Approximately 1% of the population has schizophrenia; schizophrenia is the most common psychotic disorder and often results in a chronic illness

    B. Schizophrenia is a disorder of the brain like epilepsy or multiple sclerosis

    C. Generally the individual is fairly normal early in life, experiences subtle changes after puberty, and undergoes severe symptoms in the late teens to early adulthood

    D. The vast majority of individuals develop the disorder in adolescence or young adulthood, with only 10% of cases first diagnosed in people over the age of 45

    E. The current knowledge base on the cause of schizophrenia is uncertain

    F. Several factors have been identified as having a high correlation or association with the development of schizophrenia; they include the following:

      1. Brain structure and functioning

        a. Changes in basal ganglia activity

        b. Structural brain abnormalities, such as enlarged ventricles, cerebral atrophy, decreased cerebral blood flow, and decreased brain volume

        c. Reduced glucose metabolism in the frontal and temporal lobes as seen on imaging studies (CT, MRI, and PET scans)

        d. Imbalance between neurotransmitter systems (dopamine, serotonin, PCP glutamate, norepinephrine, gamma-aminobutyric acid, and acetylcholine)

      2. Genetic factors

        a. Multiple studies have shown an increased risk for development of schizophrenia when there is a positive family history of schizophrenia

        b. The risk for the development of schizophrenia increases for those with first-degree relatives diagnosed with schizophrenia

        c. There has been no specific genetic defect identified that causes schizophrenia

      3. Psychological factors

        a. There are no specific studies that indicate that stress causes schizophrenia, but studies have shown that stress does affect relapse and exacerbation of schizophrenic manifestations

Practice to Pass

How would knowledge about a genetic predisposition to schizophrenia be helpful?

b. The existence of several factors together such as genetic predisposition to schizophrenia along with the presence of stressful events may contribute to the development of schizophrenia

4. Environmental factors

   a. Observations have suggested that exposure to infectious agents such as viruses in early infancy may contribute to the development of schizophrenia

   b. Research studies have indicated an association between schizophrenia and complications during pregnancy or labor such as oxygen deprivation, short gestation periods, and low birth weights

III. ASSESSMENT FOR SYMPTOMATOLOGY (SUBJECTIVE/OBJECTIVE)

 A. Positive symptoms indicate a distortion or excess of normal functioning: they often occur as the initial symptoms of schizophrenia and precipitate the need for hospitalization; they include the following:

1. Delusions—fixed false beliefs or ideas

   a. Paranoid type: the individual believes others are out to get him or her; the client may be hostile, suspicious, and aggressive

   b. Grandiose type: the individual has excessive feelings of importance and power over others

   c. Religious type: the individual has delusions that focus on a religious context

   d. Somatic type: the individual has delusions that are fixed on an irrational belief about his or her body

   e. Nihilistic: the client has delusions of nonexistence

   f. Persecutory: the client has delusions that others are out to get or are plotting against him or her

   g. Thought broadcasting: the individual has the delusional belief that others can hear his or her thoughts

   h. Thought insertion: the individual has the delusional belief that others have the ability to put thoughts in a person's mind against that person's will

   i. Thought control: the individual has the delusional belief that others can control a person's thoughts against one's will

   j. Ideas of reference: a cognitive distortion in which words or actions by a person other than the client that have no relationship to the client, but which the client interprets as related to him or her; also called personalization

 2. Hallucinations, usually auditory; possible **illusions**—inaccurate perception or misinterpretation of sensory impressions

3. Psychosis, which is a disorderly mental state in which a client has difficulty distinguishing reality from his or her own internal perceptions

4. Bizarre and possibly aggressive behaviors (catatonic, etc.)

5. Formal thought disorders

   a. Echolalia: repeating the words of another person for no logical reason

   b. Echopraxia: purposeless imitation of movements performed by others

   c. Clang associations: rhyming words in a sentence that make no sense

   d. Illogical thinking patterns

   e. Neologisms: invented new words that are meaningful only to that person

   f. Word salad: combination of words in a sentence that have no connection and make no sense

B. Negative symptoms indicate a loss or lack of normal functioning; they develop over time and hinder the person's ability to endure life tasks; they include the following:

1. Anhedonia: diminished ability to experience pleasure or intimacy

2. Alogia: poverty of speech and content of speech
3. Anergia: lack of energy, lack of persistence, lack of self-care
4. Avolition: lack of motivation and goals
5. Ambivalence: inability to make a decision because of conflicting emotions
6. Affect disturbances
   a. Blunted
   b. Flat; no facial expression or emotion is present
   c. Inappropriate
7. Social withdrawal accompanying anhedonia
8. Dependency
9. Lack of ego boundaries
10. Concrete thought processes
11. Sleep disturbance

Practice to Pass

What are considered nursing priorities when a client is experiencing psychosis?

IV. NURSING DIAGNOSES/ANALYSIS

A. **Risk for Violence, Self-Directed or Directed toward Others** related to lack of trust, panic-level anxiety, command hallucinations, delusional thinking, or perception of the environment as threatening

B. **Disturbed Sensory Perception** related to hallucinations, delusional thinking, withdrawal into self, or perception of the environment as threatening

C. **Disturbed Thought Processes** related to possible hereditary factors, delusional thinking, hallucinations, or inaccurate interpretation of the environment

D. **Anxiety** related to inaccurate interpretation of the environment, unfamiliar environment, repressed fear, or panic level of stress

E. **Ineffective Coping** related to inability to trust, low self-esteem, or inadequate support systems

F. **Defensive Coping** related to difficulty in perceiving reality

G. **Social Isolation** related to lack of trust, regression to earlier level of function, delusional thinking, or past experiences of difficulty in interactions with others

H. **Impaired Verbal Communication** related to inability to trust, regression to earlier level of development, or disordered and unrealistic thinking

I. **Self-Care Deficit (specify)** related to withdrawal into self, regression to earlier level of development, or perceptual or cognitive impairment

J. **Disturbed Sleep Pattern** related to repressed fears, hallucinations, or delusional thinking

K. **Chronic Low Self-Esteem** related to withdrawal into self, lack of trust, poor socialization skills, or chronic illness

V. PLANNING AND IMPLEMENTATION OF SPECIFIC TREATMENT MODALITIES

A. **Psychopharmacology** (see Table 9-1 for nursing considerations for clients on antipsychotic medications)

1. Typical antipsychotics (traditional)
   a. Initially introduced in the 1950s
   b. Also referred to as neuroleptic medications
   c. Effectively treat only the positive symptoms of schizophrenia and have no therapeutic effect on the negative symptoms
   d. Depot therapy injections available in a few traditional antipsychotic drugs for clients who have a poor adherence history
   e. Most common side effects are the extrapyramidal side effects (EPS) (see Table 9-2)

Practice to Pass

How are depot injections of antipsychotic medications helpful?

Table 9-1	Antipsychotic Drugs and Nursing Considerations
Drug Class and Name	**Nursing Considerations and Interventions**
Typical/traditional • Acetophenazine (Tindal) • Chlorpromazine (Thorazine) • Fluphenazine (Prolixin) • Haloperidol (Haldol) • Loxapine (Loxitane) • Mesoridazine (Serentil) • Molindone (Moban) • Perphenazine (Trilafon) • Thioridazine (Mellaril) • Thiothixene (Navane) • Trifluoperazine (Stelazine) • Triflupromazine (Vesprin) **Atypical (Second Generation)** • Aripiprazole (Abilify) • Clozapine (Clozaril) • Olanzapine (Zyprexa) • Olanzapine/fluoxetine (Symbyax) • Quetiapine (Seroquel) • Risperidone (Risperdal) • Sertindole (Serlect) • Ziprasidone (Geodon)	*General* 1. Assess client's response to medication and for any possible drug interactions. 2. Monitor client on antipsychotic meds for extrapyramidal side effects (EPS) and other adverse reactions. 3. Administer the Abnormal and Involuntary Movement Scale (AIMS) to assess the client on antipsychotic meds for signs of tardive dyskinesia. 4. Assess for signs of neuroleptic malignant syndrome (NMS) and access emergency care for client if NMS suspected. 5. Monitor the client's vital signs for hypotension, orthostatic hypotension, and tachycardia. 6. Monitor the client's body weight for weight gain. 7. Monitor blood glucose and lipids. 8. Monitor the client for any seizure activity. 9. Instruct the client to avoid getting overheated in the sun; use sunblock; and avoid taking hot baths. 10. Perform weekly WBC counts with clozapine because of risk of agranulocytosis
Antiparkinsonism/anticholinergic to treat extrapyramidal side effects • Benztropine (Cogentin) • Biperiden (Akineton) • Ethopropazine (Parsidol; not presently available in United States) • Procyclidine (Kemadrin) • Trihexyphenidyl (Artane) **Dopamine Agonist** Amantadine (Symmetrel) **Beta Adrenergic Blocker** Propranolol (Inderal) **Benzodiazepines** Lorazepam (Ativan) **Antihistamine** Diphenhydramine (Benadryl)	*Nursing Measures for Side Effects (Anticholinergic Symptoms)* 1. Suggest chewing sugarless gum or hard candy to offset side effect of dry mouth. 2. Suggest rinsing mouth frequently to decrease side effect of dry mouth. 3. Encourage use of stool softeners, increasing water intake, and dietary fiber to decrease side effect of constipation. 4. Suggest use of saline nasal sprays to decrease side effect of nasal congestion. 5. Instruct client to use caution due to temporary side effect of blurred vision. Vision will return to previous condition in a few weeks. 6. Instruct client to report any eye pain immediately. 7. Instruct client on need to use caution in the sun, wear sunscreen, sunglasses, and avoid becoming overheated because of side effects of photophobia and photosensitivity. 8. Instruct client to use caution with sudden changes in body positions due to possible orthostatic hypotension. 9. Monitor client for signs of urinary retention and hesitation.

Table 9-2	Extrapyramidal Side Effects from Antipsychotic Medications
Akathisia	Motor restlessness, inability to remain still; can also occur as subjective feeling
Akinesia	Absence of movement or difficulty with movement
Dystonias	Muscle spasms, spastic movements of the neck and back, can be painful and frightening for the client
Pseudoparkinsonism	Shuffling and slow gait, masklike facial expression, tremors, pill-rolling movements of the hands, stooping posture, rigidity
Tardive dyskinesia	Involuntary and abnormal movements of the mouth, tongue, face, and jaw; may progress to the limbs; irreversible condition; may occur in months after antipsychotic medication use
Neuroleptic malignant syndrome	A potentially lethal side effect of antipsychotic medication that requires emergency treatment; manifested symptoms include hyperthermia, muscle rigidity, tremors, altered consciousness, tachycardia, hypertension, and incontinence

2. Atypical antipsychotics
   a. Developed and first marketed in 1990
   b. Effective in treating the positive and negative symptoms of schizophrenia
   c. Minimal to no risk of developing EPS
   d. Decreased risk for development of tardive dyskinesia (TD)
   e. Often chosen as first line of treatment for schizophrenia
   f. Can cause weight gain
   g. Can cause metabolic abnormalities that increase risk for cardiac conditions and diabetes mellitus
3. Medications used to treat side effects of antipsychotics
   a. Antiparkinsonism (anticholinergics) to treat parkinsonism and dystonia
   b. Dopamine agonist to treat parkinsonism
   c. Antihistamine for rapid relief of acute dystonia
   d. Beta blocker to treat akathisia
   e. Anticholinergics used to prevent or manage EPS of antipsychotic medications; common anticholinergeric side effects are dry mouth, blurred vision, constipation, decreased lacrimation, photophobia, urinary hesitance, tachycardia, and nausea
   f. Benzodiazepine used to treat akathisia

B. **Individual and group interventions**
   1. Management of delusions and hallucinations
      a. Establish a trusting, therapeutic relationship with the client by being honest, supportive, and consistent
      b. Communicate empathetically in response to client's feelings
      c. Encourage the client to express feelings and thoughts
      d. Assess for signs that the client is possibly having delusions or hallucinations
      e. Communicate with the client using clear, direct statements
      f. Provide an environment with a low degree of stimulation
      g. Express to the client that you understand that he or she believes the delusion or hallucination but you do not share in the delusional belief or hallucination
      h. Avoid arguing with the client about the delusion or hallucination; acknowledge if part of the delusion is real
      i. Provide reality testing and focus on reality
      j. If the client is experiencing a visual hallucination, provide a room with adequate lighting

Practice to Pass

How might you assess for tardive dyskinesia?

2. General nursing considerations and interventions

   a. Provide an environment that is safe for the client and others
   b. Avoid any physical contact or touching of the client
   c. Encourage the client to verbalize feelings and thoughts openly
   d. Utilize therapeutic communication techniques with the client
   e. Identify support systems for the client

   f. Assess for self-destructive behaviors and provide needed precautions
   g. Provide for activities of daily living (ADLs) when the client is not able to meet those needs

   h. Provide opportunities for the client that promote socialization and decrease isolation
   i. Involve the client in setting realistic goals in the treatment plan
   j. Provide daily living skills groups for the client to participate in

C. ***Milieu therapy***: a method of psychotherapy that controls the environment of the client to provide interpersonal contacts in order to develop trust, assurance, and personal autonomy
   1. Provide for the client's safety and the safety of others in the milieu
   2. Provide a supportive environment that is structured and predictable
   3. Collaborate with the multidisciplinary team regarding the client's plan of care
   4. Collaborate with the client regarding his or her plan of care
   5. Encourage the client to participate in milieu groups and activities that promote socialization
   6. Assist client with ADLs as needed, but encourage independence as client progresses

D. **Family therapy**
   1. Involve the family to determine use of appropriate community resources
   2. Educate the family about the chronic illness of schizophrenia, implications, early signs and symptoms of relapse, disease management, medication management, and community support systems available

   3. Provide an outlet for the family to discuss its feelings and fears and explore healthy or helpful and effective coping skills
   4. Educate family that stress within the family (expressed emotion) can increase risk of client relapsing

VI. EVALUATION/OUTCOMES

A. **Evaluation of the client's treatment and progress** is an ongoing, continual process

B. **Outcome criteria are individualized for each client** and may include the following:
   1. Remain free of harm, and demonstrate absence of violence toward others
   2. Be able to establish a trusting, open relationship with therapist/nurse
   3. Report and experience no hallucinations or diminished hallucinations
   4. Report and experience no delusional thought processes
   5. Demonstrate increased socialization skills and decreased isolative behavior
   6. Demonstrate appropriate affect and improved thought processes
   7. Report the ability to experience pleasure and improved interest in activities
   8. Demonstrate an improved ability to concentrate and complete tasks
   9. Demonstrate improved speech patterns and congruent communication
   10. Adhere to medication schedule as prescribed
   11. Demonstrate no EPS or adverse reactions to medication regime
   12. Verbalize side effects and adverse reactions to report to practitioner/MD
   13. Verbalize indication, dosage, route, and schedule of medication regime
   14. Actively participate in plan of care
   15. Demonstrate ability to meet ADLs with or without assistance
   16. Demonstrate effective coping patterns
   17. Utilize appropriate community resources

Practice to Pass

Schizophrenia is generally considered a chronic condition, which needs long-term management. What are some nursing interventions that may decrease relapse potential?

C. Outcome criteria are individualized for each client's family and may include the following:

1. Be able to verbalize and identify early signs and symptoms of disease exacerbation
2. Be able to verbalize the implications of schizophrenia as a chronic illness
3. Demonstrate effective coping patterns
4. Utilize appropriate community resources
5. Be able to verbalize client's medication regime
6. Be able to verbalize and identify signs and symptoms of EPS and neuroleptic malignant syndrome (NMS)
7. Be able to verbalize how and when to access emergency care services

VII. SPECIFIC DISORDERS

A. Schizophrenia: a syndrome characterized by difficulty thinking clearly, knowing what is real, managing feelings, making decisions, or relating to others

1. The positive characteristics of schizophrenia are added behaviors not normally seen, such as delusions, hallucinations, positive formal thought disorders, bizarre behavior, and overactive affect
2. The negative characteristics of schizophrenia are the absence of normal behaviors, such as flat affect, minimal self-care, social withdrawal, and concrete thinking
3. People with schizophrenia may exhibit purposeless or ritualistic behaviors or even pace for hours on end; some have bizarre facial or body movements
4. The most common type of hallucination is auditory; the next most common type is visual
5. Delusions are false beliefs that cannot be changed by logical reasoning or evidence; it is thought that they represent dysfunction in the information-processing circuits between the hemispheres
6. People with schizophrenia frequently have ineffective social skills, which increases their sense of isolation
7. Neurobiological factors of schizophrenia include genetic defects, abnormal brain development, neurodegeneration, disordered neurotransmission, and abnormal brain structures
8. Psychiatric rehabilitation emphasizes the development of skills and supports, considers the client to be in control, and promotes choices, self-determination, and individual responsibility

B. Schizoaffective disorder: having clinical manifestations characteristic of both schizophrenia and a mood disorder, such as depression, mania, or a mixed episode

1. Client experiences symptoms of a mood disorder with one or more of the following:
   a. Delusions
   b. Hallucinations
   c. Disorganized speech
   d. Disorganized behavior
   e. Negative characteristics
2. Clients often have difficulty maintaining a job or functioning in school, experience problems with self-care, are socially isolated, and often suffer from suicidal ideation

C. Schizophreniform disorder: the essential features of schizophrenia are present with the exception that the duration is at least one month, but less than six months

D. Other psychotic disorders

1. **Delusional disorder**: the presence of non-bizarre delusions (delusions that could possibly occur in reality) that persist for at least one month; no other manifestations of psychosis are noted
2. **Brief psychotic disorder**: the presence of at least one positive symptom of schizophrenia with duration between one day and one month; the existence or absence of any stressor should be noted

3. **Shared psychotic disorder (*folie à deux*)**: a delusional system develops in the context of a close relationship between two people who share a similar delusion; the person who shares the delusion is not as impaired as the person with the disorder and delusion
4. **Substance-induced psychotic disorder**: the presence of hallucinations and delusions are a direct result of the physiological effects of a substance
5. **Psychotic disorder due to a general medical condition**: the presence of hallucinations and delusions are a direct result of the general medical condition

Case Study

As you begin your shift as the charge nurse in an acute care psychiatric unit, you are informed in shift change report of a new client admission. The client has a medical diagnosis of schizophrenia, paranoid type, and has had multiple psychiatric hospital admissions caused by poor adherence to antipsychotic medication therapy.

1. What types of symptoms might you anticipate seeing?
2. What are the priorities of care for the client?
3. What are the possible nursing diagnoses?
4. How will you approach this client to begin fostering a therapeutic relationship?
5. What options are available to decrease incidence of poor medication adherence?

For suggested responses, see pages 298–299.

POSTTEST

1 While talking with a female client diagnosed with schizophrenia, the nurse notices the client look away from the nurse and stare at the wall while making facial grimaces. What is the most appropriate intervention by the nurse?

1. End the conversation because the client is not listening.
2. Administer the ordered prn trihexyphenidyl (Artane).
3. Ask the client if she sees something on the wall.
4. Redirect the conversation to a neutral topic.

2 A client taking antipsychotic medications for treatment of schizophrenia reports feeling nervous. The nurse notices that the client is pacing the long hallway and is unable to remain still, even when in conversation with other clients. What term should the nurse use to document this occurrence?

1. Akathisia
2. Akinesia
3. Dystonia
4. Tardive dyskinesia

3 The client who has schizoaffective disorder takes both haloperidol (Haldol) and valproic acid (Depakote). When the client asks the nurse to explain what this particular combination of drugs is expected to do, what would be the best response by the nurse?

1. "Haloperidol (Haldol) makes your moods calmer and valproic acid prevents tight muscles."
2. "This combination is good for people who have problems like yours."
3. "Haloperidol improves your thinking and valproic acid stabilizes your moods."
4. "This is an old combination of drugs that helps people to keep thinking and feelings in balance."

4 A client admitted to an inpatient unit has a diagnosis of paranoid-type schizophrenia. The new mental health care worker on this unit approaches the nurse and asks about the best way to work with this client. How should the nurse respond?

1. "When possible, remain at arm's length from this client."
2. "This client is anxious. Offer back rubs at bedtime."
3. "Offer this client a hand-shake before beginning conversation."
4. "To get the client's attention, place your hand gently on the arm or hand."

5 The client has schizophrenia, residual type. A nursing care plan should give priority to which nursing diagnosis?

1. Impaired Verbal Communication
2. Self-Care Deficit
3. Social Isolation
4. Anxiety

6 The nurse observes that the client with paranoid schizophrenia appears very preoccupied. The client is pacing back and forth in the hall, periodically looking to the side, clenching the fist, and saying, "I told you to go away." At this time, the nurse should plan to do which of the following? Select all that apply.

1. Offer frequent orienting stimuli.
2. Reduce proximity to others.
3. Refrain from using non-verbal hand gestures.
4. Avoid touching the client during conversation.
5. Reassure the client of the safety of the environment.

7 The nurse is to complete an AIMS assessment of the client. When explaining this test to the client, the nurse should say that this test will help to identify if the client is beginning to have which of the following?

1. Weak muscles
2. Shaking hands and feet
3. Uncontrollable motions in the body
4. Slowed body movement

8 A client reports having blurred vision that began after beginning drug therapy with a traditional antipsychotic. What would be the best response by the nurse?

1. "You need to schedule an appointment with your eye doctor to get a new prescription for your eyeglasses."
2. "Blurred vision is a temporary side effect of your medication that usually resolves within a few weeks."
3. "You need to stop taking your antipsychotic medication and notify your doctor immediately."
4. "Blurred vision is a permanent condition as a result of your medication."

9 A client is planning to be discharged from the hospital. It is the nurse's responsibility to educate this client regarding prescribed medications. This client is taking clozapine (Clozaril). The nurse makes it a priority to teach the client to notify the physician immediately for which of the following?

1. Feelings of increased energy and interest in the environment
2. Unusual reactions to exposures to the sun
3. Interferences with the normal sleep pattern
4. Indications of any sort of infection

10 A client with chronic schizophrenia has been receiving an atypical antipsychotic for three months. The nurse concludes that the client is experiencing a reduction in negative symptoms of schizophrenia if a family member says which of the following? Select all that apply.

1. "We walked together for 15 minutes, and I could see no evidence he was 'hearing voices.'"
2. "For the past week, he has gotten up, dressed, and taken a walk early each morning."
3. "It's been more than a month since he said that he is a Martian prince."
4. "We went to a musical concert, and he smiled and applauded the musicians."
5. "I've noticed that his thoughts are better organized."

➤ *See pages 187–189 for Answers and Rationales.*

ANSWERS & RATIONALES

Pretest

1 **Answer: 4** **Rationale:** Risk for Violence is correct. Safety is always the highest priority when caring for any client. This is particularly true when the client has paranoid schizophrenia. These clients are extremely suspicious and distrusting of the environment and feel that others have harmful intent toward them. They maintain an alert and watchful hypervigilance and are at high risk for aggression and/or violence. Interrupted Thought Processes, Social Isolation, and Impaired Verbal Communication are appropriate for the client's care plan but are not given highest priority, as they are not as important as safety. **Cognitive Level:** Analyzing **Client Need:** Safety and Infection Control **Integrated Process:** Nursing Process: Diagnosis **Content Area:** Mental Health **Strategy:** Recognize that in any nursing situation, highest priority is always assigned to providing safety and maintaining basic physiologic functioning. **Reference:** Varcarolis, E., Carson, V., & Shoemaker, N. (2009). *Foundations of psychiatric mental health nursing: A clinical approach* (6th ed.). St. Louis, MO: Saunders Elsevier, pp. 331–338.

2 **Answer: 2** **Rationale:** "That must be a frightening thought; we are nurses who work at this hospital" is correct. The client is experiencing a delusion and indeed believes that the nursing staff members are secret police. Understandably, the client will be distrusting, suspicious, and frightened of all actions of the staff. The nurse should show awareness of the feelings of the client ("That must be a frightening thought.") and present reality about the role of the nursing staff ("We are nurses who work at this hospital."). "That is a strange idea; we aren't secret police" demeans the client and fails to allow the client to know the staff's role. "Being suspicious isn't easy, is it? You won't be tortured here" attempts to respond to the client's feeling and present reality, but it does not tell the patient about the role of the staff. "There is no need to be frightened; we will keep you safe" attempts to be reassuring, but it fails to give reality-based information that might assist the client to feel more comfortable with the staff. It also could suggest to the client that torture will occur but not at this location. **Cognitive Level:** Analyzing **Client Need:** Psychosocial Integrity **Integrated Process:** Caring **Content Area:** Mental Health **Strategy:** Look for an answer that both shows understanding of the client's feeling and presents reality as perceived by the nurse. **Reference:** Varcarolis, E., Carson, V., & Shoemaker, N. (2009). *Foundations of psychiatric mental health nursing: A clinical approach* (6th ed.). St. Louis, MO: Saunders Elsevier, pp. 319, 320.

3 **Answer: 2, 3, 5** **Rationale:** Three options are correct because diminished pleasure, blunted affect, and difficulty making decisions all represent a loss or lack of normal skills and functioning of the individual, which is the definition of negative symptoms of schizophrenia. First-generation antipsychotic drugs typically do not improve these symptoms but second-generation antipsychotic drugs do. Positive symptoms of schizophrenia, such as abnormal thoughts and hallucinations are symptoms that, if present, clearly and certainly indicate the presence of psychosis. **Cognitive Level:** Analyzing **Client Need:** Psychosocial Integrity **Integrated Process:** Nursing Process: Planning **Content Area:** Mental Health **Strategy:** Define, then compare and contrast positive and negative symptoms of schizophrenia. Recognize that both groups of symptoms are undesirable, so the term negative can be confusing, unless you recall that it is the absence of what the typical person would have or experience. Think carefully about this, as the terms themselves can lead to confusion unless you have a clear definition in mind. **Reference:** Varcarolis, E., Carson, V., & Shoemaker, N. (2009). *Foundations of psychiatric mental health nursing: A clinical approach* (6th ed.). St. Louis, MO: Saunders Elsevier, pp. 312–317.

4 **Answer: 3** **Rationale:** Preparing the client for immediate transfer to an emergency department is correct. This client is exhibiting signs and symptoms of possible neuroleptic-induced malignant syndrome (NMS), which is a potentially lethal side effect of antipsychotic medications that requires immediate medical care. The care cannot be delayed, as the NMS may progress rapidly and lead to client death. The client is not simply experiencing extrapyramidal effects (EPS), which would indicate the need for a prn anticholinergic. While orthostatic hypotension may occur as a side effect to many antipsychotic medications, making this the priority intervention at this time would ignore the possibility that NMS is present. Suspected NMS should be considered an immediate medical emergency. Failing to recognize the urgency of the situation and arranging for a physician's visit later in the day could put the client at grave risk for negative consequences, possibly including death. **Cognitive Level:** Analyzing **Client Need:** Pharmacological and Parenteral Therapies **Integrated Process:** Nursing Process: Implementation **Content Area:** Mental Health **Strategy:** Pay attention to the particular combination of symptoms that the client is manifesting. Look at them as a group, not individually. Recognize that in any nursing situation, highest priority is always assigned to providing safety and maintaining basic physiologic functioning. **Reference:** Varcarolis, E., Carson, V., & Shoemaker, N. (2009). *Foundations of psychiatric mental health nursing: A clinical approach* (6th ed.). St. Louis, MO: Saunders Elsevier, pp. 329, 331.

5 **Answer: 2** **Rationale:** Acknowledging that the exact cause is unclear is correct. The precise cause of schizophrenia is unknown. The general consensus is that schizophrenia results from the interaction between a variety of biological and psychosocial factors that have been correlated with schizophrenia. Research has correlated genetic factors with schizophrenia, but more research is needed. Poor parenting skills and early-age trauma have not been documented as exact causes of schizophrenia. **Cognitive Level:** Analyzing **Client Need:** Psychosocial Integrity **Integrated Process:** Teaching and Learning **Content Area:** Mental Health **Strategy:** Look for the answer that will fit in any situation. Remember that in spite of extensive research and sophisticated diagnostics, no single cause for schizophrenia has yet been established. **Reference:** Varcarolis, E., Carson, V., & Shoemaker, N. (2009). *Foundations of psychiatric mental health nursing: A clinical approach* (6th ed.). St. Louis, MO: Saunders Elsevier, pp. 309–312.

6 Answer: 1 Rationale: Attending one group meeting with a staff member within three days is correct. This option recognizes that the client is not likely to initiate interpersonal or social activity independently. It is also a measurable goal that is reasonable to achieve in a short time. Clients need to meet short-term goals during hospitalization to promote a sense of accomplishment, which may increase their self-esteem. Leading a unit community group by the time of discharge is a possible long-term goal; however, this could be an unrealistic goal for the time of discharge. Being more comfortable in group situations by three days is not written in measurable terms, even though it specifies a short time frame for accomplishment. It fails to indicate how the nurse can know that a client is "more comfortable." Enjoying participation in group therapy by the time of discharge is not written in measurable terms. It fails to indicate how the nurse can know that a client "enjoys participating." **Cognitive Level:** Analyzing **Client Need:** Psychosocial Integrity **Integrated Process:** Nursing Process: Planning **Content Area:** Mental Health **Strategy:** Look for an outcome that is stated so specifically that it could be measured by any nurse at the end of the specified time frame. **Reference:** Varcarolis, E., Carson, V., & Shoemaker, N. (2009). *Foundations of psychiatric mental health nursing: A clinical approach* (6th ed.). St. Louis, MO: Saunders Elsevier, pp. 319–321.

7 Answer: 1, 2, 4 Rationale: Aggressive outbursts, constipation, and nutritional deficiency are correct. Catatonic schizophrenia is characterized by two phases: nonresponsive hypoactivity and unpredictable hyperactivity and aggression that may be dangerous to self or others. The nurse must always anticipate that the aggressive stage may occur. Constipation is possible because of the psychomotor retardation and relative immobility of the client. This client will likely be receiving antipsychotic medications, most of which have anticholinergic side effects, including constipation. Unless the staff assists the client and allows extra time for meals, the likelihood of nutritional deficiency is increased because of the client's psychomotor retardation and inability to verbally report

any feelings of hunger. Regarding the option for ineffective coping, the client is actually experiencing impaired individual coping, as expressed through the presenting behaviors. Regarding the option for memory deficit, many clients who have had catatonic episodes are able to recall details and events occurring during a period of stupor. **Cognitive Level:** Analyzing **Client Need:** Safety and Infection Control **Integrated Process:** Nursing Process: Diagnosis **Content Area:** Mental Health **Strategy:** Form a mental picture of this client. Apply concepts of basic physiology and theoretical knowledge about manifestations of catatonic schizophrenia. **Reference:** Varcarolis, E., Carson, V., & Shoemaker, N. (2009). *Foundations of psychiatric mental health nursing: A clinical approach* (6th ed.). St. Louis, MO: Saunders Elsevier, pp. 331–336.

8 Answer: 3 Rationale: Clang associations is correct. These are association disturbances in which schizophrenic clients rhyme words in a sentence that seems nonsensical to the listener. Echopraxia is meaningless imitation of motions made by others. Echolalia is involuntary parrot-like repetition of words spoken by others. Associative looseness does not involve rhyming, but rather lack of integration or logical connection between thoughts. **Cognitive Level:** Applying **Client Need:** Psychosocial Integrity **Integrated Process:** Communication and Documentation **Content Area:** Mental Health **Strategy:** Notice that the client is speaking in a rhyming fashion. If you don't remember the meaning of each of the terms, look at the root elements in the other terms. **Reference:** Varcarolis, E., Carson, V., & Shoemaker, N. (2009). *Foundations of psychiatric mental health nursing: A clinical approach* (6th ed.). St. Louis, MO: Saunders Elsevier, pp. 287, 315.

9 Answer: 3 Rationale: Body weight is correct. Increase in body weight and body mass index (BMI) can occur very quickly when clients take olanzepine (Zyprexa). Baseline data about these should be obtained before the client begins to take this drug. Determining the client's sleep pattern is not an urgent consideration, although the nurse should recognize that daytime somnolence might be an early side effect of the olanzepine (Zyprexa). Food and fluid preferences are important considerations when the nurse teaches the client about usual side effects, but this can be done later. While some clients do have digestive disturbances while taking olanzepine (Zyprexa), this is not nearly as common as the side effect of rapid weight gain. **Cognitive Level:** Analyzing **Client Need:** Pharmacological and Parenteral Therapies **Integrated Process:** Nursing Process: Assessment **Content Area:** Mental Health **Strategy:** Think about the most common and untoward side effects associated with second-generation antipsychotics. These include hyperglycemia, weight gain, and new-onset type 2 diabetes. Recall that unwelcome weight gain frequently contributes to non-compliance. **Reference:** Varcarolis, E., Carson, V., & Shoemaker, N. (2009). *Foundations of psychiatric mental health nursing: A clinical approach* (6th ed.). St. Louis, MO: Saunders Elsevier, p. 327.

10 **Answer: 3** **Rationale:** Thought insertion is correct. This is a thought disorder of schizophrenia that is defined as the client believing that others are putting thoughts in his or her mind against the client's will. Thought broadcasting is the belief by a client that he or she can broadcast his or her thoughts to others. Thought blocking occurs when a client's thoughts stop in midstream. Thought control is the belief that others can control one's thoughts against his or her will. **Cognitive Level:** Applying **Client Need:** Psychosocial Integrity **Integrated Process:** Communication and Documentation **Content Area:** Mental Health **Strategy:** Review basic definitions of cognitive distortions common in persons with schizophrenia. **Reference:** Kneisl, C., Wilson, H., & Trigoboff, E. (2009*). Contemporary psychiatric-mental health nursing* (2nd ed.). Upper Saddle River, NJ: Prentice Hall, pp. 374, 388.

Posttest

1 **Answer: 3** **Rationale:** Asking if the client sees something on the wall is correct. This client is most likely experiencing a visual hallucination. First, it is important for nurses to know the content of the hallucination so they can assist the client to process the experience and prevent any aggressive behavior. After this intervention is completed, then the client should be oriented back to reality. Ending the conversation would not promote trust with the client or allow the nurse to assess content of the hallucination. Trihexyphenidyl will not prevent hallucinations. The nurse should not redirect the conversation until the nurse has evaluated for hallucinations. **Cognitive Level:** Analyzing **Client Need:** Psychosocial Integrity **Integrated Process:** Nursing Process: Implementation **Content Area:** Mental Health **Strategy:** Recognize that this client is responding to internal stimuli. **Reference:** Varcarolis, E., Carson, V., & Shoemaker, N. (2009). *Foundations of psychiatric mental health nursing: A clinical approach* (6th ed.). St. Louis, MO: Saunders Elsevier, pp. 314–316.

2 **Answer: 1** **Rationale:** Akathisia is correct. This is an extrapyramidal side effect of antipsychotic medications that may manifest as subjective and objective restlessness and increased motor movement. Akinesia is also an extrapyramidal side effect, but it is not shown in this client's behavior. Akinesia is decreased activity or motor movement. Dystonia is also an extrapyramidal side effect, but it is not shown in this client's behavior. Dystonia presents as sudden and often painful contractions of muscles, especially of the head and neck. Tardive dyskinesia is also an extrapyramidal side effect, but it is not shown in this client's behavior. Tardive dyskinesia presents as involuntary muscle movements, strange tics, and repetitive motor movements in persons who have taken antipsychotics for a long period of time. The situation gives no past history of the client. **Cognitive Level:** Applying **Client Need:** Pharmacological and Parenteral Therapies **Integrated Process:** Communication

and Documentation **Content Area:** Mental Health **Strategy:** Define each term for yourself and then look back at the client behaviors described in the stem of the question. **Reference:** Fontaine, K. (2009). *Mental health nursing* (6th ed.). Upper Saddle River, NJ: Prentice Hall, p. 200.

3 **Answer: 3** **Rationale:** "Haloperidol improves your thinking and valproic acid stabilizes your moods" is correct. The nurse should know that the client has the right to have information about medications being taken. This information should be accurate and given in manner that the client is likely to be able to understand. The nurse's answer should be based on the understanding that haloperidol (Haldol) is a traditional antipsychotic and that valproic acid (Depakote) is a traditional anticonvulsant that is also used for the nontraditional purpose of mood stabilization. Stating that Haloperidol makes moods calmer and valproic acid prevents tight muscles contains inaccurate information about expected drug effects. Stating that this combination is good for "people who have problems like yours" is a nonspecific response and does not provide the client with the requested information. Stating that that this is an old combination of drugs is an inaccurate statement because this sort of combination is not old—FDA approval for administering certain anticonvulsants (including valproic acid) was not approved until the early 2000s. **Cognitive Level:** Analyzing **Client Need:** Pharmacological and Parenteral Therapies **Integrated Process:** Teaching and Learning **Content Area:** Mental Health **Strategy:** Look carefully at each option for factual correctness. This will require that you know relevant information about these two drugs. **Reference:** Varcarolis, E., Carson, V., & Shoemaker, N. (2009). *Foundations of psychiatric mental health nursing: A clinical approach* (6th ed.). St. Louis, MO: Saunders Elsevier, pp. 295, 327–328.

4 **Answer: 1** **Rationale:** Staying at arm's length from the client is correct. Paranoid schizophrenic clients are very suspicious and potentially dangerous. It is best to avoid any physical contact, as well as any symbolic or actual invasion of the client's personal space because the client may feel threatened. Offering a back rub, shaking hands, and placing a hand on the client involve physical contact. It is unlikely that the client could tolerate this without becoming aggressive. **Cognitive Level:** Analyzing **Client Need:** Safety and Infection Control **Integrated Process:** Teaching and Learning **Content Area:** Mental Health **Strategy:** Recall a paranoid client you have seen in the clinical area. How do you think this client would react to each of these actions? **Reference:** Fontaine, K. (2009). *Mental health nursing* (6th ed.). Upper Saddle River, NJ: Prentice Hall, pp. 359–361.

5 **Answer: 3** **Rationale:** Social Isolation is correct. Residual-type schizophrenia manifests with socially withdrawn behavior, an inappropriate affect, and an absence of prominent psychotic symptoms. The most likely and common nursing diagnosis would be Social Isolation.

Impaired Verbal Communication, Self-Care Deficit, and Anxiety are less likely to be seen in a client with residual schizophrenia than is social isolation. **Cognitive Level:** Analyzing **Client Need:** Psychosocial Integrity **Integrated Process:** Nursing Process: Diagnosis **Content Area:** Mental Health **Strategy:** Recall prominent behaviors associated with residual schizophrenia. Then consider which nursing diagnosis would encompass these behaviors. **Reference:** Varcarolis, E., Carson, V., & Shoemaker, N. (2009). *Foundations of psychiatric mental health nursing: A clinical approach* (6th ed.). St. Louis, MO: Saunders Elsevier, pp. 334, 336.

6 **Answer: 2, 3, 4 Rationale:** Three options are correct. This client is actively responding to internal stimuli and could easily react aggressively to others, especially if experiencing command hallucinations or if responding to actual or perceived intrusions of others into the client's own personal space. The described behaviors do not suggest that this client is disoriented. Instead the nurse should recognize indications that the client is experiencing hallucinations. The client is likely to respond aggressively to moving hand gestures, which will be perceived as a physical threat. If the nurse offered verbal reassurance of the safety of the environment, it is highly unlikely that the client would feel reassured. Indeed, this action might provoke further suspiciousness, as the client's hyperalertness and mistrust will lead to misinterpretation of environmental events. **Cognitive Level:** Analyzing **Client Need:** Psychosocial Integrity **Integrated Process:** Nursing Process: Planning **Content Area:** Mental Health **Strategy:** Recall that during periods of active hallucinations, clients are more responsive to internal stimuli than to external stimuli. This can put the client and others at risk for injury. **Reference:** Kneisl, C., Wilson, H., & Trigoboff, E. (2009). *Contemporary psychiatric–mental health nursing.* (2nd ed.). Upper Saddle River, NJ: Prentice Hall, pp. 393–394.

7 **Answer: 3 Rationale:** Uncontrollable motions is correct. The AIMS (Abnormal Involuntary Movement Scale) is used to screen for signs of tardive dyskinesia, which is a possible side effect associated with long-term use of an antipsychotic, particularly of the traditional type. It is characterized by involuntary, repetitive, and often bizarre movements of the mouth, face, trunk, and extremities. It is considered irreversible, so early recognition is imperative. The AIMS test does not include assessments for muscle weakness, which would indicate acute EPS (extrapyramidal side effects) rather than tardive dyskinesia. The AIMS test excludes regular repetitive rhythmic tremors. These are indications of acute EPS (extrapyramidal side effects), not chronic tardive dyskinesia. The AIMS test does not measure slowed body movements, which would indicate acute EPS (extrapyramidal side effects), not chronic tardive dyskinesia. **Cognitive Level:** Analyzing **Client Need:** Pharmacological and Parenteral Therapies **Integrated Process:** Teaching and

Learning **Content Area:** Mental Health **Strategy:** Mentally review the major differences between tardive dyskinesia and acute EPS. **Reference:** Kneisl, C., Wilson, H., & Trigoboff, E. (2009). *Contemporary psychiatric–mental health nursing.* (2nd ed.). Upper Saddle River, NJ: Prentice Hall, pp. 855–857.

8 **Answer: 2 Rationale:** Stating that the blurred vision is temporary is correct. Blurred vision is an anticholinergic symptom/side effect that usually resolves in a few weeks. If there is no improvement with time, then the doctor should be notified. It is too early to schedule an appointment, as the client can be expected to accommodate to this side effect within a matter of days. However, if the client also complains of pain in the eye, the physician should be notified immediately, as the client may be experiencing glaucoma as a result of the pupillary dilation that caused the blurred vision. There is no indication of pain with the blurring of vision, so the nurse does not have to respond urgently. Permanent blurred vision is unusual. The client can be expected to accommodate to this side effect within a matter of days. **Cognitive Level:** Analyzing **Client Need:** Pharmacological and Parenteral Therapies **Integrated Process:** Teaching and Learning **Content Area:** Mental Health **Strategy:** Compare and contrast effects of anticholinergic drugs with anticholinergic side effects. **Reference:** Varcarolis, E., Carson, V., & Shoemaker, N. (2009). *Foundations of psychiatric mental health nursing: A clinical approach* (6th ed.). St. Louis, MO: Saunders Elsevier, pp. 328–329.

9 **Answer: 4 Rationale:** Indication of any sort of infection is correct. Agranulocytosis is the most dangerous common side effect of clozapine and can lead to death if not detected and treated early. In addition to the requirement that weekly analysis of WBCs must be completed before clozapine can be reordered, it is important that the client, family, and nursing staff understand that changes in the WBC could occur during the time period between two laboratory tests. Therefore, reporting any observations of suspected infection is an urgent priority. Feeling more energy and interest probably indicates a decrease in the intensity of negative symptoms of schizophrenia, and notification of the physician can be delayed. Sensitivity to ultraviolet rays is a potential side effect of clozapine that is generally more bothersome than dangerous. Interference with a normal sleep pattern is a problem that should be reported to the physician, but urgent reporting is not necessary. **Cognitive Level:** Analyzing **Client Need:** Pharmacological and Parenteral Therapies **Integrated Process:** Teaching and Learning **Content Area:** Mental Health **Strategy:** Note the word *critical* in the question. Look for the most potentially dangerous side effect. **Reference:** Varcarolis, E., Carson, V., & Shoemaker, N. (2009). *Foundations of psychiatric mental health nursing: A clinical approach* (6th ed.). St. Louis, MO: Saunders Elsevier, pp. 326–327.

ANSWERS & RATIONALES

10 **Answer: 2, 4** **Rationale:** Two options are correct. Improvement in motivation and volition and ability to experience pleasure indicate a reduction in negative symptoms. While getting up, dressed, and taking a walk indicates improvement, the improvement is in the positive symptoms of schizophrenia: auditory hallucinations. The statements about it having been a month since he said he is a Martian prince and about his thoughts being better organized indicate improvement in the positive symptoms of schizophrenia: delusions. **Cognitive Level:** Analyzing **Client Need:** Psychosocial Integrity **Integrated Process:** Nursing Process: Evaluation **Content Area:** Mental Health **Strategy:** Review differences between positive and negative symptoms of schizophrenia. Recall that both have a negative or unhealthy character. **Reference:** Kneisl, C., Wilson, H., & Trigoboff, E. (2009). *Contemporary psychiatric–mental health nursing.* (2nd ed.). Upper Saddle River, NJ: Prentice Hall, pp. 374–375.

References

American Psychiatric Association (2000). *Diagnosis and statistical manual of mental disorders* (4th ed., text revision). Washington, DC: American Psychiatric Association, pp. 288, 297–344.

Carpenito, L. J. (2011). *Nursing diagnosis: Application to clinical practice* (13th ed.). Philadelphia, PA: Lippincott Williams & Wilkins.

Fontaine, K. (2009). *Mental health nursing* (6th ed.). Upper Saddle River, NJ: Pearson Education.

Kniesl, C., Wilson, H., & Trigoboff, E. (2009). *Contemporary psychiatric–mental health nursing* (2nd ed.). Upper Saddle River, NJ: Pearson Education.

North American Nursing Diagnosis Association (2008). *Nursing diagnosis: Definitions and classification 2009–2011.* Indianapolis, IN: Wiley-Blackwell.

Stuart, G. (2009). *Principles and practice of psychiatric nursing* (9th ed.). St. Louis: Elsevier Science.

Townsend, M. (2011). *Essentials of psychiatric–mental health nursing* (5th ed.). Philadelphia, PA: F. A. Davis.

Varcarolis, E. & Halter, M. (2010). *Foundations of psychiatric mental health nursing: A clinical approach* (6th ed.). Philadelphia: Saunders.

10 Delirium, Dementia, and Other Cognitive Mental Disorders

Chapter Outline

Overview/Classification
Etiology
Assessment

Nursing Diagnoses/Analysis
Planning/Implementation

Evaluation/Outcomes
Specific Disorders

NCLEX-RN® Test Prep

Use the accompanying online resource, NursingReviewsandRationales, to test yourself with hundreds of NCLEX®-style practice questions.

Objectives

➤ Identify eight characteristics commonly seen in clients experiencing dementia.
➤ Describe three treatment modalities for clients with delirium and dementia.
➤ Differentiate between delirium and dementia.
➤ State examples of at least five nursing diagnoses frequently used in the management of clients with cognitive mental disorders.
➤ Describe nursing interventions that are helpful to clients experiencing delirium, dementia, and other cognitive mental disorders.

Review at a Glance

agnosia an inability to recognize familiar situations, people, or stimuli; not related to impairment in sensory organs
agraphia inability to read or write
alexia inability to identify an object or its use by sight such as a toothbrush or telephone; visual agnosia
aphasia a loss of ability to understand or use language
apraxia an inability to carry out skilled and purposeful movement; inability to use objects properly
astereognosis inability to identify familiar objects when placed in hand, such as a comb or pencil; tactile agnosia
auditory agnosia inability to recognize familiar sounds such as a ringing doorbell or telephone

catastrophic reaction overreaction toward minor stresses that occurs in demented clients
confabulation filling in of memory gaps with imaginary information in an attempt to distract others from observing the deficit
delirium an acute, usually reversible brain disorder characterized by clouding of consciousness (decreased awareness of environment) and a reduced ability to focus and maintain attention
dementia a chronic, irreversible brain disorder characterized by impairments in memory, abstract thinking, and judgment, as well as changes in personality
dysarthria problem with articulation
dysgraphia impaired ability to write

dysnomia impaired ability to name an object
executive functioning the cognitive ability to plan, sequence
hyperetamorphosis need to compulsively touch and examine every object in environment
hyperorality need to taste, chew, and examine any object small enough to be placed in mouth
perseveration phenomena repetitive behaviors such as lip licking, finger tapping, pacing, or echolalia
psychosis hallucination and/or delusions, disorganized thought process, disorganized behavior
sundown syndrome disorientation that worsens at end of day

PRETEST

1 The client is experiencing delirium in the postoperative period after open reduction internal fixation of the left hip secondary to a fracture from a fall. Which intervention will the nurse address as the highest priority?

1. Reducing anxiety
2. Maintaining adequate hydration
3. Turning and repositioning every two hours
4. Offering frequent reorienting statements

2 A client is admitted status post-hip replacement; her medical history is otherwise benign. She is placed on morphine sulfate intravenously as needed for surgical pain. Soon she begins to mumble, and becomes confused and combative. What conclusion should the nurse draw? Select all that apply.

1. The client is experiencing symptoms of delirium.
2. The recent cognitive changes, if untreated, can lead to death.
3. The client is experiencing symptoms of vascular dementia.
4. The client is at risk for injury.
5. The behavior is impulsive.

3 A client is admitted for treatment of alcohol-withdrawal delirium. It will be of high priority for the nurse to address which of the following when writing the client's care plan? Select all that apply.

1. Fluctuating level of awareness
2. Self-esteem enhancement
3. Impaired individual coping
4. Restlessness and irritability
5. Potential for seizures

4 A client in stage II of dementia of the Alzheimer's type often wanders due to confusion and becomes lost. Which priority nursing diagnosis should the nurse select to address this behavior?

1. Confusion related to impaired cognition
2. Anxiety related to fear of cognitive deficits
3. Impaired Verbal Communication related to anxiety
4. Risk for Injury related to cognitive deficits

5 The client has a diagnosis of dementia of the Alzheimer's type (DAT) and is being cared for by the spouse in the home. What self-care activity will be most important for the nurse to recommend to the spouse?

1. Regular attendance at church services
2. Periodic times of respite from caregiving
3. Participation in reminiscence therapy
4. Establishment of a predictable daily schedule

6 Which most appropriate client outcome statement would the nurse formulate for a 68-year-old female client experiencing an acute episode of delirium?

1. Have decreased confusion as evidenced by orientation to person, place, and time.
2. Remain free from self-directed violence as evidenced by agreement to a no-suicide contract.
3. Verbalize increased feelings of self-esteem as evidenced by statements acknowledging ability to perform certain tasks independently.
4. Have intact tactile senses as evidenced by ability to recognize familiar objects placed in her hand.

7 Which nursing intervention would be most effective in improving the orientation level of a 74-year-old male client with dementia?

1. Speak directly into the client's ear when telling him the day of the month and time.
2. Assure the client that his deceased spouse is expected home later in the day.
3. Keep the client's television tuned to a 24-hour news station during the daytime hours.
4. Put traditional seasonal decorations within the client's view.

8 The client diagnosed with dementia of Alzheimer's type is receiving several medications. An unlicensed assistant who is enrolled in nursing school asks the nurse, "Which medication may improve mental functioning by increasing acetylcholine?" Which medication should the nurse identify?

1. Fluoxetine (Prozac)
2. Trazodone (Desyrel)
3. Haloperidol (Haldol)
4. Donepezil (Aricept)

9 A client diagnosed with dementia secondary to vascular disease has comorbid major depressive disorder. He has a flat affect, depressed mood, and short-term memory loss. Paroxetine (Paxil) is prescribed for the depression. A family member says, "I don't remember the reason this medicine might help." What is the nurse's best response?

1. "It improves circulation to the brain."
2. "It elevates blood glucose levels in cell of brain"
3. "It works on the serotonin levels in the brain."
4. "It will increase oxygen levels in the brain."

10 A female client with stage II dementia of the Alzheimer's type is cared for at home by her daughter. Which statement by the caregiver indicates to the nurse that she understands personal coping strategies that are most likely to be useful for her mother?

1. "I need to stay with my mother 24 hours a day."
2. "I need to bathe my mother every day before breakfast."
3. "I need to postpone my vacation for a few more years."
4. "I need to spend time with my mother doing something we both enjoy."

➤ *See pages 206–208 for Answers and Rationales.*

I. OVERVIEW/CLASSIFICATION

A. *Delirium*: an acute, reversible cognitive disorder characterized by decreased consciousness of environment, decreased ability to focus and sustain attention, disorientation, memory impairment, impaired speech, altered sensory perception, problems with the sleep wake cycle, psychomotor changes, and/or emotional problems

1. Develops over a short period of time (usually hours to days) and behavior tends to fluctuate during the course of the day; can persist up to three to six months
2. Evidence from history, physical examination, and/or laboratory findings suggests that the disturbance is caused by the direct physiological consequences of a general medical condition
3. Client tends to act out of impulse
4. If untreated can lead to seizures, stupor, coma, and death
5. Types of delirium
    a. Delirium due to ... (indicate general medical condition)
    b. Substance-intoxication delirium (indicate substance)
    c. Substance-withdrawal delirium (indicate substance)
    d. Delirium due to multiple etiologies
    e. Delirium not otherwise specified
6. Delirium may or may not be accompanied by **psychosis**
7. Prevalence in general population is 0.4%, in adults greater than 55, prevalence is 1.1%
8. Delirium is commonly seen in intensive care units, geriatric units, medical surgical units, geriatric psychiatry units, emergency departments, alcohol/drug treatment centers, oncology units, and in general, hospitalized clients

B. ***Dementia***: a chronic, usually progressive irreversible brain disorder characterized by impairments in memory, deterioration in language/speech, motor dysfunction, sensory deficits, diminished ability to perform activities of daily living, disturbance in executive functioning, reduced or absence of abstract thinking, and impaired judgment

   1. Chronic development of multiple cognitive deficits manifested by memory impairment (must have memory impairment for a diagnosis to occur) in addition to one or more of the following cognitive disturbances:
      a. **Aphasia**, a loss of the ability to understand or use language speech
      b. **Apraxia**, an inability to carry out skilled and purposeful movement; the inability to use objects properly
      c. **Agnosia**, an inability to recognize familiar situations, people, or stimuli; not related to impairment in sensory organs
      d. Disturbance in **executive functioning** (i.e., planning, organizing, sequencing, abstracting)
   2. Course is insidious and progressive, characterized by gradual onset and continuing cognitive decline
   3. Cognitive deficits cause a significant impairment in social, occupational, and/or vocational functioning and represent a significant decline from previous level of functioning
   4. May or may not be accompanied by behavioral changes, psychosis, and/or mood changes
   5. Types of dementia
      a. Dementia of the Alzheimer's type
      b. Vascular dementia (formerly multi-infarct dementia)
      c. Dementia due to other general medical conditions (indicate medical condition)
      d. Substance-induced persisting dementia (indicate substance)
      e. Dementia due to multiple etiologies
      f. Dementia due to substance withdrawal (indicate substance)
      g. Dementia not otherwise specified

C. **Amnestic disorders**
   1. Development of memory impairment characterized by inability to learn new information or inability to recall previously learned information
   2. Can be transient lasting for one month or less, or chronic lasting for more than one month
   3. Diagnosis is not made if problems with memory occurred exclusively during a state of delirium
   4. Diagnosis is not made if cognitive deficits are present that are representative of dementia
   5. Causes significant impairment in social occupational and/or vocational functioning that represents a significant decline from a previous level of functioning
   6. Types of amnestic disorders
      a. Amnestic disorder due to … (indicate the general medical condition)
      b. Substance-induced persisting amnestic disorder (indicate substance)
      c. Amnestic disorder not otherwise specified

D. **Other cognitive disorders**
   1. Cognitive dysfunction caused by a direct physiological effect of a general medical condition that does not meet criteria for any of the specific delirium, dementia, or amnestic disorders
   2. Cognitive disorders not otherwise specified
      a. Mild neurocognitive disorder: diagnosed secondary to results of neuropsychological testing or clinical assessment
      b. Postconcussional disorder: occurs after head trauma

Practice to Pass

A 74-year-old client is hospitalized for a fractured hip and is not scheduled for surgery until early the next morning. The client is alone, with no family available. She is administered morphine for pain. As the sun goes down, she is disoriented × 2, has memory loss, difficulty sleeping, and screams and yells. Identify two to three possible explanations for the behavior.

II. ETIOLOGY

    A. Delirium is caused by pathophysiological effects of medical problems, substances, and or multiple etiologies; the precise effect on the brain is dependent on etiology, and may be due to hypoxia and/or neurotransmission dysregulation

    B. Dementia due to general medical conditions: pathophysiological effects are dependent on precise etiology of dementia; cause is related to pathophysiological insult or changes to cerebral tissue/neuronal function; examples include the following:

      1. Decreased cerebral blood flow: i.e., cardiac dysrhythmias or arrest, shock, hypertension, congestive heart failure, cerebrovascular attack, transient ischemic attacks, pulmonary embolism, systemic lupus erythematosus

      2. Brain hypoxia: i.e., chronic obstructive pulmonary disease, asthma, emphysema, anemia, carbon monoxide poisoning

      3. Vitamin deficiency: (deficiencies in thiamine, niacin, and/or folic acid) i.e., caused by alcoholism, pernicious anemia, Wernicke's disease, Korsakoff's syndrome

      4. Infections: i.e., sepsis, subacute bacterial endocarditis, pneumonia, urinary tract infection, human immunodeficiency virus

      5. Endocrine and metabolic disorders: i.e., hypoglycemia, insulin shock, hypothyroidism, adrenal insufficiency, electrolyte imbalances, acidosis, alkalosis

      6. Hepatic and renal failure: i.e., hepatic encephalopathy; end-stage renal disease

      7. Neurological degeneration: i.e., Alzheimer's disease, Creutzfeldt-Jakob disease, Parkinson's disease, Huntington's chorea, multiple sclerosis

      8. Autoimmune disorders: i.e., temporal arteritis, systemic lupus erythematosus

      9. Traumatic brain injury

      10. Brain tumors: i.e., benign or malignant carcinomas

    C. Substance-induced cognitive disorders

      1. Prescribed medications: i.e., antiepileptics, neuroleptics, anxiolytics, antidepressants, cardiovascular medications, antineoplastics, hormones; chemotherapeutic agents

      2. Exposure to toxic substances: i.e., lead, aluminum, heavy metals

      3. Substance use/abuse: i.e., alcohol, cannabis, cocaine, hallucinogens, anxiolytics, opioids

      4. Withdrawal states: reduction or abrupt termination in use of substance, i.e., alcohol, sedatives, hypnotics, anxiolytics, or illicit drugs

Practice to Pass

A client has just been admitted to the emergency department and is manifesting with confusion, combativeness, and restlessness. What information should you obtain first? Identify one to two screening tools you might use on the client.

III. ASSESSMENT

    A. Delirium has a sudden onset and an identifiable cause

      1. A positive diagnosis of delirium includes the following:

        a. A thorough history and physical and medical evaluation

        b. An abnormal electroencephalogram (EEG) confirming cerebral dysfunction

        c. Several examinations should be done throughout the day to detect fluctuations in levels of consciousness that characterize the syndrome

        d. Abnormal laboratory and/or diagnostic testing (i.e., x-ray, MRI, CAT scan) that identify underlying etiology of delirium

        e. Rule out of other disorders that may mimic the symptoms of delirium (i.e., acute stress disorder, mood disorders, anxiety disorders, psychotic disorders)

      2. Assessment of signs and symptoms

        a. Fluctuating levels of consciousness (i.e., alternating periods of coherence with periods of confusion); disorientation worsens at the end of the day, referred to as **sundown syndrome**

        b. Alternating patterns of hyperactive (typical of drug withdrawal) to hypoactive (typical of metabolic imbalance) states

    c. Hyperactive responses
        1) Autonomic hyperactivity: i.e., increased blood pressure, pulse, dilated pupils
        2) Restlessness, picking at clothes or bed linen, irritability, euphoria
        3) Calling out for help, striking out at others, bizarre and destructive behavior, combativeness, anger, profanity

    d. Hypoactive responses
        1) Lethargy, apathy, withdrawn behavior
        2) Reduced alertness or awareness of environment

    e. Affective changes: may be labile, manifested by mood swings such as anger, euphoria, apathy, agitation, depression, anxiety

    f. Cognitive changes
        1) Disorganized thought process such as frightening delusions
        2) Diminished ability to focus attention, easily distracted
        3) Disorientation to person, place, and/or time
        4) Impairment in recent and remote memory (recent memory loss is more common)
        5) Alteration in sensory perception such as illusions, hallucinations (i.e., auditory, visual, gustatory, tactile, olfactory)

    g. Sleep pattern disturbances
        1) Vivid/terrifying dreams or nightmares
        2) Excessive sleepiness during the day
        3) Inability to sleep at night

    h. Speech/language problems
        1) Dysarthria: problem with articulation
        2) Dysnomia: impaired ability to name an object
        3) Dysgraphia: impaired ability to write
        4) Aphasia: difficulty getting ideas to words

B. Dementia

  1. A positive diagnosis of dementia must include the following:
    a. A thorough history and physical and medical evaluation
    b. Memory impairment is required for diagnosis (usually recent and remote) and one or more of the following: aphasia, apraxia, agnosia, problems with executive functioning
    c. Abnormal laboratory and/or diagnostic testing (i.e., x-ray, MRI, CAT scan) to identify underlying etiology of dementia
    d. Rule out other disorders that may mimic the symptoms of dementia (i.e., amnestic disorder, schizophrenia, major depressive disorder)

  2. Assessment of signs and symptoms
    a. Affective changes: client may be extremely sensitive to stressors, affect may be labile and can include anger, euphoria, apathy, agitation, depression, anxiety
    b. Cognitive changes
        1) If psychotic, disorganized thought process such as frightening delusions
        2) Diminished ability to focus attention, easily distracted
        3) Disorientation to person, place, and/or time
        4) Impairment in recent and remote memory
        5) If psychotic, alteration in sensory perception such as illusions, hallucinations (i.e., auditory, visual, gustatory, tactile, olfactory), or may have agnosia (difficulty recognizing objects)
        6) Problems with executive functioning: i.e., inability to plan, work, budget, drive
        7) Inability to use tools: i.e., washing machine, dishwasher, oven
    c. Sleep pattern disturbances
        1) Vivid/terrifying dreams or nightmares
        2) Excessive sleepiness during the day
        3) Inability to sleep at night

    d. Speech/language problems
      1) Aphasia
      2) Vague and empty speech (i.e., says it, thing)
      3) Mutism
      4) Echolalia (repeating words said by others)
      5) Slurred speech
    e. Motor activity problems
      1) Apraxia: problems with dressing, drawing, cooking
      2) Problems with gait (i.e., unstable, wobbly, prone to falls)
    f. Behavioral problems
      1) Boundary violations
      2) Inappropriate jokes, disinhibited behavior

C. Specific progressive stages of dementia of Alzheimer's type (may similarly occur in other dementia disorders) in persons with Alzheimer's disease, the disorder usually progresses over a period of years from Stage 1 to Stage 3

  1. Stage 1: mild (typically lasts one to three years)
    a. Difficulty performing complex tasks related to a decline in recent memory; forgetfulness, missed appointments; clients has insight into and are frightened by their confusion
    b. Declining personal appearance, inappropriate dress for weather
    c. Lack of spontaneity in verbal and non-verbal communication
    d. Disoriented to time but can remember people and places
    e. Decreased concentration, increased distractibility, impaired judgment

  2. Stage 2: moderate (lasting approximately two to ten years)
    a. Poor impulse control with frequent outbursts and tantrums; labile emotions; **catastrophic reactions** or overreactions to minor stresses occur frequently in demented clients
    b. Wandering or aggressive behavior, psychotic episodes such as hallucinations and/or delusions
    c. Aphasia, initially the inability to "find words" progresses to a limitation of the use of as few as six words
    d. **Hyperorality**, the need to examine, taste, and masticate (chew) any object small enough to be placed in the oral cavity
    e. **Perseveration phenomena**, repetitive behaviors such as lip licking, finger tapping, pacing, and/or echolalia
    f. **Confabulation**, the filling in of memory gaps with imaginary information in an attempt to distract others from observing the deficit
    g. **Agraphia**, the inability to read or write
    h. Agnosia, the inability to recognize familiar situations, people, or stimuli; can occur as auditory, visual, or tactile impairments
      1) **Auditory agnosia** is the inability to recognize familiar sounds such as a ringing doorbell or telephone
      2) **Astereognosis**, or tactile agnosia, is the inability to identify familiar objects such as a comb or pencil when placed in the hand
      3) **Alexia**, or visual agnosia, is the inability to identify an object or its use by sight such as a toothbrush or telephone

  3. Stage 3: severe (lasting eight to ten years before death occurs)
    a. Kluver-Bucy syndrome develops, which includes the continuation of hyperorality and the development of binge eating

Practice to Pass

A client with dementia secondary to Huntington's chorea is admitted to the geriatric psychiatric unit secondary to behavioral issues (he is combative) and manifests psychotic features (visual hallucinations and delusions). Explain what medications you might administer for mood, psychosis, and/or anxiety.

      b. Hyperetamorphosis, the need to compulsively examine and touch every object in the environment

      c. Progressive deterioration in motor ability including inability to walk, sit up, or smile

      d. Progressive decrease in response to environmental stimuli leading to total non-responsiveness or vegetative state

      e. Severe decline in cognitive function; losing ability to recognize others or even self

      f. May scream spontaneously or be able to say only one word; frequently becomes mute

  D. Screening tools for cognitive disorders

    1. Folstein Mini-Mental State Examination: an organic screening tool useful for differentiating dementia from functional states (see Box 10-1 for sample items)

      a. Total score of 30 points

      b. Score of 9–12 indicates a high likelihood of organic illness

    2. Cognitive Performance Scale: a subscale from the nursing home Minimum Data Set

      a. Ranges from 0 (cognitively intact) to 6 (very severe cognitive impairment)

      b. Items assessed on the MDS include comatose, short-term memory, decision-making ability, making self understood, eating ability, and self-performance

    3. Geriatric Depression Screening Scale

      a. Useful screening tool specifically developed for older adults to screen for possible depression (symptoms can mimic dementia)

      b. A 15- or 30-item questionnaire with dichotomous "yes" or "no" answers; easy to administer in approximately 15 to 20 minutes; certain items are reverse-scored for more accurate assessment

      c. Results indicate absence of or mild depression (0 to 10), moderate depression (11 to 20) or severe depression (21 to 30) (when using the longer 30-item questionnaire)

  E. Differentiating between delirium, dementia, and depression

    1. Delirium may coexist with dementia, making accurate assessment and appropriate treatment difficult; see Table 10-1 for comparisons between delirium and dementia

    2. Because depression can be overlooked in older adults or interpreted as early dementia, see Table 10-2 for comparisons between dementia and depression

---

Box 10-1	**Orientation to Time**
Sample Items from the Mini-Mental State Examination (MMSE)	"What is the date?"

Orientation to Time
"What is the date?"

Registration
"Listen carefully, I am going to say three words. You say them back after I stop. Ready? Here they are...
HOUSE (pause), CAR (pause), LAKE (pause). Now repeat those words back to me."
[Repeat up to 5 times, but score only the first trial.]

Naming
"What is this?" [Point to a pencil or pen.]

Reading
"Please read this and do what it says." [Show examinee the words on the stimulus form.] CLOSE YOUR EYES

Table 10-1   **Comparisons between Delirium and Dementia**

Delirium	Dementia
Onset is usually sudden; acute development	Onset is insidious and progressive; chronic development
Caused by temporary, reversible disturbance in brain function	Caused by irreversible alteration of brain function
Duration: hours to days	Duration: months to years
EEG: diffuse slowing of fast cycles related to state of excitement	EEG: normal or mildly slow
Disturbed attention, learning, and thinking, poor perception	Impaired memory, both recent and remote
Disorientation, impairments in judgment, abstract thinking, and learning	Impaired memory (recent memory affected before remote memory)
Orientation: fluctuates throughout day; periods of lucidity; sundown syndrome (worsens at night)	Progressively loses orientation to person, place, and time—loses time orientation first, then place, then person; sundown syndrome
Hallucinations, delusions, illusions	Change in personality; normal peculiarities are exaggerated: suspicious—paranoid, compulsive—rigid, orderliness
Labile affect	Labile affect; prone to apathy, depression, withdrawal, stubbornness in attempt to cope with surroundings and decreased abilities
Act on impulse, loss of usual social behavior	Decreased inhibitions; restlessness, agitation, especially if coerced; inflexible—routine important, anxiety, rage, despair
Coping mechanisms—none, no psychological impairment	Uses denial and repression—confabulation to make up for memory loss
Normal or mild misnaming of objects	Aphasia, agnosia, agraphia in later stages
Nursing Interventions	*Nursing Interventions*
Maintain nutrition and fluid balance, could be life-threatening	Not usually life-threatening
Restrain only when necessary since it increases agitation and fear; safety is a priority; one-on-one observation	Individualized attention, consistent social interaction, group activities, exercise, stimulation of senses, active during the day
Repetitive orientation, don't reinforce hallucinations; lighted room, family members present	Lighted room, personal belongings, clear simple instructions; find out source of anxiety, try to alleviate—coping mechanisms to defend self become emphasized during anxiety

Table 10-2   **Comparisons between Dementia and Depression**

Dementia	Depression
Onset slow and progressive, difficult to pinpoint onset	Onset relatively rapid, can be traced to distressing event or situation
Recent memory is impaired, attempts to hide cognitive losses with confabulation	Readily admits to memory loss; other cognitive impairments may or may not be present; can recall recent events
Affect is shallow and labile	Depressed mood is pervasive
Attention and concentration may be impaired	Attention and concentration usually intact
Unable to recognize familiar people and places, may get lost easily, disoriented to time	Oriented to person, place, and time
Approximate "near miss" answers are common, tries to answer	"Don't know" answers are common, refuses to participate in activities, prefers to be left alone
Changes in personality (from cheerful and easy-going to angry to suspicious)	Personality remains stable
Struggles to perform ADLs, is frustrated as a result	Apathetic to performing ADLs, loses interest in appearance
Appetite and sleep patterns may not be affected	Changes in appetite, weight, and sleep pattern

IV. NURSING DIAGNOSES/ANALYSIS

A. Priority nursing diagnoses for persons with cognitive impairment

1. Acute Confusion related to alcohol or drug abuse, medication ingestion, fluid and electrolyte imbalances, infection

2. Risk for Injury or Risk for Trauma related to aggressive behavior, labile emotions, impaired judgment, illusions, delusions, hallucinations, and/or wandering

3. Anxiety related to fear of cognitive and behavioral deficits

4. Disturbed Thought Processes related to distractibility, decreasing judgment, memory loss, delusions

5. Bathing/hygiene/dressing/grooming/feeding Self-Care Deficit related to inability to sequence skills necessary to perform these skills, agitation, confusion, delusions and/or hallucinations

6. Impaired Verbal Communication related to aphasia, agraphia, agnosia

7. Disturbed Sleep Pattern related to fear, anxiety, sundowning, agitation, inability to sleep

8. Disturbed Sensory Perception related to illusions and/or hallucinations (olfactory, gustatory, tactile, visual, auditory)

B. Priority nursing diagnoses for persons with dementia (in addition to the above)

1. Compromised/disabling Ineffective Family Coping related to changing roles, physical exhaustion, financial problems

2. Risk for and/or Caregiver Role Strain related to lack of respite resources or support from significant others, unpredictable illness course, insufficient finances, aggressive behavior, or emotional outbursts of client

3. Disturbed Sensory Perception (specify visual/auditory/tactile/gustatory, olfactory) related to biochemical imbalances

4. Disturbed Self-Esteem related to loss of independent functioning, loss of capacity for remembering, loss of capability for effective verbal communication

5. Risk for Violence: Self-Directed or Directed at Others related to confusion, agitated state, suicidal ideation, delusions, hallucinations, and/or illusions

6. Imbalanced Nutrition Less Than Bodily Requirements related to confusion, agitation, refusal to eat, no memory of eating

7. Risk for Fluid and Electrolyte Imbalance related to confusion, refusal to drink, agitation, no memory of need to drink fluids or last time of fluid intake

V. PLANNING AND IMPLEMENTATION

A. Specific treatment modalities

1. Psychopharmacology for treatment of underlying disorder

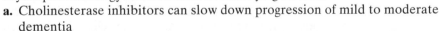

   a. Cholinesterase inhibitors can slow down progression of mild to moderate dementia

   1) Tacrine (Cognex) effects can be seen in six weeks; can cause elevation in liver enzymes; discontinue therapy if occurs

   2) Donepezil (Aricept) slows deterioration of mild to moderate dementia without serious liver toxicity attributed to tacrine

   3) Rivastigmine (Exelon)

   4) Galantamine (Reminyl); side effects include nausea and diarrhea

   b. NMDA (n–methyl–D–aspartate) receptor modulator: memantine (Namenda), decreases glutamate transmission by blocking NMDA receptors

2. Treatment of target symptoms

   a. Treatment of anxiety

   1) Lorazepam (Ativan) has less drug accumulation and leads to less confusion than longer acting anxiolytics; monitor for sedation and potential for falls

Practice to Pass

Compare and contrast the three stages of Alzheimer's disease.

2) Trazodone (Desyrel) can decrease agitation and aggression without decreasing cognitive performance; because of sedating effects, can also help with sleep

3) Buspirone (Buspar) is not sedating and has fewer side effects; preferable to benzodiazepines; can take up to four weeks to be effective

b. Treatment of depression

1) Selective serotonin reuptake inhibitors (SSRIs) are better tolerated in older adults than tricyclic antidepressants, which have high anticholinergic and cardiac side effects

2) SSRIs include fluoxetine (Prozac), paroxetine (Paxil), sertraline (Zoloft), nefazodone (Serzone)

3) Typical antidepressant mirtazapine (Remeron) facilitates sleep and stimulates appetite so is useful for clients with insomnia and decreased appetite

c. Treatment of psychosis/behavioral disturbances

1) Antipsychotics effective in the treatment of psychosis related to cognitive dysfunction are the typical antipsychotic olanzapine (Zyprexa) and the atypical antipsychotic haloperidol (Haldol)

2) Antipsychotics should initially be prescribed in low doses

3) The typical antipsychotic haloperidol can cause tardive dyskinesia, extrapyramidal, and anticholinergic side effects

d. Treatment of agitation/behavioral disturbances

1) Mood stabilizers can facilitate a reduction in behavioral disturbances and agitation

2) Effective mood stabilizers are carbamazepine (Tegretol), valproic acid (Depakote), and gabapentin (Neurontin)

B. Behavior modification

1. Physical restraints should be used only as a last resort for persons who are a danger to self or others; agency-specific policy regarding restraints must be adhered to

2. Safety: sensor devices alert staff when a client is wandering, either out of bed, chair, room, or unit; the client should be placed on one-to-one nursing care when a danger to self or others

3. Reality orientation: reorient client to reality when applicable (sometimes not effective in late stages), place labels on objects in the environment, use large-print calendars and clocks, discuss meaningful topics such as significant life events (i.e., family, work, hobbies), place pictures of family members in room, play music that client can relate to

4. Therapeutic communication: do not argue with client; do not argue with delusional systems and/or hallucinations; communicate in a calm, quiet voice with simple, clear instructions; set limits on untoward behavior in a firm, non-judgmental manner

5. Decreasing agitation: distract client from activity that is contributing to agitation, (i.e., take client on short walk, involve client in art, dancing, television); medicate client with anxiolytics as prescribed before escalation in agitation occurs

6. Sensory stimulation: allow client to touch various objects such as fabric, buttons, thread, pets (pet therapy); do not allow client to be overstimulated, as this can be stressful and contribute to exacerbation of untoward behaviors

C. Group and individual therapies

1. Reminiscence (life review therapy): occurs one on one or in a group; reminiscence facilitates discussion of topics that deal with specific life transitions (i.e., childhood, adolescence, marriage, childbearing, grandparenting, retirement), and/or can help trigger memories of pets, music, favorite foods, special occasions; may trigger positive or negative memories

2. Validation therapy: interaction with clients on a topic they initiate, in a place and time where they feel most secure; facilitates reality orientation; the underlying

feelings of concern should be addressed by the nurse (i.e., "You miss your husband," "You must be feeling lonely here"); emotional support should be given to client as necessary; this type of orientation/validation is geared towards person and place rather than time

D. **Milieu therapy** (see Box 10-2)

1. Special care units (are environmentally designed and specifically programmed to serve needs of residents with Alzheimer's disease and related dementias)

2. Design components of special care unit

   a. Safe, secure, specially adapted physical environment to accommodate wandering behavior inside and outside (circular unit design, secure walkway and patio)

   b. Personalized rooms with clients own furniture and familiar belongings

   c. Clean, well-maintained, well-lit environment with windows (safety)

   d. Stimuli from birdcage, fish aquarium, or other pets

   e. Location adjacent to child daycare programs so that multigenerational interaction occurs

3. Structured programs and activities that provide quality interaction between staff, residents, and families, such as art therapy, music therapy, spiritual groups, pet therapy, dance, exercise

4. Caring, consistent, well-trained multidisciplinary staff; special training programs that lead to certification in caring for clients with dementia are available and encouraged

5. Interdisciplinary care: psychiatry, nursing, physical therapy, occupational therapy, speech therapy, dietary, social work, working as a team to improve quality of life for clients in all areas

E. **Community resources**

1. Refer family to Alzheimer's association or other dementia-related organizations

2. Encourage family/significant other to utilize respite care resources

Practice to Pass

You are the nurse manager of a special care unit for clients with dementia. The wife of a newly admitted client approaches you and says, "I can't take care of him all by myself any longer, but I feel that I am betraying him by placing him in a nursing home." How would you respond?

Box 10-2	The following interventions should be incorporated into the care of confused clients:
Nursing Interventions for Clients with Cognitive Impairment	• Provide simple, clear instructions focusing on one task at a time. • Break tasks into very small steps. • Speak slowly and in a face-to-face position when communicating with clients known to have a hearing loss. Shouting causes distortion of high-pitched sounds and can frighten the client. • Allow the client to have familiar objects around him or her to maintain reality orientation and enhance self-worth and dignity. • Discuss topics that are meaningful to the client such as significant life events, family, work, hobbies, and pets. • Refrain from arguing or convincing client that delusions, illusions and/or hallucinations are not real. • Provide a simple, structured environment with consistent personnel to minimize confusion and provide a sense of security and stability in the client's environment. Stimuli should be balanced. • Encourage reminiscence and discussion of life review by sharing things such as picture albums, personal objects, and familiar music. • Discuss family traditions and holidays, memories of school, courtship, dating rituals, children, grandchildren, favorite pets, and other significant past events. • Encourage family/caregivers to express feelings, particularly frustration and anger. Encourage family/caregiver to seek respite care when needed. • Provide a list of community resources and support groups available to assist in decreasing stress and role strain for the family/caregiver.

3. Refer family to social services when necessary for resources, short-term/long-term counseling, legal/ethical concerns
4. Referral to hospice services when indicated (i.e., Stage 3 of Alzheimer's disease)

F. **Meeting life-sustaining nutritional and fluid management needs**
1. Weigh client daily, calculate BMI
2. Calculate client's daily caloric intake when applicable
3. Offer small frequent meals rich in carbohydrates and protein (six small meals if client cannot tolerate three large meals per day)
4. Offer nutritious finger foods such as sandwiches, crackers, cheese, and fruit
5. Offer drinks that are high in vitamins, minerals, and electrolytes throughout the day
6. Assess fluid and electrolyte status
7. Monitor urinary output every eight hours
8. Monitor laboratory studies as indicated for dehydration: blood urea nitrogen (BUN), creatinine, hematocrit, and lithium levels
9. Monitor laboratory studies as indicated for nutritional balance: pre-albumin, albumin, ferritin, hemoglobin, and hematocrit levels
10. Assess bowel movements daily for frequency and consistency, obtain order for laxatives or stimulants when indicated
11. Assess for abdominal pain or discomfort
12. Administer high-fiber foods unless contraindicated
13. Offer frequent fluids to maintain hydration, encourage 2000 mLs in 24 hours unless contraindicated
14. Monitor and record daily input and output

VI. EVALUATION/OUTCOMES

A. **Client will remain free of injury** as evidenced by absence of being lost from wandering, falls, fractures, bruises, contusions, or burns
B. **Client will participate in self-care** (i.e., feeding, grooming, dressing) at optimal level with appropriate degree of supervision and guidance to maintain independence
C. **Client will communicate basic needs** with the use of visual and/or verbal clues
D. **Caregivers will demonstrate adaptive coping strategies** for dealing with the stress of the caregiver role
E. **Client will interact with others** in group activities and maintain anxiety level at a minimum in response to frustrating/stressful situations
F. **Client will sleep** five to seven hours per night and nap one to two hours per day
G. **Client will maintain adequate nutrition and hydration**

VII. SPECIFIC DISORDERS

A. **Labels for specific disorders** are those identified in the *Diagnostic and Statistical Manual of Mental Disorders 4th Edition Text Revision* (APA, 2000); descriptions are adapted and summarized
B. **Delirium** (APA, 2000)
1. Due to (general medical condition): there is evidence from history, physical assessment, or laboratory test results that the disturbance is directly caused by a general medical condition (e.g., delirium due to hepatic encephalopathy)
2. Substance-intoxication delirium: symptoms developed during substance intoxication or medication use (e.g., alcohol intoxication delirium)
3. Substance-withdrawal delirium: symptoms developed during, or shortly after, a withdrawal syndrome (e.g., alcohol withdrawal delirium)
4. Delirium due to multiple etiologies: symptoms developed because of a general medical condition plus substance intoxication or medication side effect

   5. Delirium not otherwise specified (NOS): symptoms are suspected to be caused by a general medical condition or substance use, but there is insufficient evidence to establish a specific etiology

C. Dementia (APA, 2000)

   1. Dementia of the Alzheimer's type (DAT): cognitive deficits are not caused by other central nervous system conditions known to cause progressive deficits in memory or cognition (e.g., cerebrovascular disease, Parkinson's disease, Huntington's disease, subdural hematoma, normal-pressure hydrocephalus, brain tumor) or systemic conditions known to cause dementia (e.g., hypothyroidism, vitamin deficiencies, hypercalcemia, neurosyphilis, HIV infection) or substance-induced conditions (e.g., dementia of the Alzheimer's type with early onset; with depressed mood)

   a. Late onset dementia of the Alzheimer's type: occurs in people over age 65; characteristic findings are loss of nerve cells and the presence of plaques on neurons and tangles on neuron fibers (see Figure 10-1)

   b. Early onset dementia: occurs in people under age 65

   c. Diagnosis is usually made by ruling out causes for clients' symptoms; neuroimaging is used to see brain atrophy

   2. Vascular dementia (formerly multi-infarct dementia): focal neurological signs and symptoms or laboratory test results indicative of cerebrovascular disease are judged to be etiologically related to the disturbance (e.g., vascular dementia, uncomplicated)

   3. Dementia due to other general medical conditions: physiological evidence that the disturbance is directly the result of HIV disease, head trauma, Parkinson's disease,

Figure 10-1

Neuron with neurofibrillary tangles seen in Alzheimer's disease

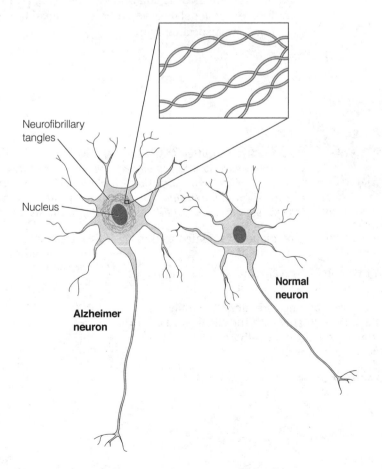

Neurofibrillary tangles

Nucleus

Alzheimer neuron

Normal neuron

Huntington's disease, Pick's disease, Creutzfeldt-Jakob disease, hypothyroidism, brain tumor, or vitamin deficiency (e.g., dementia due to HIV disease)

4. Substance-induced persisting dementia: physiological evidence that the deficits are caused by the persisting effects of substance use (e.g., a drug of abuse, a medication) (e.g., alcohol-induced persisting dementia)

5. Dementia due to multiple etiologies: physiological evidence that the disturbance has more than one etiology (e.g., head trauma plus chronic alcohol use, dementia of the Alzheimer's type with subsequent development of vascular dementia)

6. Dementia not otherwise specified (NOS): clinical presentation of dementia for which there is insufficient evidence to establish a specific etiology

D. **Amnestic disorders** (APA, 2000)

1. Amnestic disorder due to (general medical condition): there is evidence from history, physical assessment, or laboratory findings that the disturbance is directly caused by a general medical condition (e.g., amnestic disorder due to head trauma)

2. Substance-induced persisting amnestic disorder: physiological evidence that the memory disturbance is related to the persisting effects of drug abuse or medication use (e.g., alcohol-induced persisting amnestic disorder)

3. Amnestic disorder not otherwise specified: clinical presentation of amnesia for which there is insufficient evidence to establish a specific etiology

E. **Cognitive disorder** not otherwise specified (APA, 2000)

1. Mild neurocognitive disorder: impairment in cognitive functioning as evidenced by neuropsychological testing or clinical assessment accompanied by objective evidence of a general medical condition or central nervous system dysfunction

2. Postconcussional disorder: following a head trauma, impairment in memory or attention with associated symptoms

Case Study

An 85-year-old female client was admitted to the hospital two weeks ago with laboratory test that reveal a urinary tract infection and dehydration. She is placed on intravenous fluids and intravenous antibiotics. She manifests intervals of disorientation, confusion, combativeness, and memory impairment, particularly at night. She has pulled her IV and indwelling urinary catheter out twice on your shift. She has blood in her urine, and is not receiving her antibiotics/fluids as needed due to this behavior.

1. Identify two nursing diagnoses related to the behavioral care of the client.

2. List two outcome/evaluation criteria that might be appropriate for the client.

3. A sitter (one-on-one care) and the family are not available to stay with the client. Would you or would you not physically restrain the client. Explain your answer.

4. List and describe at least four nursing interventions aimed at promoting safety and security for the client.

5. What follow-up assessments will you make to continue to monitor her status?

For suggested responses, see pages 299–300.

POSTTEST

1 A confused wheelchair-bound client diagnosed with dementia of Alzheimer's type is homebound. Although she has no contact with men, she says to the home health nurse, "I have a date tonight for the Valentine's dance." What is the most appropriate response by the nurse?

1. "You're confused again. There isn't a dance tonight and this isn't Valentine's Day."
2. "I didn't think your spouse was still living. Who is your date with?"
3. "I think you need some more medication. I'll be right back with your shot."
4. "Today is January 11th. Tell me about some of the other dances you've been to."

2 The nurse is teaching a family caregiver how to help a family member with stage 1 dementia secondary to Alzheimer's disease complete activities of daily living. Which information should be included in the teaching?

1. Perform ADLs for the client.
2. Have the client plan a schedule for ADLs.
3. Give the client ample time to perform the ADLs as independently as possible.
4. Tell the client that the ADLs must be finished by 9:00 a.m.

3 When working with a client who has dementia, the primary intervention by the nurse is to ensure which of the following?

1. Client is offered dietary choices to stimulate appetite.
2. Client meets other clients with dementia to prevent social isolation.
3. Client discusses feelings of fear and loss to prevent low self-esteem and anxiety.
4. Client remains in a safe and secure environment to prevent injury.

4 A female client is going to be admitted to the geriatric psychiatric unit with a diagnosis of dementia secondary to stage 2 Alzheimer's disease (AD). The psychiatric emergency room nurse providing the admission report informs the unit nurse she has behavioral disturbances, primarily aggressive. The admitting nurse anticipates which of the following? Select all that apply.

1. The client probably cannot recognize herself in the mirror.
2. The client will consistently socialize with other clients on the unit.
3. The client needs constant supervision.
4. The aggressive behavior may be secondary to depression.
5. The client will be wheelchair-bound.

5 A delirious client was recently released from soft bilateral wrist and ankle restraints. Suddenly, the client begins to beat the sheets and yell, "Get those bugs away from me! They're all over! Get them!" What is the best initial response by the nurse?

1. "What kind of bugs are on you?"
2. "Those are just little bugs, they won't hurt you."
3. "You're seeing bugs because you are sick, but I don't see any bugs on you."
4. "Just hold very still and the bugs will crawl away."

6 The nurse is caring for a female client on the inpatient psychiatric unit who has dementia. When the nurse asks who her support persons are, she says her husband takes care of her. Her history and physical indicate that she has been widowed for six years. The nurse concludes she is confabulating and draws which conclusions?

1. The client is untruthful about her husband.
2. The client's response may be due to her inability to remember an answer.
3. Confabulation is also known as amnesia.
4. Disturbed sleep often causes confabulation.
5. Confabulation is a means for persons with dementia to make up for their cognitive losses.

7 The client has a medical diagnosis of dementia. The nurse observes that when anyone speaks loudly or harshly to the client, the client cries out, retreats to bed, shivers, and covers the head. When documenting and giving intershift report, how should the nurse should refer to the client's behavior?

1. Pseudodementia
2. Pseudodelirium
3. Catastrophic reaction
4. Sundown syndrome

8 A client with dementia has been admitted to a nursing home. Which nursing intervention will help the client maintain optimal cognitive function?

1. Discuss pictures of children and grandchildren with the client.
2. Play word games and do crossword puzzles with the client.
3. Watch the evening news on the television with the client.
4. Provide the client with a list of tasks to perform each day.

9 The nurse wishes to improve the hydration status of the confused client. Which action should the nurse take?

1. Place a pitcher of water at the bedside.
2. Offer fruit juice, soft drinks, or water every two hours while awake.
3. Instruct all staff members to stop by and offer fluids frequently.
4. Instruct a family member to sit with the client and offer fluids frequently.

10 A client who scores 11 out of 30 on the Mini-Mental State Examination asks the nurse what this score might mean. The nurse's response will convey that this score suggests a high likelihood of which of the following?

1. Educational deficiencies
2. Bipolar disease
3. Brain dysfunction or disease
4. Low self-esteem

➤ *See pages 208–210 for Answers and Rationales.*

ANSWERS & RATIONALES

Pretest

1 **Answer: 2** **Rationale:** Physiological and safety needs take precedence over psychological needs. Therefore, of the options given, assuring adequate hydration is the highest priority. If hydration is not maintained, the delirium will intensify, and the client will become at risk for various physiological complications, ultimately even death. Anxiety and fear are common experiences when the client is delirious. When present, they complicate management of delirium. However, these are psychological experiences and have lesser priority than basic physiological or safety needs. Turning and repositioning is very important to prevent future problems, but this physical measure is not a basic requirement for maintaining life.

Maintaining adequate hydration is critical to continuation of life and, therefore, takes priority. The client who is delirious is generally disoriented, and the nurse should make frequent attempts to reorient the client. However, providing basic safety and maintaining basic physiologic needs are always of highest priority. **Cognitive Level:** Analyzing **Client Need:** Physiological Adaptation **Integrated Process:** Nursing Process: Planning **Content Area:** Mental Health **Strategy:** Ask the question, "What's the worst thing that could happen to this client?" The answer is, of course, "The client could die." Use this common sense approach to answer this question. **Reference:** Varcarolis, E., & Halter, M. (2010). *Foundations of psychiatric mental health nursing: A clinical approach* (6th ed.). St. Louis, MO: Saunders Elsevier, p. 64.

2 **Answer: 1, 2, 4, 5** **Rationale:** Four options are correct. The onset of delirium is acute versus progressive. The client is manifesting changes in behavior that are acute. Death can result if delirium is not treated. Due to the confusion and combativeness the client could be at risk for injury (i.e., pull IV out, try to get out of bed, hit hand on side rail). Many untoward behaviors (i.e., combativeness) in clients with delirium are impulsive, and so sometimes unpredictable. The onset of dementia is progressive versus acute. **Cognitive Level:** Analyzing **Client Need:** Psychosocial Integrity **Integrated Process:** Nursing Process: Assessment **Content Area:** Mental Health **Strategy:** It is important to differentiate the onset of dementia versus delirium since behaviors may be similar. Also, assessment of potential for injury is imperative because clients with delirium, due to impulsiveness, are at risk for injury. **Reference:** Stuart, G.W., (2009). *Principles and Practice of Psychiatric Nursing* (9th ed.). St. Louis, MO: Mosby, Elsevier, pp. 390, 391.

3 **Answer: 1, 4, 5** **Rationale:** Because the physical consequences of alcohol withdrawal can be lethal, they take precedence over psychological concerns. Clients with delirium associated with alcohol withdrawal typically fluctuate between hyperalertness and under-reactivity to the environment, which is unpredictable and can occur rapidly. Presenting signs and symptoms of delirium caused by withdrawal from alcohol include hyperactive behaviors such as restlessness and irritability. When coupled with unpredictable changes in level of awareness and impaired judgment, these symptoms place the client at risk for injury. Clients in active withdrawal from alcohol are at high risk for seizures. One reason for using benzodiazepines as the cross-tolerant agents for medically supervised withdrawal is that most of them have anticonvulsant effects. Physical consequences of alcohol withdrawal can be lethal and take precedence over any psychological considerations, including self-esteem enhancement. Impaired coping can be addressed if needed once physiological status is stabilized. **Cognitive Level:** Analyzing **Client Need:** Psychosocial Integrity **Integrated Process:** Nursing Process: Planning **Content Area:** Mental Health **Strategy:** Recall that delirium occurs because of disruptions in physiologic processes. The correct options will then be easy to determine. **Reference:** Kneisl, C., Wilson, H., & Trigoboff, E. (2009). *Contemporary psychiatric-mental health nursing* (2nd ed.). Upper Saddle River, NJ: Prentice Hall, pp. 270–271.

4 **Answer: 4** **Rationale:** Wandering behavior poses a potential risk for injury or trauma because clients experiencing dementia get lost easily and are unable to retrace their steps back to their starting point. Although the nursing diagnoses in the other options apply, maintaining the safety of these clients is of utmost importance. **Cognitive Level:** Applying **Client Need:** Psychosocial Integrity **Integrated Process:** Nursing Process: Diagnosis **Content Area:** Mental Health **Strategy:** Look beyond the presenting

behaviors of wandering and confusion and identify the risks associated with the behaviors. **Reference:** Kneisl, C., Wilson, H., & Trigoboff, E. (2009). *Contemporary psychiatric-mental health nursing* (2nd ed.). Upper Saddle River, NJ: Prentice Hall, p. 254.

5 **Answer: 2** **Rationale:** It is most important for the nurse to recognize that this spouse, like others providing care to persons with DAT, is at high risk for caregiver role-strain. Having to provide constant care to a person with declining cognitive and physical capacity can exhaust and overwhelm the caregiver. The nurse should not assume that the spouse's spiritual belief system includes worship in a church. The nurse should assess the spouse's belief system before making any recommendation for spiritual support. Reminiscence therapy is more likely to be useful to the client in early stages of dementia. While it may be useful to the spouse as part of anticipatory grieving, it is most important to recognize the high risk for caregiver role-strain. While a predictable daily routine may be generally helpful to the spouse, it is most necessary for the client. **Cognitive Level:** Applying **Client Need:** Health Promotion and Maintenance **Integrated Process:** Nursing Process: Planning **Content Area:** Mental Health **Strategy:** Consider who is the client in the question. **Reference:** Varcarolis, E., & Halter, M. (2010). *Foundations of psychiatric mental health nursing: A clinical approach* (6th ed.). St. Louis, MO: Saunders Elsevier, p. 437.

6 **Answer: 1** **Rationale:** Clients experiencing acute episodes of delirium will have periods of lucidity and will regain full orientation when the underlying cause of the delirium is identified and treated. Suicidal ideation may be seen with dementia but is not usually associated with delirium. When the client is delirious, injury is more likely to be the result of impulsive, non-intentional acts. Low self-esteem is commonly seen with dementia but is not usually found with delirium. Tactile agnosia may be seen with dementia but is not usually associated with delirium. **Cognitive Level:** Applying **Client Need:** Physiological Adaptation **Integrated Process:** Nursing Process: Planning **Content Area:** Mental Health **Strategy:** Compare and contrast usual presenting behaviors associated with delirium and dementia to determine the correct option. **Reference:** Varcarolis, E., & Halter, M. (2010). *Foundations of psychiatric mental health nursing: A clinical approach* (6th ed.). St. Louis, MO: Saunders Elsevier, p. 429.

7 **Answer: 4** **Rationale:** When attempting to increase the level of orientation of the client with dementia, non-verbal stimuli may be more effective than verbal stimuli. It is important that decorations be traditional, as the client is more likely to have intact remote memory that allows for recognition of objects from the distant past. The nurse should not assume that the client with dementia has a hearing deficit; what is present is a cognitive deficit. It will be more important for the nurse to speak simply and to repeat reorienting stimuli frequently. Except in emergency situations where client safety is compromised, the nurse should avoid giving the client with dementia untruthful or nonrealistic information (such as a deceased spouse is expected home later). Instead of reorienting the client, the news station would likely increase disorientation because the client would not be able to process the events in a normal cognitive manner. Additionally, constant stimulation would probably be overtaxing to the client. **Cognitive Level:** Analyzing **Client Need:** Physiological Adaptation **Integrated Process:** Nursing Process: Implementation **Content Area:** Mental Health **Strategy:** Recognize that sometimes a simple solution and a simple answer stand out from all the rest. This is one example of that notion. **Reference:** Kneisl, C., Wilson, H., & Trigoboff, E. (2009). *Contemporary psychiatric-mental health nursing* (2nd ed.). Upper Saddle River, NJ: Prentice Hall, p. 256.

8 **Answer: 4** **Rationale:** Donepezil (Aricept) is a cholinesterase inhibitor that appears to slow down cognitive deterioration in individuals with mild to moderate dementia. When the activity of cholinesterase is inhibited, the amount of acetylcholine in the synapse is increased. Fluoxetine is a selective serotonin reuptake inhibitor that has antidepressant action. Trazodone is a tetracyclic antidepressant. Haloperidol is an antipsychotic agent. **Cognitive Level:** Applying **Client Need:** Pharmacological and Parenteral Therapies **Integrated Process:** Teaching and Learning **Content Area:** Mental Health **Strategy:** Identify the classification and general uses of each medicine the client is receiving. **Reference:** Varcarolis, E., & Halter, M. (2010). *Foundations of psychiatric mental health nursing: A clinical approach* (6th ed.). St. Louis, MO: Saunders Elsevier, p. 445.

9 **Answer: 3** **Rationale:** Short-term memory loss is a sign of depression in the older adult that can be caused by a deficit of serotonin in the brain. Paroxetine (Paxil) blocks the reuptake of serotonin resulting in elevated levels of serotonin in the brain. Also, the nurse should keep the communication as simple as possible because the listeners may not know or understand human anatomy or commonly used medical expressions. The other three options convey inaccurate information about the effects of an antidepressant. **Cognitive Level:** Analyzing **Client Need:** Pharmacological and Parenteral Therapies **Integrated Process:** Teaching and Learning **Content Area:** Mental Health **Strategy:** Recall classification systems of antidepressants. Identify the drug class for paroxetine (Paxil). The name of the class will give you the answer to this question. **Reference:** Varcarolis, E., & Halter, M. (2010). *Foundations of psychiatric mental health nursing: A clinical approach* (6th ed.). St. Louis, MO: Saunders Elsevier, p. 710.

10 **Answer: 4** **Rationale:** Spending non-stressful time with the client helps diminish feelings of resentment, isolation, and alienation in the caregiver. Since remote memories are less diminished than recent memories, there is also

the possibility that it will also increase the client's self-esteem by allowing reminiscence of past pleasurable life events. Close supervision of the client should be provided at all times to enhance safety. However, if one caregiver remains with the client 24 hours a day, that person is at high risk for developing caregiver role-strain with feelings of resentment, isolation, and alienation. Regular periods of respite are necessary to help prevent this occurrence in caregivers. While assistance to personal hygiene and establishing a routine are important when providing care to the person with dementia, there is no prescribed time that personal hygiene should occur. Regular periods of respite are necessary for caregivers. **Cognitive Level:** Analyzing **Client Need:** Health Promotion and Maintenance **Integrated Process:** Caring **Content Area:** Mental Health **Strategy:** Notice that this question is focused on the caregiver, not the client. **Reference:** Fontaine, K., & Fletcher, C. (2009). *Mental health nursing* (6th ed.). Upper Saddle River, NJ: Prentice Hall, p. 562.

Posttest

1 **Answer: 4** **Rationale:** Using a method of reality orientation that increases self-worth and personal dignity is correct. It also allows client reminiscence, which is useful to persons with dementia as their remote memories are more intact than recent ones. By telling the client there isn't a dance and it isn't Valentine's Day, the nurse is attempting to present reality, but in a non-therapeutic manner. The statement is made in a demeaning and belittling manner. The nurse should present reality and provide orienting stimuli in a manner that preserves the client's self-esteem. Saying "I didn't think your spouse was still living" and asking who the date is with promotes further disorganization in thinking and orientation in this client with dementia. The client's statement indicates disorientation and disorganized thinking that is very common in persons with dementia. There is nothing to suggest that the client's behavior requires a prn medication (such as aggression toward others). **Cognitive Level:** Analyzing **Client Need:** Psychosocial Integrity **Integrated Process:** Communication and Documentation **Content Area:** Mental Health **Strategy:** Look for an option that presents reality and provides orienting stimuli in a manner that preserves the client's self-esteem. **Reference:** Kneisl, C., Wilson, H., & Trigoboff, E. (2009). *Contemporary psychiatric-mental health nursing* (2nd ed.). Upper Saddle River, NJ: Prentice Hall, pp. 255–256.

2 **Answer: 3** **Rationale:** Clients with early dementia should be allowed to provide their own ADLs as independently as possible for as long as possible. They will need extra time to perform tasks. It is premature to provide ADLs to the client with early dementia. This will likely be necessary at a later stage of the illness. Having the client develop a written schedule for ADLs may be overwhelming to the client and increase confusion and uncooperativeness. Giving the client a deadline by which time the ADLs must be completed may be over-whelming and, therefore, increase confusion and/or uncooperativeness. **Cognitive Level:** Analyzing **Client Need:** Psychosocial Integrity **Integrated Process:** Teaching and Learning **Content Area:** Mental Health **Strategy:** Recognize the interdependent relationship between self-esteem and independent functioning. **Reference:** Kneisl, C., Wilson, H., & Trigoboff, E. (2009). *Contemporary psychiatric-mental health nursing* (2nd ed.). Upper Saddle River, NJ: Prentice Hall, pp. 156–157.

3 **Answer: 4** **Rationale:** Client safety and security are nursing priorities for clients with the disorientation, confusion, and memory deficits seen in dementia. Dietary choices will not stimulate appetite. Additionally, recall that clients with dementia should not be expected to make choices, as this can overwhelm them. Client safety and security are nursing priorities for clients with dementia rather than social isolation or low self-esteem or anxiety. **Cognitive Level:** Analyzing **Client Need:** Psychosocial Integrity **Integrated Process:** Nursing Process: Implementation **Content Area:** Mental Health **Strategy:** Recall Maslow's hierarchy of needs or some other system that you know to be useful to assist with prioritizing. **Reference:** Fontaine, K. (2009). *Mental health nursing* (6th ed.). Upper Saddle River, NJ: Prentice Hall, pp. 564–565.

4 **Answer: 3, 4** **Rationale:** The client needing constant super-vision and the aggression being secondary to depression are correct. Stage 2 AD clients must be supervised at all times due to behavior problems and memory impair-ment that may place the client at danger to self or oth-ers. Constant supervision is necessary. The underlying etiology of aggressive symptomology in clients with stage 2 aggressive behaviors may be secondary to depression. The other three options are incorrect. Non-recognition of self occurs in stage 3 AD. Clients in stage 2 AD have impaired social skills which are variable. The inability to walk occurs in stage 3 AD. **Cognitive Level:** Analyzing **Client Need:** Psychosocial Integrity **Integrated Process:** Nursing Process: Assessment **Content Area:** Mental Health **Strategy:** Differentiating cognitive and motor symptoms of AD stages 1, 2, and 3 are imperative to the assessment process when determining appropriate nursing diagnosis. **Reference:** Stuart, G.W. (2009). *Principles and Practice of Psychiatric Nursing* (9th ed.). St. Louis, MO: Mosby, Elsevier, p. 393.

5 **Answer: 3** **Rationale:** The client is experiencing tactile hallucinations. The most appropriate response is "You're seeing bugs because you are sick, but I don't see any bugs on you," which orients the client to the reality of being sick and reassures the client of safety. By making statements that essentially agree that the bugs exist (the other three options), the nurse is commu-nicating that the hallucinated objects are real. This could make the client feel even more frightened. **Cognitive Level:** Analyzing **Client Need:** Psychosocial Integrity **Integrated Process:** Communication and Documentation **Content**

Area: Mental Health **Strategy:** Recognize the client's fear and the attendant need for safety. **Reference:** Varcarolis, E., & Halter, M. (2010). *Foundations of psychiatric mental health nursing: A clinical approach* (5th ed.). St. Louis, MO: Saunders Elsevier, p. 430.

6 **Answer: 2, 5** **Rationale:** Two options are correct. Confabulation is due to memory impairment. Confabulation is a means for clients with dementia to compensate for what they can't remember. Three options are incorrect. Confabulation is not lying. Confabulation is not known as amnesia; the defini-tion of amnesia is significant memory loss. Disturbed sleep is not a cause of confabulation. **Cognitive Level:** Analyzing **Client Need:** Psychosocial Integrity **Integrated Process:** Nursing Process: Assessment **Content Area:** Mental Health **Strategy:** Recall the definition of confabulation and how it relates to a client with dementia's memory skills. **Reference:** Stuart, G.W. (2009). *Principles and practice of psychiatric nursing* (9th ed.). St. Louis, MO: Mosby, Elsevier, p. 394.

7 **Answer: 3** **Rationale:** Catastrophic reaction is the human response of overreacting to minor stresses that often occurs in demented clients. Pseudodementia (a medical diagnosis) is a reversible disorder that mimics dementia. Pseudodelirium (a medical diagnosis) is characterized by symptoms of delirium without any identifiable organic cause. Clients with dementia rather than delirium also often experience extreme agitation at the end of the day, probably as a result of tiredness and fewer orienting stimuli such as planned activities and contact with people. This human response of restless and agitated behavior worsens at night and is commonly referred to as sundown syndrome. **Cognitive Level:** Applying **Client Need:** Physiological Adaptation **Integrated Process:** Communication and Documentation **Content Area:** Mental Health **Strategy:** Remember that the nurse diagnoses and reports human responses. The nurse does not establish medical diagnoses. **Reference:** Varcarolis, E., & halter, M. (2010). *Foundations of psychiatric mental health nursing: A clinical approach* (6th ed.). St. Louis, MO: Saunders Elsevier, pp. 501–502.

8 **Answer: 1** **Rationale:** Recent memory loss is a common problem found in dementia; therefore, the client may be frustrated when constantly confronted with evidence of failing memory. Pictures of family members can encour-age a discussion of remote memories that will help the client feel less anxious while promoting a sense of plea-sure from discussing past experiences. The three incor-rect options rely on recall of recent memories rather than remote memories and can cause increased anxiety and confusion. **Cognitive Level:** Applying **Client Need:** Psychosocial Integrity **Integrated Process:** Nursing Process: Implementation **Content Area:** Mental Health **Strategy:** Think of elders you have known. Identify areas of their lives that they enjoyed discussing. **Reference:** Fontaine, K. (2009). *Mental health nursing* (6th ed.). Upper Saddle River, NJ: Prentice Hall, p. 562.

ANSWERS & RATIONALES

9 Answer: 2 Rationale: When working with a confused client, the most effective nursing action is simple, direct, and unambiguous. This option assigns responsibility to the nurse and specifies the frequency of the nursing intervention. The nurse should vary the type of fluid offered and limit the number of choices for the client to make since making choices can be confusing to the client. The nurse should not assume that the client will drink water placed at the bedside. The nurse should actively offer the water to the client at regularly planned intervals. Instructing all staff members to stop by and offer fluids frequently does not show a planned sequence for offering fluids. The term frequently does not have universal meaning. Further, no one person has responsibility to offer the fluids. Instructing a family member to sit with the client and offer fluids frequently is incorrect because it removes the responsibility from the nurse to the family. It also does not specify a time period for offering the fluids. The family's presence may be helpful to both the nurse and the client but the responsibility for increasing hydration should remain with the nurse. **Cognitive Level:** Applying **Client Need:** Physiological Adaptation **Integrated Process:** Nursing

Process: Implementation **Content Area:** Mental Health **Strategy:** Remember that even when clients are not confused, the best intervention is simple, direct, and specific. **Reference:** Varcarolis, E., & Halter, M. (2010). *Foundations of psychiatric mental health nursing: A clinical approach* (6th ed.). St. Louis, MO: Saunders Elsevier, p. 427.

10 Answer: 3 Rationale: A Mini-Mental State Examination score of less than 20 usually indicates the presence of dementia or delirium and requires further investigation. When responding verbally to the client, it is important that the nurse use simple words, rather than medical terms. The Mini-Mental State Examination does not measure education, bipolar disorder, or self-esteem. These components are investigated in a Mental Status Examination. **Cognitive Level:** Applying **Client Need:** Psychosocial Integrity **Integrated Process:** Teaching and Learning **Content Area:** Mental Health **Strategy:** Compare and contrast the components of the Mental Status Examination and the Mini-Mental Status Examination. **Reference:** Kneisl, C., Wilson, H., & Trigoboff, E. (2009). *Contemporary psychiatric-mental health nursing* (2nd ed.). Upper Saddle River, NJ: Prentice Hall, pp. 165, 241.

References

American Psychiatric Association (2000). *Diagnostic and statistical manual of mental disorders* (4th ed. text revision). Washington, DC: American Psychiatric Association, pp. 35–80.

Fontaine, K. (2009). *Mental health nursing* (6th ed.).Upper Saddle River, NJ: Pearson Education.

Kniesl, C.,Wilson, H., & Trigoboff, E. (2009). *Contemporary psychiatric–mental health nursing* (2nd ed.). Upper Saddle River, NJ: Pearson Education.

LeMone, P. Burke, K., & Bauldoff, G. (2011). *Medical-surgical nursing: Critical thinking in patient care* (5th ed.). Upper Saddle River, NJ: Pearson Education.

North American Nursing Diagnosis Association (2008). *Nursing diagnosis: Definitions and classification 2009–2011.* Indianapolis, IN: Wiley-Blackwell.

Stuart, G. (2009). *Principles and practice of psychiatric nursing* (9th ed.). St. Louis: Elsevier Science.

Townsend, M. (2011). *Essentials of psychiatric–mental health nursing* (5th ed.). Philadelphia, PA: F.A. Davis.

Varcarolis, E., & Halter, M. (2010). *Foundations of psychiatric mental health nursing: A clinical approach* (6th ed.). Philadelphia: Saunders.

Substance Use Disorders

11

Chapter Outline

Overview	Nursing Diagnoses/Analysis	Evaluation/Outcomes
Etiology	Planning and	Dual Disorder Issues
Assessment	Implementation	Family Issues

Objectives

➤ Identify at least six causative factors associated with substance abuse or dependence.

➤ Identify five behavior patterns of substance use of clients with substance abuse.

➤ Differentiate between psychological and physical dependency.

➤ State examples of at least five nursing diagnoses frequently used for clients exhibiting clinical symptoms of substance abuse or dependency.

➤ Describe four treatment modalities for acute intoxication and withdrawal.

➤ Formulate a plan of care for a client with a substance use disorder.

➤ Identify expected outcomes for the client who has a substance use disorder.

NCLEX-RN® Test Prep

Use the accompanying online resource, NursingReviewsandRationales, to test yourself with hundreds of NCLEX®-style practice questions.

Review at a Glance

abstinence a term that indicates someone has quit or stopped an addictive behavior; is not synonymous with recovery or healing from addiction

craving a psychological "hungry" feeling to engage in addictive behavior even if an individual was not originally planning to use, or thinking about using the substance or engaging in the addictive behavior

dependence a diagnostic term that means an individual's substance use patterns meet three of the seven criteria needed to make the diagnosis of dependence

intoxication symptoms that occur with excessive use of alcohol or other drug

physical dependence a physiological adaptation to a drug; withdrawal can occur only when an individual acquires physical dependence

recovery a term that means someone is abstinent and working a program of personal growth and self-discovery

relapse a term used to describe someone who has returned to active addictive behavior

substance abuse the purposeful use, for at least one month, of a drug that

results in adverse effects to one's self or others

substance dependence occurs when drug use is no longer under control and continues despite adverse effects

tolerance reduced response to a drug's action; it can be biologically inherited or developed gradually over time

withdrawal a condition that occurs after a person who has used a substance regularly and heavily has recently decreased or stopped use, and now demonstrates a pattern of signs and symptoms that in general are the opposite of the acute effects of the drug

PRETEST

1 A nurse is teaching a group of clients about addiction. One client says he can stop drinking whenever he wants. The nurse concludes that this client does not yet understand that addiction is a disease in which individuals primarily lose ability to do which of the following?

1. Control addictive and impulsive behaviors.
2. Recognize that addictive behavior is harmful to themselves and others.
3. Act sober even if they are not.
4. Think logically about their addictive behaviors.

2 As part of assessment activities to determine if the client is alcohol dependent, the nurse needs to conduct a CAGE assessment with the client. Which question asked by the nurse would be consistent with the structure of CAGE? Select all that apply.

1. "Have you ever counted the number of drinks consumed?"
2. "Have you ever felt that you needed to cut down on your drinking?"
3. "Have you ever been annoyed by comments made about your drinking?"
4. "Have you ever found yourself gulping drinks before going out?"
5. "Have you ever had a morning 'eye-opener' to calm your nerves?"

3 After orienting the client to the addiction treatment unit, the nurse suggests that the client invite his 13-year-old son to the family sessions. The client questions why the son needs to participate, because he has not seen his father drunk. What is the best response by the nurse?

1. "Your son probably knows that you are an alcoholic."
2. "Your son has probably seen changes in you when you were drinking."
3. "It's good that you have concern for your underage son."
4. "Thirteen-year-olds are old enough to start learning about the effects of alcohol."

4 The nurse conducts an in-service session about impaired nursing practice. The nurse evaluates that the teaching was effective when one of the nurses says that the most influential risk for impaired nursing practice is which of the following?

1. Having grown up in a dysfunctional family
2. Feeling that nurses' knowledge about drugs protects them from drug dependency
3. Thinking that professionals are not at high risk for substance dependency
4. Having a tendency to involve self in codependent professional and personal relationships

5 A male client comes to day treatment surrounded by an intense odor of alcohol. The client staggers when walking but insists that that he has not consumed any alcohol. The nurse concludes that this behavior constitutes which of the following?

1. Denial
2. Rationalization
3. Transference
4. Countertransference

6 A female alcohol-dependent client who has cardiomyopathy tells the nurse that she is certain that her family and friends are against her. The client goes on to say, "They stay on my back about my drinking and say I could die from it." What would be the best response by the nurse?

1. "Anyone saying this to you must have a problem with his or her own drinking."
2. "Although their intentions are good, they have no right to judge another person's drinking."
3. "Do you think they may be jealous that you can drink more than they can?"
4. "Perhaps they have noticed that your drinking creates consequences for you."

7 A client who is recovering from alcoholism presents in the psychiatric unit and tells the admitting nurse she is very depressed and has a hard time staying sober. The nurse concludes that the most likely treatment sequence for this client will be which of the following?

1. Depression before the sobriety issue
2. Sobriety issue before the depression
3. Sobriety issue and depression at the same time
4. Depression after the sobriety issue has been resolved

8 As part of the clinical experience, a student nurse is required to attend an Alcoholics Anonymous (AA) meeting and write a report about what was learned. What information would the student include in the report about the twelve-step program? Select all that apply.

1. People learn to change negative attitudes and behaviors into positive ones.
2. Once an individual learns how to be sober, he or she can graduate from attending meetings.
3. Once an individual has achieved sobriety, he or she continues to be at risk for relapse into drinking.
4. Acceptance of being an alcoholic will prevent urges to drink, since it represents giving up one's denial.
5. A Higher Power will protect individuals if they feel like using.

9 The nurse working in the maternal care area is reinforcing physician health teaching about the risks of substance use during pregnancy. When questioned by the client, the nurse should reply that which drugs are most likely to lead to significant physical, cognitive, and developmental problems for any infant?

1. Benzodiazepines
2. Hallucinogens
3. Alcohol
4. Cocaine

10 Having requested it as part of a comprehensive treatment program, the client is to receive disulfiram (Antabuse). Which statement should the nurse include when teaching the client about this drug?

1. "Inhaling fumes from paints and wood stains may cause a disulfiram reaction."
2. "Eating inadequately cooked seafood may lead to disulfiram resistance."
3. "Taking disulfiram will reduce your physical craving for alcohol."
4. "If you consume alcohol while taking disulfiram, rapid intoxication will occur."

➤ *See pages 227–229 for Answers and Rationales.*

I. OVERVIEW

A. *Substance abuse* is defined as the purposeful use, for at least one month, of a drug that results in adverse effects to oneself or others

B. *Substance dependence* occurs when the use of the drug is no longer under control and continues despite adverse effects; the client experiences tolerance and withdrawal

1. A medical and spiritual illness with well-defined signs and symptoms including denial and relapse

2. Disease progression and course of illness is predictable and treatable
3. Treatment focus is **abstinence** (voluntarily going without drugs), medications as appropriate, education, lifestyle change, and increasing self-awareness and personal growth

Box 11-1	**Frequently Abused Controlled and/or Illegal Substances**
Substances of Abuse	**1.** Alcohol **2.** Sedatives **3.** Narcotics **4.** Cannabis **5.** Amphetamines **6.** Cocaine **7.** Hallucinogens **8.** Inhalants

Source: Fontaine, K. L. (2009). *Mental health nursing* (6th ed.). Upper Saddle River, NJ: Prentice Hall, p. 380.

C. Statistics
1. Substance use disorders in the United States cost over $300 billion a year
2. Alcoholism is a major health problem, one that is responsible for 100,000 deaths annually in the United States
3. 7.5% of the population is dependent on a substance
4. 10% of people are said to have alcoholism

D. Types of substance use/dependence disorders
1. Addictive substances are characterized by preoccupation with and compulsion to engage in an activity (see Box 11-1 for a list of addictive substances)
    a. Depressants (opiate/opioids/sedatives/hypnotics)
    b. Stimulants
    c. Cannabinoids/hallucinogens
    d. Inhalants
2. Definitions of substance use disorders

    a. *DSM-IV-TR* clinical syndromes
        1) Intoxication (state of experiencing acute effects of a substance)
        2) Withdrawal (manifestations associated with cessation of a substance)
        3) Abuse (purposeful excessive use of a harmful substance)
        4) Dependence
    b. The American Society of Addiction Medicine (ASAM) defines substance dependence as a *primary*, chronic relapsing *disease* with genetic, psychosocial, and environmental factors influencing it; it is characterized by continuous periodic *impaired control* over the substance, *preoccupation* with the substance, use of the substance despite *adverse consequences*, and distortions in thinking—most notably denial; inherent in the definition are the concepts of **tolerance**, **withdrawal**, **physical dependence**, and psychological dependence
    c. American Nurses Association and National Nurses Society on Addictions (ANA and NNSA) define addiction as an illness characterized by compulsion, loss of control, and continued pattern of abuse despite perceived negative consequences; obsession with a dysfunctional habit; the dysfunctional patterns include patterns of alcoholism, drug abuse, misuse of tobacco, eating disorders, excessive gambling or spending, and certain compulsive sexual disorders

E. Medical theory of addiction: Jellinek's four phases of alcoholism
1. Prealcoholic phase
    a. Distinct symptoms that the social drinker does not experience
    b. Drinking to cope with emotions
    c. Lack of recognition that tension is caused by drinking
    d. Tolerance develops

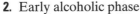

Practice to Pass

Your client's son arrives intoxicated to visit his medically ill father on the unit. The client is concerned, starts crying, and asks you for your assistance. How would you respond?

2. Early alcoholic phase
   a. Begins drinking in secret
   b. Gulps first few sips
   c. Attachment to alcohol present
   d. Access to alcohol involved in planning all social activities
   e. Tolerance develops (needing more alcohol to get the same effect)
   f. Continues engaging in drinking despite negative consequences
   g. Feels guilty about drinking
   h. Becomes isolated and withdrawn
   i. Has mood swings, diminished self-esteem
   j. Uses denial and rationalization
3. Crucial phase
   a. Beginning of disease process and psychological dependence
   b. Intermittent loss of control ensues when drinking (uses more than intended); binge drinking occurs
   c. Preoccupation with use develops
   d. Use of defense mechanisms
   e. Experiences craving and other triggers to use
   f. Concern over drinking expressed by others
   g. Anger, alienation of family and friends; client may exhibit aggression
   h. Drops all nondrinking socialization, including friends who don't drink
   i. Activities of daily living (ADLs) suffer: sleep, appetite, and energy problems present
   j. Family issues surface: alienation, anger, role and relationship problems
4. Chronic phase
   a. Drinks to blackout/pass-out/incapacitation
   b. Cognitive, physical, and emotional health deterioration
   c. Reverse tolerance may develop (less quantity than previously required to bring intoxication)
   d. Life falls apart; may experience psychosis

II. ETIOLOGY

A. **Brain structures involved in substance dependence**
   1. Ventral tegmental area
   2. Nucleus accumbens
   3. Mesolimbic dopaminergic pathways
   4. Endogenous opioid and serotonin system
   5. Neurotransmitters and receptor sites
B. **Process of brain reward system (BRS) activation**
   1. All drugs affect the cells in some way, either increasing or decreasing some cellular activities
   2. Use of mood-altering substances or engaging in addictive behaviors causes increased availability of dopamine/serotonin/opioid peptides and facilitates other neurotransmitter (gamma-aminobutyric acid, glutamate, acetylcholine) dysregulation
   3. Short-term euphoric response is generated by this activity, which eventually leads to the symptoms of addictive thinking, denial, and impaired control
   4. Euphoric response engenders the immediate and profound desire for re-administration (**cravings** that are like a psychological "hunger," triggers, and urges)
   5. The positive immediate short-term euphoria overshadows any long-term consequences associated with engaging in addictive behaviors
   6. Continued use leads to development of tolerance
   7. Experience of tolerance leads to increased dose and frequency of use

8. Physical dependence and withdrawal syndrome may develop
9. Psychological dependence develops

C. **Genetic/biologic risk**
1. No one specific marker is responsible for substance abuse—the more risk factors, the greater the risk for developing the disease
2. Genetics: twin studies demonstrate a 30 to 50% vulnerability for substance abuse, sons and daughters of people with alcoholism have a four and three times higher tolerance and occurrence of alcoholism over sons and daughters of parents who do not have alcoholism
3. Biology: genetic vulernabilities may affect brain responses

D. **Psychosocial risk**
1. Personality traits: individuals with certain personality traits are thought to be susceptible to the reinforcing effects of engaging in substance abuse leading to dependence
    a. Antisocial: lack of responsiveness to people, places, and things in their environment; persons with antisocial personality traits experience a positive response to the psychoactive properties of engaging in substance use
    b. Introversion: feelings of inadequacy or low self-esteem are mediated by the euphoric effect of engaging in substance use
    c. Impulsiveness: impulsivity is reinforced because of the inability to anticipate impending negative consequences of use
2. Developmental failures: individuals who have lived with painful experiences are at risk to self-medicate or misuse their medication
    a. Abuse survivors—may experience disturbances in their sense of self
    b. Lack of nurturance in childhood—may lead to an inability to self-soothe
    c. Coping skills deficit
    d. Positive coping skills may not have been learned in the person's family of origin
    e. The learning of positive coping skills may have been inhibited because of the positive reinforcing effect of euphoria when using a substance to cope with feelings

E. **Dual disorders risk**
1. Approximately 30 to 40% of individuals with a psychiatric disorder develop substance dependence
    a. Individuals with psychiatric disorders are at risk for developing addictive disorders
    b. Initially drugs and alcohol may have been used to help individuals deal with being depressed, being anxious, or having painful memories
    c. With continued use dependence develops for individuals at risk
2. Individuals with addiction are at risk for developing psychiatric disorders
    a. Substance use can induce the development of psychiatric illness as the nucleus accumbens and the ventral tegmental area (plays a role in cognition, motivation, and learning) and the neurotransmitter system (plays a role in mood regulation) are affected
    b. Any one of a number of psychiatric disorders can develop
3. Individuals with substance abuse may be misdiagnosed as some disorders mask dependence (see Table 11-1)
    a. Mood disorders
    b. Anxiety disorders
    c. Adjustment disorders
    d. Sleep disorders

Table 11-1 The Process of Dual Diagnosis: Differences among Substance Dependence, Anxiety, Depression, and Chronic Pain

Dynamics	Substance Dependence	Anxiety	Depression	Chronic Pain
Contributing factors to the development of disease	Alcohol and other drug use Changes in brain chemistry and function Biology Environment Psychosocial Factors	Alcohol and other drug use Changes in brain chemistry and function Biology Environment Psychosocial factors	Alcohol and other drug use Changes in brain chemistry and function Biology Environment Psychosocial factors	Persistent nonmalignant medical problem with resultant pain Persists beyond expected time for healing Psychosocial factors
Symptoms	Sleep/appetite disturbance Tolerance/withdrawal/progression Loss of control of substance use and behavior; preoccupation with use Continued use despite negative consequences Denial: distortions in thinking, feeling, and behavior Physical, interpersonal, social occupational, legal, and spiritual problems Hospitalization, incarceration, thoughts of suicide Feelings of helplessness/hopelessness	Muscle tension and overactive bodily responses: pounding heart, panic, trembling Hypervigilance Distortions in thinking, feeling, and behavior Avoidance of feared situations Physical, interpersonal, social, occupational, legal, and spiritual problems Hospitalization, immobilization, thoughts of suicide Feelings of helplessness/hopelessness	Appetite disturbance and sleep, decreased energy level Sad or irritable mood Loss of pleasure or interest in most enjoyable activities Distortions in thinking, feeling, and behavior Physical, interpersonal, social, occupational, legal, and spiritual problems Hospitalization, immobilization, thoughts of suicide Feelings of helplessness/hopelessness	Tolerance/withdrawal Medication misuse Anxiety, worry, frustration Sad or irritable mood Distortions in thinking, feeling, and behavior Loss of pleasure or interest in most enjoyable activities Physical, interpersonal, social, occupation, legal, and spiritual problems Hospitalization, immobilization, thoughts of suicide Feelings of helplessness/hopelessness
Recovery components	Abstinence: medications to help stop using mood-altering substances Social support: 12-step group Cognitive restructuring Relaxation training Education: disease/recovery process Practice recovery skills Coping skills training Psychotherapy: group therapy/group counseling Exercise/nutrition/sleep Changes in negative lifestyle habits	Nonaddictive anti-anxiety medications Social support Cognitive restructuring Relaxation training Education: disease/recovery process Practice recovery skills Coping skills training Psychtherapy: group therapy/group counselin Exercise/nutrition/sleep Changes in negative lifestyle habits	Antidepressant medication Social support Cognitive restructuring Relaxation training Education: disease/recovery process Practice recovery skills Coping skills training Psychotherapy: group therapy/group counseling Exercise/nutrition/sleep Changes in negative lifestyle habits	Nonaddictive pain medications Social activity Cognitive restructuring Relaxation training Education: disease/recovery process Practice recovery skills Coping skills training Group support/group counseling Exercise/nutrition/sleep Changes in negative lifestyle habits

       e. Personality disorders

       f. Antisocial disorders

       g. Psychotic disorders

       h. Chronic pain

       i. Disorders of delirium, dementia, amnesia, and other cognitive disorders

    4. Individuals with dual diagnoses and who are intoxicated are at increased risk of suicide

    5. Treatment for dual diagnoses is more successful if both illnesses are treated concurrently

F. Environmental risk

    1. Social learning theory: use of substances is a learned behavior

       a. Normalized behavior: engaging in substance use is influenced by exposure to peer pressure, role models, societal norms

       b. Culture: engaging in substance use is influenced by culture; certain cultural groups have use patterns that put them at risk for developing dependence (e.g., those of northern European descent have a higher rate of alcoholism than those of southern European descent)

    2. Profession: health care professionals (HCPs) are at risk to develop substance use disorders because the high stress and pressure of their jobs and availability of substances

       a. The impaired nurse: nurses are at risk for developing addictive disorders

          1) 10% of nurses working in most specialties and 15% of nurse anesthetists develop addiction

          2) Nursing practice is impaired when an individual is unable to meet the requirements of the professional code of ethics and standards of practice because of cognitive, interpersonal, or psychomotor skills affected by conditions of the individual (psychiatric illness, excessive alcohol or drug use) in interaction with the environment

       b. Risk factors for vulnerability

          1) Access to drugs

          2) Long hours

          3) Tremendous responsibility

          4) Job-related stress

          5) Family history of substance dependence

       c. Signs and symptoms of the nurse who abuses or is dependent on drugs and alcohol

          1) Increased irritability with clients and colleagues

          2) Mood swings, may be shifting rapidly; might be calm after taking drugs

          3) Withdrawn, isolated: wants to work night shift; avoids informal staff get-togethers

          4) Purposely waits until alone to open the narcotic cabinet

          5) Late for work; misses work; elaborate excuses for missing work

          6) Work quality decreases

          7) Charting is illegible

          8) Signs out more narcotics than other nurses on the unit

       d. System response

          1) Signs that a nurse is abusing/dependent on substances must be reported to nursing management

          2) In most states, there is opportunity for supportive intervention rather than loss of licensure if the impaired nurse seeks treatment and follows the monitoring recommendation from the Board of Nursing in the state in which he or she practices

III. ASSESSMENT

A. **Substance use disorders**: patterns of abuse and dependence are gathered from a standardized screening and assessment tool and nursing baseline assessment

1. Screening/assessment tools
   a. CAGE
      1) Have you ever done the following?
         a) Attempted to *Cut back* on your alcohol?
         b) Been *Annoyed* by comments made about your drinking?
         c) Felt *Guilty* about your drinking?
         d) Had an *Eye-opener* in the morning to calm your nerves?
      2) A positive answer for two of the screening questions indicates a need for further assessment
   b. Michigan Alcoholism Screening Test (MAST)
   c. Addiction Severity Index (ASI)

B. **Nursing admission assessment data** that focuses on use of substances
   1. Physical assessment/systems review
      a. Blackout or lost consciousness: blacking out or passing out can be related to a person's use of alcohol or other substances
      b. Changes in bowel movement: persons using alcohol and/or drugs frequently can experience changes in bowel movement; changes range from diarrhea because of drinking to constipation from using pain medications frequently; withdrawal from narcotics can cause diarrhea
      c. Weight loss or weight gain: persons using alcohol or drugs regularly may experience weight loss/gain and/or poor nutritional balance
      d. Experiencing stressful situation: stress can precipitate an increase in drinking; stress can also result from drinking or using drugs regularly
      e. Sleep problems: persons using alcohol and/or other drugs experience a variety of sleep problems; one may start using alcohol to promote sleep, but once someone develops tolerance, sleep is more difficult
      f. Chronic pain: persons experiencing chronic pain may use drugs and/or alcohol to self-medicate
      g. Concern over substance use: if friends and relatives worry about substance use, it is generally because there is something to be concerned about
      h. Cutting down on alcohol consumption (or drug use, prescription medication use, gambling, or addictive behavior): if one feels that he or she must cut down, it is usually because there are problems
   2. Personal family assessment: persons with positive family history are at risk for developing an addictive disorder
   3. Chemical use assessment: key elements
      a. Identify type of substance used
      b. Date of last substance use
      c. Pattern and frequency of substance use
      d. Amount
      e. Age at onset
      f. Age of regular use
      g. Changes in use patterns
      h. Periods of abstinence in history
      i. Previous withdrawal symptoms
      j. Ask about each substance or behavior separately
      k. Ranges of substances can be ingested into the body in numerous ways; remember that about 30 to 40% of alcohol users also use another substance
      l. Legal problems to related to substance use

Practice to Pass

An elderly client is confused about the reason why she was transferred to the inpatient addictions unit. She says she only has two drinks a night. What additional assessment data do you need before you can respond to her concern?

Practice to Pass

A client is not experiencing pain relief from the Darvocet that you administered 90 minutes ago. What are you concerned about?

4. Medication assessment
   a. Ask about pain-relief medications, laxatives, cold medications, sleep and/or stay awake medications, and/or anxiety/nerve control medications
   b. Prescribed dose is now not enough to control pain/anxiety even though it might have helped at the beginning
   c. Runs out of medication early and needs a refill early
   d. Pain medication that is used for physical pain is now used for emotional pain
   e. Medication is used for dealing with "stress" or stressful events
   f. More medication was taken than intended
   g. Laxatives are used regularly because the pain medications cause constipation or because the individual has difficulty having bowel movements without the use of laxatives
   h. Cold tablets or cough syrup are taken more frequently than expected
5. Over-the-counter (OTC) or nutritional supplement assessment: use of any herbal, vitamin, or OTC products to help with sleep, weight loss, staying awake, giving more energy, stabilizing mood and/or improving mood, or making client feel a certain way
6. Social history assessment: persons experiencing physical, sexual, or emotional abuse may medicate internal distress by using mood-altering substances
7. Laboratory value assessment: laboratory values that may be abnormal in substance abusers:
   a. Gamma glutamyl transferase (GGT)
   b. Aspartate aminotransferase (AST)
   c. Alkaline phosphatase (AK)
   d. Lactate dehydrogenase (LDH)
   e. Mean corpuscular volume (MCV)
   f. Urine toxicology and blood screen for drugs of abuse is an essential component of substance use evaluation (e.g., blood alcohol level or BAL >0.08%)

IV. NURSING DIAGNOSES/ANALYSIS

A. **Risk for Injury**: potential for complications of substance withdrawal
B. **Risk for Suicide**: losses, poor self-concept, hopelessness
C. **Imbalanced Nutrition**: less than body requirements: poor nutritional intake
D. **Deficient Fluid Volume**: poor fluid intake, possible vomiting and diarrhea
E. **Risk for Injury**: potential for relapse

F. **Dysfunctional Family Process**: substance dependence disorder
G. **Deficient Knowledge**: substance dependence disorder
H. **Anxiety**: patterns and consequences of substance abuse
I. **Ineffective Coping**: inability to accurately appraise stressors, choose practical responses, and/or use available resources
J. **Ineffective Denial**: an attempt to disavow the knowledge or meaning of an event to reduce anxiety/fear to the detriment of health
K. **Disturbed Self-Esteem**: negative self-evaluation and feelings about self or self-capacities, which may be directly or indirectly expressed
L. **Disturbed Sleep Pattern**: time-limited disruption of sleep (natural, periodic suspension of consciousness) amount and quality
M. **Chronic Pain**: pain that has a duration of greater than six months
N. **Ineffective Health Maintenance**: inability to identify, manage, or seek out help in order to achieve or maintain recovery

O. **Hopelessness:** state in which an individual sees limited/no alternatives/personal choices available and is unable to mobilize energy on own behalf

P. **Powerlessness:** a perception that one's own action will not significantly effect an outcome; a perceived lack of control over or influence on a current situation or immediate happening

Q. **Spiritual Distress:** disruption in the life principle that pervades a person's entire being and that integrates and transcends a person's biological and psychosocial nature (NANDA, 2008)

V. PLANNING AND IMPLEMENTATION

A. **Nursing care in acute stages of substance use**
 1. Care of the client during intoxication
    a. Focus is on safety
    b. Interventions
       1) Maintain safe environment
       2) Orient to time, place, and person
       3) Maintain adequate nutrition and fluid balance; administer thiamine and folic acid supplements
       4) Monitor for beginning of withdrawal signs and symptoms
    c. Outcome: client remains safe during periods of intoxication
 2. Care of the client experiencing withdrawal from mood altering substances: focus is safe withdrawal process
    a. Interventions
       1) Maintain safe environment
       2) Create a low-stimulation environment
       3) Monitor vital signs and withdrawal symptoms
          a) Nausea/vomiting
          b) Tremor
          c) Paroxysmal sweats
          d) Anxiety
          e) Agitation
          f) Tactile disturbances
          g) Auditory disturbances
          h) Visual disturbances
          i) Headache or fullness in head
          j) Disorientation and sensorium
       4) Some clients who might be opiate-dependent may be managed long term with the use of methadone; the methadone may be initially prescribed for withdrawal but then the client will be maintained on a certain daily dose; contrary to popular belief many people who are maintained on methadone do very well with recovery
       5) The nurse must be careful in assessing the chronic pain client for withdrawal as some of the pain that the client is experiencing is related to his or her chronic pain and is not an acute withdrawal symptom
       6) While female clients may have been initially screened for pregnancy, they should be screened later in the episode of care to be sure that any medication use potentially harmful to the fetus is minimized; alcohol is the most harmful drug of all and the most harmful to the fetus of any drug
       7) Monitor for delirium tremens, psychotic symptoms, and suicide/seizure risk

        8) Administer the withdrawal medication: antiepileptics; benzodiazepines; sedative vitamins; or other medications as ordered; thiamine helps to prevent confusion and other mental status changes

           a) Benzodiazepines are the drug of choice for alcohol or benzodiazepine withdrawal

           b) It is preferable to give the longer-acting agent so the tapering process is smoother for the client with a longer acting medication

        9) Maintain adequate nutrition and fluid intake

        10) Maintain normal comfort measures

        11) Monitor for covert substance use during detoxification period

        12) Provide emotional support and reassurance to client and family

        13) Provide reality orientations and address hallucinations in a therapeutic manner

        14) Advise client of the depressive uneasy feelings and the fatigue that is usually experienced during withdrawal

        15) Begin to educate the client about the disease of addiction and the initial treatment goal of abstinence

    b. Outcome

        1) Safe withdrawal from drugs and alcohol

        2) Oriented to reality

        3) Begin to develop motivation and commitment for abstinence and **recovery** (abstinence plus working a program of personal growth and self-discovery)

B. Nursing care in the rehabilitative stages of abuse

  1. Focus is on teaching about the disease/recovery process and building on the client's motivation for abstinence, lifestyle change, and recovery

  2. Interventions

    a. Assist client to complete detoxification from all substances; monitor for suicide and/or seizure risk

    b. Promote abstinence from all substances

    c. Administer medications for enhancing abstinence, treatment of mood/anxiety, and/or thought disorders as applicable

    d. Assist clients to put structure and discipline back into their lives

    e. Facilitate hope

    f. Teach disease/recovery dynamics

    g. Teach about how the disease has impacted the roles and functions for the individual and the family

    h. Provide therapeutic interaction/group counseling to do the following:

        1) Process losses (i.e., loss of independence)

        2) Discuss memories and flashback

        3) Address shame and guilt

        4) Educate about disease/recovery

        5) Facilitate acceptance of illness

    i. Teach and encourage practice of recovery skills

        1) Encourage daily commitment to sobriety and recovery

        2) Build/utilize sober support networks (i.e., AA or other 12-step groups)

        3) Teach the importance of honesty and making amends

        4) Encourage daily prayer/mediation

        5) Teach drink refusal skills and managing cravings

        6) Enhance coping/communication/problem-solving skills

        7) Practice asking for help

        8) Recognition of signs of impending **relapse** (return to substance use behavior)

           a) Hungry

           b) Angry

           c) Lonely

           d) Tired

           e) Having thoughts about using but not telling anyone

           f) Slipping back into using old defensive mechanisms as opposed to honesty and openness

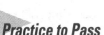

j. Help the client to develop an emergency plan, which is a list of things the client would do and people he or she would call if he or she felt like using or actually used

k. Demonstrate how to utilize affirmations, slogans, and the serenity prayer

l. Initiate random breathalyzers and urine drug screens to objectively assess for sobriety/substance use

     1) Breathalyzers are an inexpensive way to do random checks to see if individuals are coming to program sober; because many clients have high tolerance it is difficult to determine if they have been drinking

     2) Random urine drug screen test provides the client with objective evidence of sobriety or use (urine collection procedure: instruct the client not to turn on the water or flush the toilet until the specimen is given to the nurse)

m. Clients with eating disorders will need to work with the dietitian and family physician about increasing/decreasing caloric intake and discontinuing laxative use; clients will need to increase their daily water and fiber intake

n. Clients who have experienced multiple relapses and seem to have severe addiction may not have a goal of immediate total abstinence; their goals may be to increase the number of sober days within a specific period of time or reduce the number of drinks/money gambled at one sitting; this goal is developed from the Harm Reduction Model, which basically says "there certainly is a beneficial effect to the general public if someone reduces the number of drinks each time they drink"; while this is not an ideal goal for clients it certainly makes sense to decrease risk of more serious consequences

C. Treatment modalities and nursing interventions

  1. Medical model: teach the disease and recovery dynamics

  2. Assist the client to comply with treatment recommendations

  3. Assist with dual diagnosis treatment

  4. Detoxification/abstinence medications

    a. Disulfiram (Antabuse): usual dose is 250 mg/day

     1) Prevents breakdown of alcohol

     2) Person who drinks alcohol becomes very sick (flushing, weakness, nausea/vomiting)

     3) Teach about monitoring for use of alcohol in products/food containing alcohol

     4) Can elevate liver enzymes

    b. Naltrexone (ReVia): usual dose is 50 mg/day orally

     1) Prevents or diminishes cravings/euphoric effect of engaging in addictive behavior (i.e., alcohol/drugs/gambling)

     2) Can elevate liver enzymes

    c. Acamprosate calcium (Campral)

     1) Helps clients abstain from alcohol

     2) Acts as a glutamate receptor modulator to restore neuronal balance between excitation and inhibition

Practice to Pass

A client who was just discharged from outpatient services on 250 mg of disulfiram a day calls to say she is breaking out in a red rash all over her face. The client stated she was cleaning light fixtures. What is your concern and what will you advise the client to do?

   d. Antidepressant/anti-anxiety medication
   1) Enhances and stabilizes mood and diminishes anxiety
   2) Teach about the decreased effectiveness of the medication if there is use of mood-altering substances
   3) To discontinue medication it should be tapered slowly
   4) Avoid use of benzodiazepines in clients with dependence unless part of a withdrawal management protocol

! **Practice to Pass**

A young teen was just admitted to your addiction program; she is not happy to be here and feels she is too young to be an alcoholic. She "drinks the same amount as everyone else" she knows and believes she was just unlucky to be involved in a traffic accident. What education will you provide to the client? What approach will you use?

5. The 12-step model
   a. Teach that there is no effective cure for addiction
   b. Encourage 12-step involvement
   c. Regular meeting attendance diminishes ambivalence and promotes acceptance about never engaging in addictive behaviors again
   d. Key elements of 12-step framework are acceptance, surrender, processing grief, higher power, and power of the group
6. Cognitive behavioral model
   a. Develop and use positive coping skills
   b. Implement specific skill training
   1) Assertiveness
   2) Drink refusal
   3) Problem solving
   4) Cognitive restructuring
   5) Mood management
   6) Anger problems
   7) Social skills
   8) Listening-communication skills
   c. Identify and change behaviors associated with substance abuse and dependence (i.e., going into the liquor store to buy soft drinks)
7. Relapse prevention model
   a. Identify situations and factors that contribute to relapse
   b. Increase positive self-efficacy expectations about the ability to achieve abstinence
   c. Increase coping skills
   d. Become a member of a relapse prevention group
8. Motivational enhancement/stages of change
   a. Utilize various types of reflective listening and other specialized communication strategies to help build a client's commitment to change
   b. Express empathy; ambivalence is a normal part of the change process
   c. Help to develop discrepancy between the way the clients see themselves and the way they really are
   d. Avoid getting into arguments over things, especially labels
   e. Be alert to resistance; resistance is a sign to change strategies
   f. Support the client's self-efficacy
9. Assess the client's stage of change and apply nursing interventions according to the stage of change the client is in
   a. Precontemplation: "We are blind to our problems"
   b. Contemplation: "We are not ready to change"
   c. Determination/preparation: "We are getting ready to change"
   d. Action: "We are learning how to change; we are doing it"
   e. Maintenance: "We make changes stick"

VI. EVALUATION/OUTCOMES

    A. Completes the withdrawal process safely

    B. Makes a commitment to stopping substance use and participates in the treatment process

    C. Learns about the dynamics of substance dependence and the recovery skills necessary to recover from this disease

    D. Begins to identify the consequences of the substance use or addictive behaviors

    E. Begins to practice some recovery behaviors while in treatment

    F. Begins to accept having a substance abuse disorder and the inability to use this substance in the future

    G. Identifies coping behaviors to address cravings, thoughts, and triggers to substance use

VII. DUAL DISORDER ISSUES

    A. Focus is on teaching that each disorder is an illness that requires co-occurring treatment and building on the client's motivation for abstinence, remissions of mental illness, lifestyle change, and the recovery process

    B. Additional interventions

        1. Discuss the physiological aspects of mental illness and substance abuse and of the interaction effects

        2. Teach that psychiatric medications are nonaddictive and can enhance recovery

        3. Medication teaching includes focus on the fact that drinking or drug use will interfere with the efficacy of the psychiatric medication and that medication use and drinking should not mix

VIII. FAMILY ISSUES

    A. Anger/alienation of the substance dependent person

    B. Teach disease dynamics

        1. Family rules/communication

        2. Family members' dysfunctional behaviors and denial about the substance dependence of their family member

    C. Problematic coping skills

    D. Mood adjustment problems

    E. Codependency and low self-esteem: behaviors or characteristics of the family members of clients with alcoholism

    F. Learning and practicing recovery dynamics and skills

        1. Self-love and self-care

        2. Utilizing support groups (i.e., Alcoholics Anonymous)

        3. Establishing healthy relationships/boundaries

        4. Daily prayer/meditation

        5. Improved coping/problem solving

        6. Asking for help

        7. Confronting dysfunctional beliefs and learning how to change them

        8. Affirmations, slogans, serenity prayer

    G. Processing anger and losses/memories

        1. Confronts substance abuser about the consequences of his or her use and how it affected the family

        2. Processing emotional distance between family members

        3. Processing loss of "helper/competent" role now that the recovering family member is taking back some of his or her lost family roles

Case Study

A client in her early 20s comes to the emergency department complaining of rapid heart rate and states she has passed out a couple of times recently. You suspect her symptoms are related to substance use.

1. What additional information will you gather from this client?

2. What body system will you focus your nursing assessment on?

3. What laboratory values would help you determine if substance use played a role in the development of your client's symptoms?

4. The client's symptoms are related to substance use. What information will you use to differentiate which substance the client may be abusing?

5. What nursing interventions will you need to deliver to this client?

For suggested responses, see pages 300–301.

POSTTEST

1 The nurse instructs the client about addiction. The nurse determines that the client understands the information given when the client makes which statements? Select all that apply.

1. "Addiction is a moral problem."
2. "Addiction is a medical illness."
3. "Addiction is a behavioral habit."
4. "Addiction is an emotional attachment."
5. "Addiction is difficult to cure."

2 A client says, "I have a very small drink every morning to calm my nerves and stop my hands from trembling." The nurse concludes that this client is describing which of the following?

1. An anxiety disorder
2. Tolerance
3. Withdrawal
4. Alcohol abuse

3 The emergency department client is admitted following a blow to the head sustained in a motor vehicle accident. The blood alcohol level (BAL) is 0.35% and the client is walking without stumbling and talking rationally about the accident. What alcoholic phenomenon should the nurse recognize?

1. Alcohol withdrawal syndrome
2. Intolerance
3. Psychological dependence
4. Alcohol dependency

4 A client with a long history of relapsing from cocaine dependence states that in spite of having a desire to be sober, thoughts of reusing cocaine continue to occur. The nurse decides to educate the client about the role the Brain Reward System (BRS) plays in addiction. The nurse considers that the teaching has been effective if the client makes which statement about the BRS?

1. "Reinforces the value of having positive role models."
2. "Offers a means of mediating job stress and pressure."
3. "Reduces physiologic and psychological cravings."
4. "Facilitates cravings and triggers for reusing."

5 A client asks the nurse to provide information about the detoxification process and withdrawal from a benzodiazepine. The nurse should inform the client that the process will involve which of the following?

1. Rapid reduction in amount and frequency of the drug normally used
2. Abrupt discontinuation of the drug commonly used
3. Gradual downward reduction in dosage of the drug commonly used
4. Planned, progressive addition of an antipsychotic drug

6 When the nurse is caring for a client experiencing delirium tremens, what is the most important nursing intervention?

1. Present psycho-education on the dangers of drug and alcohol use.
2. Encourage the client to develop a relapse prevention plan.
3. Administer anti-craving medications.
4. Provide withdrawal care based on unit protocol.

7 A client detoxifying from alcohol requires medications to treat the withdrawal. The nurse observes coarse hand tremors and diaphoresis. How should the nurse first react to this observation? Select all that apply.

1. Assess level of consciousness.
2. Explain the concepts of withdrawal to the client.
3. Administer ordered thiamine and folic acid.
4. Determine the most recent blood alcohol level.
5. Assess vital signs.

8 A nurse is teaching a group of community health colleagues about the use of naltrexone (ReVia) in treating alcoholism. The nurse interprets that the teaching was effective if the colleagues state that naltrexone (ReVia) is used to do which of the following?

1. Prevent withdrawal symptoms.
2. Reduce number of blackouts.
3. Reduce craving for alcohol.
4. Manage heightened anxiety.

9 Adolescent alcoholic clients often relapse into drinking because they feel pressured by their peers. Which skill training should the nurse plan for these clients in order to assist them in relapse prevention?

1. Critical-thinking skills
2. Drinking-refusal skills
3. Problem-solving skills
4. Communication skills

10 A client is admitted to a medical unit for treatment of chest pain. A family member reports a client history of chemical abuse. The client is ambivalent about the recommendation for treatment made by an addiction consulting team. What would be an appropriate nursing diagnosis for the client?

1. Dysfunctional Family Processes: Alcoholism
2. Ineffective Therapeutic Regimen Management
3. Risk for Injury
4. Decisional Conflict

➤ *See pages 229–231 for Answers and Rationales.*

ANSWERS & RATIONALES

Pretest

1 **Answer: 1 Rationale:** Controlling addictive and impulsive behaviors is correct. The key symptom of addiction is impaired control, or the inability to control, or regulate, one's addictive behavior. In addition to loss of control, the addicted person is not able to view the addictive behaviors realistically or logically, and frequently uses the defense mechanisms of denial, rationalization, and projection. While persons with addiction do not change their behavior because of negative consequences suffered (recognizing that addictive behavior is harmful), it is not that they do not recognize the consequences. Rather, they continue the addictive behavior in spite of consequences experienced. Acting sober when intoxicated is an addictive behavior. **Cognitive Level:** Applying **Client Need:** Psychosocial Integrity **Integrated Process:** Teaching and Learning **Content Area:** Mental Health

Strategy: You might find it easier to answer this question if you reword it for yourself and then look for the things that are true about addiction. **Reference:** Varcarolis, E., Carson, V., & Shoemaker, N. (2009). *Foundations of psychiatric mental health nursing: A clinical approach* (6th ed.). St. Louis, MO: Saunders Elsevier, pp. 402–403.

2 **Answer: 2, 3, 5 Rationale:** The "C" in the CAGE mnemonic represents cutting down, not counting. The "G" in the CAGE mnemonic represents guilt, not gulping drinks. Feeling a need to cut down on drinking indicates the "C," cutting down or reducing alcohol. Annoyance represents the "A," being annoyed at what others say about the drinking. As for having a morning "eye-opener," the "E" is when the client needs a drink in the morning or upon awakening. **Cognitive Level:** Applying **Client Need:** Psychosocial Integrity **Integrated Process:** Nursing Process: Assessment **Content Area:** Mental Health **Strategy:** Notice the words *would be consistent* in the stem of this question. This tells you that the correct answer is a correct item in the options. Analyze each option and select the one that is part of that set of questions. **Reference:** Vidabeck, S. (2011). *Psychiatric-mental health nursing* (5th ed.). Philadelphia, PA: Lippincott Williams & Wilkins, p. 227.

3 Answer: 2 Rationale: Stating that the son has probably seen changes in the client when drinking presents reality to the client in a matter-of-fact, informative way and creates an opportunity for the nurse to help the client see that the parent-child relationship has no doubt been impacted by the addiction. Stating that the son probably knows the client is an alcoholic applies a label to the client (an alcoholic), although the information it is conveying is accurate. Telling the client it's good that he has concern for his son offers approval or praise and allows the client to feel like a protective and good parent, instead of a parent whose behavior has impacted negatively on the son. Stating that the son is old enough to learn about the effects of alcohol removes the personal focus that is necessary to help the addicted parent recognize the impact of the addiction on the son. **Cognitive Level:** Analyzing **Client Need:** Psychosocial Integrity **Integrated Process:** Communication and Documentation **Content Area:** Mental Health **Strategy:** Choose the answer that is most accurate, informative, and respectful of the client. **Reference:** Fontaine, K. (2009). *Mental health nursing* (6th ed.). Upper Saddle River, NJ: Prentice Hall, pp. 401–402.

4 Answer: 2 Rationale: Feeling that nurses' knowledge about drugs protects them from drug dependency is correct. The most significant risk factors that lead nurses to abuse drugs and become drug dependent are (1) exposure to substances, (2) knowledge about specific effects of certain drugs, and (3) belief that knowledge about drugs will allow them to use drugs and alcohol safely. Some nurses have grown up in a dysfunctional family, but this does not put them at more risk than those in the general public who have similar backgrounds. Most nurses know that health care providers and professionals are at a high risk for drug dependency, but they deny that this could happen to them as they feel protected by their knowledge about drugs. Some nurses may have problems with codependence, but this does not put them at more risk than those in the general public who have similar problems. **Cognitive Level:** Analyzing **Client Need:** Psychosocial Integrity **Integrated Process:** Teaching and Learning **Content Area:** Mental Health **Strategy:** Identify what is different about the environment and knowledge levels of nurses and non-nurses. This will help guide you to the correct option. **Reference:** Kneisl, C., Wilson, H., & Trigoboff, E. (2009). *Contemporary psychiatric-mental health nursing* (2nd ed.). Upper Saddle River, NJ: Prentice Hall, p. 350.

5 Answer: 1 Rationale: Denial is correct. It would not be unusual for a client who has severe addiction to come to day treatment intoxicated and deny it. Denial would cause a client to insist he or she is not intoxicated or doesn't have a problem with alcoholism despite concrete evidence of the problem. Rationalization is a frequently used defense mechanism of the alcoholic individual, but if it were being used, the client would offer an explanation for the odor of alcohol (such as "I spilled a bottle of cologne as I was getting dressed.") Transference is the unconscious process of displacing feelings for significant people in the past onto the nurse in the present relationship. Countertransference is the nurse's emotional reaction to clients based on feelings for significant people in the nurse's past. **Cognitive Level:** Applying **Client Need:** Psychosocial Integrity **Integrated Process:** Nursing Process: Assessment **Content Area:** Mental Health **Strategy:** Recall the common trio of defense mechanisms used by substance dependent individuals. Look for a behavioral example of one of them. **Reference:** Kneisl, C., Wilson, H., & Trigoboff, E. (2009). *Contemporary psychiatric-mental health nursing* (2nd ed.). Upper Saddle River, NJ: Prentice Hall, p. 352.

6 Answer: 4 Rationale: Suggesting that the family and friends have noticed that her drinking creates consequences is correct. It indicates one of the areas of the CAGE questionnaire that deals with expressed concern from others about client's drinking. The other three options would support the client's belief that others are against her or have no right to be concerned about her. Specifically, each option would support the client's denial, projection, or rationalization. **Cognitive Level:** Applying **Client Need:** Psychosocial Integrity **Integrated Process:** Nursing Process: Implementation **Content Area:** Mental Health **Strategy:** Look for areas of commonalty between options. Look for the one that is different. In this case, it is the most matter-of-fact and least opinionated statement. **Reference:** Kneisl, C., Wilson, H., & Trigoboff, E. (2009). *Contemporary psychiatric-mental health nursing* (2nd ed.). Upper Saddle River, NJ: Prentice Hall, p. 353.

7 Answer: 3 Rationale: Sobriety issue and depression at the same time is correct. This client will likely be dually diagnosed with alcoholism and depression. The nurse should recognize that current standards of addiction practice call for the substance abuse disorder and the psychiatric disorder to be treated simultaneously. The other three options do not recognize that in instances of dual diagnosis, current standards of addiction practice call for the substance abuse disorder and the psychiatric disorder to be treated simultaneously. **Cognitive Level:** Applying **Client Need:** Psychosocial Integrity **Integrated Process:** Nursing Process: Planning **Content Area:** Mental Health **Strategy:** Notice that this client has two problems, one of which (alcoholism) is considered a long-term problem that can be managed but never fully recovered from. **Reference:** Varcarolis, E., Carson, V., & Shoemaker, N. (2009). *Foundations of psychiatric mental health* *nursing: A clinical approach* (6th ed.). St. Louis, MO: Saunders Elsevier, pp. 15–16.

8 **Answer: 1, 3** **Rationale:** Two options are correct. AA teaches that a client with alcoholism can never safely return to social drinking and that total abstinence is the only course in treating the addiction. When sobriety has been achieved, people don't "graduate"; they stay and help others achieve sobriety. Acceptance and Higher Power are active concepts in AA, but practicing these principles does not remove urges to drink and does not guarantee sobriety. **Cognitive Level:** Understanding **Client Need:** Health Promotion and Maintenance **Integrated Process:** Teaching and Learning **Content Area:** Mental Health **Strategy:** Recall that alcoholism is considered a chronic disease that is characterized by remissions and exacerbations. **Reference:** Fontaine, K. (2009). *Mental health nursing* (6th ed.). Upper Saddle River, NJ: Prentice Hall, p. 395.

9 **Answer: 3** **Rationale:** Alcohol use during pregnancy causes dysmorphic prenatal and postnatal difficulties and central nervous system dysfunction. These problems range from subtle cognitive-behavioral impairments to fetal alcohol syndrome, both of which predispose the infant to later academic and behavioral problems, as well as mental illness. Since alcohol is so widely used, many people do not recognize its dangers, as they either do not consider it a drug or think that it is a safe drug. The other three options indicate substances that can cause significant health problems for the infant, but these problems are not as pervasive as those associated with the mother's using alcohol during pregnancy. **Cognitive Level:** Analyzing **Client Need:** Physiological Adaptation **Integrated Process:** Teaching and Learning **Content Area:** Mental Health **Strategy:** Think about the nature of the drugs listed and their potential effects to make a selection. Do not be misled by the fact that alcohol is a drug that can be obtained legally without a prescription. **Reference:** Fontaine, K. (2009). *Mental health nursing* (6th ed.). Upper Saddle River, NJ: Prentice Hall, p. 407.

10 **Answer: 1** **Rationale:** Stating that inhaling fumes from paints and wood stains may cause a disulfiram reaction is correct. The adverse reaction of disulfiram (Antabuse) will occur if the person taking this drug ingests, inhales, or absorbs alcohol, even in very small doses (such as inhaling vapors from paints or woodstains, or oral ingestion in products such as mouthwash). These reactions include throbbing headache, tachycardia, diaphoresis, and respiratory distress. Death can occur. This drug is not used often, but the nurse should know about its uses and dangers. While eating improperly cooked seafood might lead to gastric distress and/or liver problems, uncooked seafood does not precipitate a disulfiram reaction. Disulfiram does not reduce the craving for alcohol, but opioid antagonists, such as naltrexone (ReVia) do. Disulfiram works on the classical principle of conditioned avoidance. If the individual drinks

alcohol while taking disulfiram, intensely unpleasant and dangerous physical reactions can occur. The effect of disulfiram (Antabuse) when combined with alcohol is not intoxication. Instead, the individual experiences intensely unpleasant and dangerous physical reactions. **Cognitive Level:** Analyzing **Client Need:** Pharmacological and Parenteral Therapies **Integrated Process:** Teaching and Learning **Content Area:** Pharmacology **Strategy:** Recall the principles of operant conditioning and integrate that with your knowledge of the expected drug effect. **Reference:** Varcarolis, E., Carson, V., & Shoemaker, N. (2009). *Foundations of psychiatric mental health nursing: A clinical approach* (6th ed.). St. Louis, MO: Saunders Elsevier, pp. 425–426.

Posttest

1 **Answer: 2, 3, 4** **Rationale:** Three options are correct. Alcoholism was officially listed as a disease in 1956, and Jellinek's identification of the four phases of disease progression in 1960 reinforced the disease concept ("addiction is a medical illness"). Addiction includes behavioral habits and emotional attachment, but it is seen first as a medical disease. Although alcoholism has been recognized as a disease for approximately 50 years, many members of the general public continue to view addiction as a moral weakness. Addiction experts do not consider that addiction can be cured. Instead, they consider it a chronic medical disease that can be managed. **Cognitive Level:** Analyzing **Client Need:** Psychosocial Integrity **Integrated Process:** Teaching and Learning **Content Area:** Mental Health **Strategy:** Remember that treatment approaches for alcoholism include both biomedical and biosocial models. **Reference:** Varcarolis, E., Carson, V., & Shoemaker, N. (2009). *Foundations of psychiatric mental health nursing: A clinical approach* (6th ed.). St. Louis, MO: Saunders Elsevier, pp. 405–408.

2 **Answer: 3** **Rationale:** Withdrawal is correct. Taking a drink in the morning to steady one's nerves is a sign of physical dependence and is done to avoid withdrawal symptoms. Tremors are one of the ten symptoms of alcohol withdrawal listed in the Clinical Institute Withdrawal Assessment of alcohol symptoms. People with anxiety may have tremors, but the tremors would occur throughout the day. Tolerance is not indicated because the client does not describe needing to have a larger drink in order to prevent symptoms. This client has clearly progressed from alcohol abuse to alcohol dependency. **Cognitive Level:** Applying **Client Need:** Physiological Adaptation **Integrated Process:** Nursing Process: Assessment **Content Area:** Mental Health **Strategy:** Think about persons that you know and consider to be normal drinkers. Have you ever seen them engage in an early morning drink of alcohol? If your answer is affirmative, then recognize that this person is probably not a normal drinker. **Reference:** Varcarolis, E., Carson, V., & Shoemaker, N. (2009). *Foundations of*

ANSWERS & RATIONALES

psychiatric mental health nursing: A clinical approach (6th ed.). St. Louis, MO: Saunders Elsevier, pp. 410–417.

3 **Answer: 4** **Rationale:** Alcohol dependency is correct. At a blood level of 0.35%, the non-physically-dependent, non-tolerant drinker would be confused, ataxic, and either semi-comatose or comatose. Death is expected when the BAL reaches approximately 0.50%. The situation suggests that this client has been drinking regularly over a long period of time and is now experiencing tolerance to alcohol (needing an increasing amount of alcohol to bring about the desired effect). Tolerance can only develop once the person is physically dependent on alcohol. This client is not acutely intoxicated, even though the BAL exceeds the normal level for intoxication (0.08% to 0.10%). This client's body now accepts unusually high concentrations of alcohol (tolerance) and has adapted to the presence of the alcohol (physical dependence). There is no evidence of withdrawal symptoms, such as anxiety, tremulousness, and marked elevations in vital signs. No information is given that would allow recognition of psychological dependence, which can come very early in the drinking history and precede physical dependence and tolerance. **Cognitive Level:** Analyzing **Client Need:** Physiological Adaptation **Integrated Process:** Nursing Process: Assessment **Content Area:** Mental Health **Strategy:** Review statistics about blood alcohol levels (BAL) and effects on behavior. Take note of the client's absence of usual behaviors associated with a BAL of 0.35%. **Reference:** Varcarolis, E., Carson, V., & Shoemaker, N. (2009). *Foundations of psychiatric mental health nursing: A clinical approach* (6th ed.). St. Louis, MO: Saunders Elsevier, p. 403.

4 **Answer: 4** **Rationale:** Facilitating cravings and triggers for reusing is correct. Cravings appear to be the result of pleasurable memories engendered from the psycho-activating effect of engaging in addictive behaviors. Substances of abuse alter the brain's reward system by artificially boosting dopamine effects, which keep the pleasure circuit firing. It's true that environment and role models influence use patterns but this is not part of the BRS phenomenon. As for offering a means of mediating job stress and pressure, it is true that people employ addictive behaviors to self-medicate stress and pressure experienced, but this is not part of the BRS phenomenon. Reducing physiologic and psychological cravings indicates that the BRS is a positive phenomenon that assists with drug abstinence. Instead, the BRS is a negative phenomenon that assists with maintaining or returning to the substance use pattern. **Cognitive Level:** Applying **Client Need:** Physiological Adaptation **Integrated Process:** Nursing Process: Evaluation **Content Area:** Mental Health **Strategy:** Think of the BRS as a hungry animal that is very difficult to satiate. **Reference:** Fontaine, K. (2009). *Mental health nursing* (6th ed.). Upper Saddle River, NJ: Prentice Hall, pp. 384–385.

5 **Answer: 3** **Rationale:** Gradual reduction in dosage of the drug commonly used is correct. Medically supervised withdrawal from benzodiazepines generally involves gradual downward titration of doses of the drug commonly used. Rapid or abrupt discontinuation of a benzodiazepine is physiologically dangerous and can lead to death. Planned, progressive addition of an antipsychotic is incorrect because most antipsychotics lower the seizure threshold and are, therefore, not appropriate for clients in active benzodiazepine withdrawal because they would increase the risk of seizure activity. **Cognitive Level:** Applying **Client Need:** Physiological Adaptation **Integrated Process:** Teaching and Learning **Content Area:** Mental Health **Strategy:** Compare protocols for alcohol withdrawal and benzodiazepine withdrawal. Identify areas of commonality and reasons for same. **Reference:** Fontaine, K. (2009). *Mental health nursing* (9th ed.). Upper Saddle River, NJ: Prentice Hall, p. 382.

6 **Answer: 4** **Rationale:** Providing withdrawal care based on unit protocol is correct. Alcohol withdrawal delirium (delirium tremens, or DTs) is a physiologically dangerous process with potentially fatal consequences. Various medical approaches are used to treat it, and the nurse's care must fit into the protocol of the particular agency. Priority is assigned to the client's physical needs during this major withdrawal phenomenon. Beginning education about the disease (presenting psycho-education) and encouraging development of a relapse prevention plan are not appropriate at this time because the client is in physiologic peril. These options can be appropriate after the withdrawal period has ended. Administering anti-craving medications is not the highest current priority, as the client is actively withdrawing from alcohol and can be at risk physiologically. **Cognitive Level:** Analyzing **Client Need:** Reduction of Risk Potential **Integrated Process:** Nursing Process: Implementation **Content Area:** Mental Health **Strategy:** Remember that alcohol withdrawal delirium is considered a medical emergency and can lead to death if not properly treated. **Reference:** Kneisl, C., Wilson, H., & Trigoboff, E. (2009). *Contemporary psychiatric-mental health nursing*. (2nd ed.). Upper Saddle River, NJ: Prentice Hall, p. 331.

7 **Answer: 1, 5** **Rationale:** Assessing level of consciousness and vital signs are correct. The nurse should recognize possible signs of autonomic hyperactivity that is a part of alcohol withdrawal delirium. If the vital signs (also a part of autonomic hyperactivity) are elevated and the level of consciousness decreased, the client will require a prn dose of the cross-tolerant drug that is being used as part of the withdrawal protocol. Because the client is in active withdrawal, this is not the time to teach the client (explaining the concepts of withdrawal). The priority is on maintaining physiologic functioning and environmental safety. Thiamine and folic acid may be ordered for the client who is withdrawing from alcohol, but they are used to treat complications of alcoholism, not to manage the acute symptoms of withdrawal. This can only be done with a drug that is cross-tolerant with alcohol. Determining the most recent blood alcohol level is inappropriate, as it would not provide current data. The nurse should be able to recognize and respond to the clinical signs of increasing intensity of withdrawal symptoms. **Cognitive Level:** Analyzing **Client Need:** Physiological Adaptation **Integrated Process:** Nursing Process: Implementation **Content Area:** Mental Health **Strategy:** Review the concepts of physical dependency, autonomic hyperactivity, and cross-tolerance. **Reference:** Kneisl, C., Wilson, H., & Trigoboff, E. (2009). *Contemporary psychiatric-mental health nursing* (2nd ed.). Upper Saddle River, NJ: Prentice Hall, p. 354.

8 Answer: 3 Rationale: Reducing craving for alcohol is correct. Naltrexone (ReVia) is a narcotic antagonist that is useful for treating alcohol-dependent persons with high levels of craving and somatic symptoms. It works by blocking opiate receptors and reducing or eliminating the alcohol craving. Naltrexone does not prevent withdrawal symptoms. Since it is a narcotic antagonist, and narcotics and alcohol are both CNS depressants, it is possible that naltrexone (ReVia) could precipitate withdrawal symptoms in an individual who has had recent intake of alcohol. Naltrexone (ReVia) is not expected to prevent or reduce alcoholic blackouts or to directly manage anxiety. **Cognitive Level:** Analyzing **Client Need:** Pharmacological and Parenteral Therapies **Integrated Process:** Teaching and Learning **Content Area:** Mental Health **Strategy:** Review the concept of cross-tolerance. Determine how it might relate to naltrexone's being used to treat alcoholism. **Reference:** Varcarolis, E., Carson, V., & Shoemaker, N. (2009). *Foundations of psychiatric mental health nursing: A clinical approach* (6th ed.). St. Louis, MO: Saunders Elsevier, pp. 423, 426–427.

9 Answer: 2 Rationale: Drinking-refusal skills is correct. The quality of an adolescent's recovery environment can be helpful or hurtful to someone attempting to maintain sobriety. Friends or acquaintances may encourage a recovering person to use. The recovering adolescent may want to refuse, but may not know how. Behavioral rehearsal, saying "no thanks" to an offer to engage in addictive behavior, can increase a recovering person's confidence. Critical thinking skills will not help the adolescent to refuse a drink. Problem-solving skills and communication skills may be useful but not as helpful as skills directly related to refusing to drink. **Cognitive Level:** Applying **Client Need:** Psychosocial Integrity **Integrated Process:** Nursing Process: Planning **Content Area:** Mental Health **Strategy:** Consider the tremendous impact that peer pressure has on adolescents. **Reference:** Fontaine, K. (2009). *Mental health nursing* (6th ed.). Upper Saddle River, NJ: Prentice Hall, p. 404.

10 Answer: 4 Rationale: Decisional Conflict is correct. The definition of decisional conflict is uncertainty about a course of action to be taken when choice among competing actions involve risk, loss, or challenge to personal life values. In Dysfunctional Family Processes: Alcoholism may apply, but it is more appropriate for the family than the individual. Ineffective Management of Therapeutic Regimen implies that the client has already made a commitment to recovery. Since the client probably abuses or is dependent on alcohol, risk for injury may be present. However, what is shown in the stem of the question is behavior that indicates decisional conflict. **Cognitive Level:** Applying **Client Need:** Psychosocial Integrity **Integrated Process:** Nursing Process: Diagnosis **Content Area:** Mental Health **Strategy:** Look carefully at the information that is given in the stem. Do not assume that risk for injury, which is often a correct response, is correct in this instance. **Reference:** Kneisl, C., Wilson, H., & Trigoboff, E. (2009). *Contemporary psychiatric-mental health nursing* (2nd ed.). Upper Saddle River, NJ: Prentice Hall, p. 353.

References

American Psychiatric Association (2000). *Diagnosis and statistical manual of mental disorders* (4th ed. text revision). Washington, DC: American Psychiatric Association, pp. 288, 297–344.

Carpenito, L. J. (2011). *Nursing diagnosis: Application to clinical practice* (13th ed.). Philadelphia, PA: Lippincott Williams & Wilkins.

Fontaine, K. (2009). *Mental health nursing* (6th ed.). Upper Saddle River, NJ: Pearson Education.

Kneisl, C., Wilson, H., & Trigoboff, E. (2009). *Contemporary psychiatric–mental health nursing* (2nd ed.). Upper Saddle River, NJ: Pearson Education.

North American Nursing Diagnosis Association (2008). *Nursing diagnosis: Definitions and classification 2009–2011.* Indianapolis, IN: Wiley-Blackwell.

Stuart, G. (2009). *Principles and practice of psychiatric nursing* (9th ed.). St. Louis: Elsevier Science.

Townsend, M. (2011). *Essentials of psychiatric–mental health nursing* (5th ed.). Philadelphia, PA: F. A. Davis.

Varcarolis, E., & Halter, M. (2010). *Foundations of psychiatric mental health nursing: A clinical approach* (6th ed.). Philadelphia: Saunders.

12 Family Violence and Sexual Assault

Chapter Outline

Overview of Violence
Theories of Violence

Violence in Special
Populations

Sexual Violence or Assault

NCLEX-RN® Test Prep

Use the accompanying online resource, NursingReviewsandRationales, to test yourself with hundreds of NCLEX®-style practice questions.

Objectives

➤ Differentiate between the different types of violence.
➤ Identify characteristics of the victim and characteristics of the perpetrator of violence.
➤ Analyze the clinical manifestations secondary to violence toward others.
➤ Determine appropriate nursing diagnoses applicable to clients who experience violence.
➤ Formulate a plan of care for a client who has experienced violence.
➤ Identify expected outcomes for clients who have experienced violence.

Review at a Glance

abuse a pattern of behavior manifested by the perpetrator whereby the underpinnings are due to the need to obtain complete power and control over the victim; power and control are obtained through psychological/emotional, financial, and/or physical control; causes feelings of anxiety, fear, guilt, hopelessness, helplessness, depression

assault threat of violence towards another

battering repeated violence that causes injury to another person

child abuse any act that causes neglect, psychological/emotional harm, physical harm, and/or sexual harm to a child or adolescent under the age of 18

elder abuse physical harm, psychological/emotional harm, or sexual harm to a person over the age of 65, commonly inflicted by family members

family violence violence that is inflicted on one family member by another; may be emotional/psychological, physical, financial, and/or sexual

incest sexual relations between a child or adolescent (under 18 years of age) with a relative or surrogate relative

intimate partner violence (IPV) violence towards an intimate partner intended to intimidate or degrade; can be emotional/psychological, physical, financial, and/or sexual

mandatory reporting laws laws that require the reporting of violence against a child, elder, or vulnerable adult

Munchausen's syndrome by proxy a form of abuse where the caregiver deliberately feigns psychological or physical symptoms in another person who is under their care; the perpetrator does this for emotional (not financial) gain

neglect a condition in which a caregiver does not provide age-appropriate basic needs for the individual in his or her care; can be physical, emotional, economic, social, medical, and/or educational

perpetrator the person who commits an act of abuse/violence against another

posttraumatic stress disorder (PTSD) psychiatric disorder that occurs after a traumatic event (onset typically first occurs three months after the trauma) characterized by intrusive and recurrent distressing memories of the event, recurrent distressing dreams or

nightmares of the event, sense of reliving the experience (i.e., illusions, hallucinations, delusions, dissociation), psychological distress when exposed to cues that resemble the event, physiological reactivity, and hypervigilence

rape forced sexual intercourse

sexual assault forceful genital, anal, or oral penetration of the victim by any object, including a penis (term includes rape)

shaken baby syndrome syndrome resulting from violent shaking of infants to preschool age that results in whiplashlike closed head/neck injuries, neurological consequences, and/or disability and death

stalking threat or harassment of one person to another (i.e., following someone, sending unwanted gifts, showing up at a person's place of work or home, defaming character, and/or internet/cell phone harassment)

victim person who suffers from maltreatment or violence from another

PRETEST

1 An 18-month-old client is scheduled for a minor surgical procedure. The client has numerous large bruises of different stages over the back and buttocks. The mother states that the child must have fallen down while playing alone outside but cannot provide specific information about these incidents. How should the nurse evaluate this situation?

1. Possible child abuse
2. Immature parenting
3. Normal findings in an 18-month-old
4. Indications of tissue fragility

2 A newly licensed nurse asks an experienced nurse about theories related to violent behaviors towards others. The experienced nurse should respond by making which statements? Select all that apply.

1. "The underpinnings of social learning theory lay in the idea that violent behavior is related to the perpetrator's need for control and power."
2. "There is no etiological basis for violent behavior towards others."
3. "Poor impulse control may be one reason for violent behavior."
4. "Feminist theory states that it is due to the physiology of the male gender."
5. "The male response theory states that women provoke men, and that women are responsible for the abuse."

3 A five-year-old girl is brought to the clinic for symptoms of a urinary tract infection (UTI). The nurse's assessment reveals bruises in the child's genital and rectal areas. The mother reports that she had left the little girl with her boyfriend the night before. The nurse's first priority with this client is to take which action?

1. Obtain a urine sample to confirm a UTI.
2. Teach the mother about symptoms of UTI.
3. Report suspected sexual abuse to protective services.
4. Assess the child for other health problems.

4 A client comes to the emergency department with a broken wrist and severe bruises inflicted by a beating by the intimate partner. The client states an intention to remain in the relationship at this time. What is the most appropriate response by the nurse?

1. "You need to leave the relationship."
2. "I will call a lawyer for you if you wish."
3. "Let's develop a safety plan for repeated violence."
4. "Here is a list of services that can help you."

5 A nurse is teaching a class on domestic violence to high school students. Which statement by a student would indicate to the nurse that further teaching is needed?

1. "Violence often begins in a dating relationship."
2. "The abuser will often apologize and promise to stop."
3. "If you are educated and have money, abuse does not happen."
4. "Abusers are often excessively jealous and possessive."

6 The nurse is caring for a female client who comes to the emergency room with bruises on the face, a cracked tooth and back pain. She voices concern about the safety of her pets and children, and her ability to enroll in her college as she plans. The nurse replies by explaining which of the following? Select all that apply.

1. She is correct that her pets may be at risk for injury or death from her spouse.
2. Her pets are safe; there is no correlation between interpersonal violence and injury to pets.
3. Her children are safe; there is no correlation between spousal violence and injury to children.
4. It is probable that her husband may try to sabotage her career goals.
5. She is correct that her children may be at risk for abuse.

7 A five-year-old child has been removed from the home because of sexual abuse by the stepfather. When teaching the child's mother about possible consequences the child might experience, which of the following should the nurse include?

1. Since the child was removed from the home at an early age, no long-term consequences are expected.
2. Because the abuser was someone well known by the child, the situation will be less traumatic for the child.
3. The child is at current risk for developing depression and will remain so in the future.
4. Once an adult, the child should be counseled not to have children, as the child will become an abuser.

8 A 15-year-old female student visits the school nurse's office asking about date rape and pregnancy. She confides to the nurse that her boyfriend forced her to have sex against her will. The most appropriate initial intervention of the nurse would be to do which of the following?

1. Administer a pregnancy test.
2. Teach safe sex practices.
3. Teach methods of birth control.
4. Identify the student's immediate concerns and feelings.

9 A pregnant female comes to the emergency department with bruises on her arms and abdomen after a fight with her boyfriend. What is most important for the nurse to address when teaching this client?

1. Risks of pregnancy complications caused by abuse
2. Assertiveness training to deal with the boyfriend
3. Childbirth classes to prepare for the birth
4. Instructions on the use of resources available to her

10 A pediatric client has severe injuries to the abdomen. The nurse should suspect child abuse if the parents do which of the following?

1. Delay seeking treatment for the child's injuries.
2. Give a very detailed description of the events prior to the injuries.
3. Exhibit an anxious and concerned attitude.
4. Encourage the child to explain the injuries.

➤ *See pages 250–251 for Answers and Rationales.*

I. OVERVIEW OF VIOLENCE

A. Definition of terms

1. **Abuse**: the willful infliction of physical violence, neglect, emotional/psychological violence, financial abuse, and/or sexual assault on another person
2. Violence: the physical force exerted for the purpose of dominating, controlling, lowering self-esteem, and taking away individual choice

3. **Family violence**: violence that occurs within a family system; is often used interchangeably with abuse; it includes neglect, psychological/emotional abuse, financial control, and/or sexual assault
4. **Perpetrator** (or abuser): the person who inflicts violence on another person
5. **Victim**: the person who is the recipient of abuse

B. Violence is one of the fastest-growing public health problems today

1. It cuts across all socioeconomic lines
2. It occurs in all age groups and relationship types
3. Drug and/or alcohol use/abuse by the perpetrator is often involved
4. Societal factors that contribute to violence
   a. Divorce and blended families
   b. Lack of nuclear family for support
   c. Social isolation
   d. Economic strain

5. Elders are living longer and becoming more dependent on others for care
6. Emergency department is often the first or only place of the victim's interface with the health system
7. Clients may present with injuries or somatic (bodily response) symptoms
8. Violent behavior is often cyclic and escalates in frequency and intensity over time
9. Victim may blame self in an attempt to control the situation
10. Victim may try to protect the perpetrator or be reluctant to identify the perpetrator
11. Nurses must be alert to the possibility of abuse, particularly if injuries are unexplained or explanation does not match clinical picture
12. **Mandatory reporting laws** require nurses and other health care providers to report suspected violence in all states; there are civil and criminal penalties for not reporting

C. **Types of violence**
1. Physical violence: physical harm or injury caused by beating, hitting, cutting, shooting, burning, or raping; **assault** is a threat of violence; **battering** is repeated physical violence
2. **Sexual assault**: pressured or forced sexual contact, including sexually stimulated talk or actions, inappropriate touching or intercourse, incest, and/or **rape** (forced sexual intercourse or forced penetration of objects)
3. Emotional or psychological violence
   a. Intimidation with the intent to instill fear
   b. Social isolation of an individual
   c. Violation of personal rights such as holding the victim(s) hostage, taking away care keys, locking the victim out of his/her home, not allowing the use of the phone/computer
4. Economic abuse: financial exploitation by restricting access to credit cards or money (i.e., putting victim on strict allowance), food, clothing, and/or transportation, and/or preventing the pursuit of work/career
5. **Neglect**: withholding or failing to provide proper personal care in any of the following areas:
   a. Physical: not providing needed food, clothing, and/or shelter
   b. Emotional: not providing needed love and nurturance
   c. Medical: not providing needed medical (i.e., prescriptions) and/or dental care
   d. Education: failure to enroll child in school, allowing consistent tardiness and/or truancy
   e. Abandonment: leaving children alone without age-appropriate supervision

D. **Victims: occur across the lifespan**
1. Children and adolescents
2. Siblings
3. Partners (heterosexual and homosexual)
4. Elders

E. **Physiological responses to violence**
1. Multiple injuries: especially to head, face, throat, trunk, and/or sexual organs
2. Unexplained bruises, lacerations, abrasions, head injuries, fractures, burns
3. Malnutrition and/or dehydration
4. Stress-related somatic responses such as headaches, nausea, vomiting, diarrhea, stomach pains, menstrual problems, chronic pain, insomnia, hyperinsomnia
5. Permanent disability from injury (i.e., paralysis, neurological damage)

F. **Psychological responses to violence**
1. Fear, hypervigilant responses
2. Lowered self-esteem, loss of sense of self
3. Anxiety, depression, suicidal threats and/or suicidal ideation

  4. Helplessness, hopelessness, and powerlessness
  5. Development of eating disorders (i.e., anorexia nervosa, bulimia nervosa)
  6. Difficulty problem solving and/or difficulty decision making, memory loss

  7. Acute stress syndrome, onset is typically two days to four weeks after traumatic event; if symptoms continue to occur, the diagnosis of PTSD is made
  8. Posttraumatic stress disorder (PTSD): can be acute or chronic; onset is typically three months after traumatic event

G. Etiology/psychopathology
  1. Characteristics of victims of violence
     a. Low self-esteem, feelings of helplessness and hopelessness
     b. Feelings of powerlessness, guilt, and shame
     c. May protect perpetuator and accept responsibility for abuse
     d. May blame self in an attempt to maintain a sense of control over situation
     e. May use defense mechanisms of denial, repression, suppression
  2. Characteristics of perpetrators
     a. Use threats and intimidation to control the victim
     b. Often suffered from abuse, neglect, or severe discipline as a child (intergenerational effect of family violence)
     c. Projection is primary defense mechanism: blames others or circumstances for own problems, does not genuinely take responsibility for behavior
     d. Impulsive, immature, has low self-esteem and poorly developed sense of self
     e. Have unmet dependency needs; may be extremely jealous of partner without any real justification for jealousy
     f. May be an extreme disciplinarian who believes in physical punishment
     g. Poor parenting skills (as role-modeled per parents) and developmentally inappropriate high expectations of the child/children
     h. Concerned about child's gender and/or performance prior to birth
     i. May have had difficult pregnancy and/or labor and delivery
     j. May manifest alcohol and/or other substance abuse problems
     k. Have unrealistic high expectations of others' behavior
     l. Are generally law abiding and only a danger to family
  3. Characteristics of family systems where violence occurs
     a. Socially isolated
     b. Multigenerational transmission: family history of abuse
     c. Rigid family rules and boundaries
     d. Use and abuse of power by family authority figure
     e. Drug and alcohol use prevalent in perpetrator; victim may begin to use to self-medicate
     f. Generalized anxiety and fear in the household
     g. Secrecy; family members make excuse for perpetrator's behavior; work at hiding the "family secret"

II. THEORIES OF VIOLENCE

  A. There is no single theory about the etiologies of violent behaviors; it is likely that numerous factors contribute to the behavior(s)
  B. Some current theories include the following:
     1. Neurobiological
        a. Biologists believe aggression is inherent in humans and regulated by hormones such as testosterone; increased levels affect aggression
        b. Neurophysiologists believe behavior is related to imbalances of neurotransmitters, such as serotonin

2. Social learning theory
   a. Violence is a learned behavior, learned by observation, modeling, and direct experience
   b. Intergenerational transmission; poor parenting skills contribute to it
   c. A culture that accepts and promotes violence and media that desensitizes through repeated exposure to violence both play a role
   d. Violence is part of our socialization process
3. Psychological or interpersonal theories
   a. Etiology lies in the personality of the perpetrator
   b. Perpetrator may do the following:
      1) Manifest with a psychiatric illness such as personality disorder (i.e., sociopathic personality disorder)
      2) Demonstrate poor impulse control and inability to control anger
      3) Poor coping skills
      4) Have low self-esteem and fears of abandonment
      5) Have suffered early emotional deprivation
4. Feminist theories
   a. The sexist structure of society contributes to violence
   b. Women are controlled and subordinated by power and privilege of males
   c. Violence is about gender and power
   d. Power inequities between victim and perpetrator contribute to violence
   e. Devaluation of women by society contributes to violence
5. Sociologic: societal issues promote violence
   a. Unemployment
   b. Poverty
   c. Crime
   d. Teen pregnancy
   e. Isolation

III. VIOLENCE IN SPECIAL POPULATIONS

A. **Child abuse**: maltreatment or violence against children; physical, emotional, sexual, or psychological damage done to a child
   1. Violence can range from mild to severe physiological injury (or injuries), psychological damage, disability, and death
   2. Children who observe family violence demonstrate an increase in behavioral and emotional problems more than children/adolescents that do not
      a. These children/adolescents are at increased risk for cognitive deficits
      b. These children/adolescents are at increased risk for becoming batterers themselves
   3. Witnessing violence has negative psychological effects on children
   4. Adolescents who commit homicide have often been severely and violently mistreated
   5. Types of violence
      a. Physical violence: inflicting injury to a child that can range from minor to severe injury, disability or death; see Table 12-1 for signs of physical violence to a child
      b. Emotional or psychological violence: psychological harm done by demeaning and/or intimidating treatment that undermines a child's sense of self, safety, and/or competence; see Box 12-1 for behavioral signs of emotional violence
      c. Physical neglect: harm or threatened harm to a child's health or welfare by a parent or guardian through failure to provide adequate food, clothing, shelter, proper supervision, or medical treatment; see Box 12-2 for signs of physical neglect

Table 12-1	Physical and Behavioral Signs of Physical Violence in Children
Physical Signs	**Behavioral/Psychological Signs**
Bruise in various stages of healing, often on head and neck	Behavioral extremes aggressive to passive Depression Suicidal threats/ideation Fear of parents or caregiver
Bite marks	Extreme rage or passivity
Burns in shape of objects or glove-like from immersion in hot liquids	Apprehension when other children cry Lack of trust Verbal reports of abuse
Fractures, scars, or serious internal injuries	
Lacerations Welts that may show a pattern	Hyperactivity, distractibility, or hypervigilance
Bald spots from hair being pulled	Disorganized thinking, self-injurious, or suicidal behavior Low academic achievement
	Social withdrawal
	Running away from home or illegal behaviors
	Cheating, lying, low academic performance
	Poor relationships with peers
	Inappropriately dressed for weather
	Regressive behaviors (such as enuresis, encopresis)

Box 12-1

Behavioral Signs of Emotional Maltreatment in Children

Behavior inappropriate for age, either precocious or regressed
Anxiety
Behavioral extremes
Self-destructive behaviors
Inappropriate affect
Vandalism, cheating, lying, stealing
Excessive self-soothing behaviors such as thumb-sucking and rocking
Anorexia nervosa or bulimia nervosa

Box 12-2

Signs of Physical Neglect in Children

Inappropriately dressed for season, poorly fitting and/or soiled clothing
Malnourished, always hungry, hoarding or stealing food
Medical problems such as infected sores or poor dental health
Delinquent behaviors—stealing or drug use
Poor school performance, tardiness, truancy
Social withdrawal, few friends
Listless and tired
Poor hygiene
Failure to thrive in infants

    d. Emotional neglect: chronic failure to provide a nurturing supportive environment needed for age-appropriate growth and development; parental signs of emotional neglect include the parent ignoring the child's presence or rebuffing child's attempts to interact; ignoring social, educational, or recreational needs; or denying the child opportunity to receive positive reinforcement
  6. Sibling violence: harm inflicted on a child by a sibling
    a. Most unrecognized type of violence against children
    b. May be emotional/psychological, physical, and/or sexual

   c. Parents may perceive sibling violence as part of normal part of growth and development
   d. Children/adolescents physically abused by parents are more likely to strike siblings
7. Child/adolescent sexual assault: involvement of a child or adolescent in sexual activity that they do not fully comprehend and so cannot truly consent to it
   a. Two types of sexual assault exist:
      1) Assault by a non-relative
      2) **Incest**, sexual assault by a relative(s) or surrogate relative(s) with a child or adolescent before the age of 18
   b. See Table 12-2 for physical and behavioral indicators of child sexual assault
   c. Child sexual assault can have long-term emotional/psychological and/or behavioral effects; these may include the following:
      1) Posttraumatic stress disorder (see Chapter 5)
      2) Risky sexual behaviors, sexual problems in adulthood
      3) Difficulties trusting others
      4) Anxiety and panic attacks
      5) Major depressive disorder
      6) Tobacco, alcohol, and/or other substance abuse problems
      7) Eating disorders, primarily bulimia nervosa
      8) Self-destructive behaviors such as high-risk behaviors and self-mutilation (i.e., cutting or burning self)
   d. An exploiting relationship usually develops over time; the perpetrator will initially groom the child/adolescent (i.e., bribe with gifts, money) and eventually win the child's /adolescent's confidence and trust
   e. Perpetrator imposes/demands secrecy with threats of harm to child and/or family if secrecy is violated
   f. The earlier in childhood the sexual assault occurs, the more profound the psychological/emotional damage to the child
   g. If the perpetrator is found to be a trusted friend or relative, the violation of trust is traumatic to victim and all family members

---

Table 12-2 Physical and Behavioral Signs of Child Sexual Assault

Physical Signs	Behavioral Signs
Frequent urination or dysuria	Overly sexualized behavior
Sexually transmitted disease (genital areas or throat)	Seductive and/or advanced sexual knowledge for age Promiscuity and/or prostitution
Pain or difficulty walking or sitting	Fear of a particular person or place Compulsive masturbation
Foreign matter in bladder, rectum, urethra, or vagina	Precocious sexual play Sexually abuse of another child
Sleep problems: insomnia or nightmares	
Rashes or itching in genital area	Unexplained gifts or money from questionable sources
Bruises, edema, or pain in genital	Drop in school attendance/performance
Bruises, edema, or pain in rectal area	Sudden onset of enuresis Excessive anxiety
Scarred labia or rectal fissures	Compulsive showering/bathing Running away from home
Pregnancy	Depression
	Suicide threats or ideation Self-destructive behaviors (i.e., head banging, cutting)

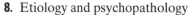

Practice to Pass

You are caring for a young child who is a suspected victim of sexual abuse by a parent. What physical and psychological data would you assess for the child and the parents?

8. Etiology and psychopathology
    a. Characteristics of individuals who sexually assault children
        1) 90% of perpetrators were severely sexually assaulted as children
        2) Are experiencing stressful life situations
        3) Have few support systems; are socially isolated
        4) Are lacking in adaptive coping mechanisms
        5) Have unusually high expectations of the child
        6) Demonstrate poor impulse control
        7) May abuse alcohol and/or other substances
    b. Characteristics of incestuous family systems (family systems theory)
        1) Father is domineering, impulsive, and physically violent
        2) Mother is passive and submissive, may be battered by spouse
        3) System is closed to outsiders; rigid family boundaries

        4) Enmeshed family system: individual boundaries are poorly defined and characterized by excessive dependence on other family members for physical and emotional/psychological needs
        5) Role reversal may take place, whereby child is the caregiver of the parent(s)
    c. See Box 12-3 for risk factors that predispose individuals to maltreat children
9. Assessment of the child experiencing physical or emotional violence
    a. Observe for physical, emotional/psychological, and behavioral signs as previously outlined in Table 12-1
    b. Be concerned if parent/caregiver delays seeking medical treatment for injuries
    c. Note vague and/or inconsistent accounts of events regarding injuries
    d. Injuries manifested do not reflect caregiver's report of cause
    e. Note resistance to leaving child alone with health care provider
    f. Assess relationship of child to caregiver (signs and symptoms of age-appropriate bonding)
    g. Assess for **shaken baby syndrome**
        1) Caused by violent shaking of a neonate, infant, and/or young child
        2) Respiratory distress and retinal bleeding are key indicators; it is a medical emergency
    h. Be alert to **Munchausen's syndrome by proxy**: injuries or illness induced in child/adolescent by caregiver in order to meet caregiver's emotional needs
        1) Gain attention, feel a sense of importance, and/or receive positive reinforcement from health care providers (i.e., "what a great mother you are")
        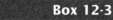
        2) Core features include traveling to seek health care from multiple providers, recurrent hospitalizations, and pathological lying

Box 12-3	Suffered abuse or neglect themselves
Risk Factors That May Predispose Individuals to Abuse Children	Hostile, blaming others
	Low self-esteem
	Impulsive, immature
	Prenatal issues (i.e., depression, unwanted pregnancy, fear of difficult labor and delivery or difficult labor and delivery)
	Burdened by caring for parents
	High expectations of others' behaviors
	Overwhelmed by care needs of others
	Unmet emotional needs of their own
	Substance abuse problems
	Experience increased socioeconomic stress
	Family pattern of violence
	Need to maintain and/or have power and control

10. Priority nursing diagnoses
    a. Pain (emotional/psychological and physical) due to the infliction by parent/ guardian with the intent to cause harm (victim)
    b. Post-Trauma related to having been the victim of physical and/or emotional abuse
    c. Social Isolation related to inadequate support systems or being prevented from interacting with peers or others
    d. Disturbed Self-Esteem related to unmet dependency needs, repeated abuse, dysfunctional family system, or not being valued by parents or guardian
    e. Fear related to repeated psychological/emotional and/or physical abuse

    f. Ineffective Family Coping related to inadequate support systems and/or poor parenting skills
11. Planning and implementation
    a. Report abuse to child protective services; be objective when reporting
    b. Provide medical and pharmacological treatment for injuries when applicable
    c. Encourage child/adolescent to discuss emotional feelings; child may be reluctant
    d. Reassure child/adolescent that he or she is not to blame
    e. Assess parents'/caregivers' ability to cope with situation
    f. Use a non-punitive approach when communicating with parents/caregivers
    g. Provide parent education, including information on normal growth and development, anger management, appropriate discipline methods, and parenting skills
    h. Refer caregiver to community resources (i.e., Parents Anonymous, parenting classes)
12. Evaluation
    a. Ongoing evaluation of child's safety
    b. Parent/caregiver verbalizes an understanding of behaviors related to normal growth and development
    c. Parent/caregiver verbalizes an understanding of resources available for anger management, parenting classes
    d. Ongoing evaluation of parent's ability to cope with situation, and follow through with goals to improve parenting skills

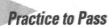

Practice to Pass

You are caring for the family of a young child who has been physically abused by the parents. To whom are you legally obliged to report the incident? What are potential consequences of not reporting child abuse as a health care provider? Discuss nursing interventions for the family.

B. **Intimate Partner Violence (IPV)**
    1. Description: may be emotional/psychological, financial, physical, and/or sexual; violence towards an intimate partner (i.e., girlfriend, boyfriend, spouse) that is intended to intimidate, degrade, control, and/or cause injury to the partner; **stalking** is also a form of violence
    2. Victims

        a. Can occur in any racial/ethnic, socioeconomic, and educational background
        b. Violence can occur within heterosexual, gay, or lesbian relationships
        c. Recipients of violence may be male or female
        d. Most frequent violence is male to female
            1) 95% reported injuries related to IPV are in women
            2) 50% of female homicides are committed by intimate partners
            3) 53% of males who are violent to partners are also violent to their children

        e. Victims of IPV are 15 times more likely to abuse alcohol or drugs
        f. Are five times more likely to commit suicide than the average population
    3. Patterns of interpersonal violence
        a. Can be psychological/emotional, financial, physical, and/or sexual
        b. First incidence of violence often occurs in dating relationship
        c. Attacks escalate in frequency and severity over time

        d. Cycle of violence may be weekly, and/or several times a year
        e. The abuse occurs: perpetrator to victim

     f. The perpetrator feels guilt—not about the abuse, but because of risk of getting caught

     g. The perpetrator makes excuses for the behavior

     h. Psychological/emotional violence is devastating due to constant threats of violence or death, a chronic fear instillation

     i. Perpetrator may make threats of taking children (or gaining custody), injuring or killing family pets, or having victim committed for mental health treatment

4. Psychological responses

     a. Victim of violence may leave perpetrator and return several times in an attempt to do the following:

          1) Get perpetrator to change his or her behavior

          2) Test own abilities to cope and survive

          3) Test children's response to leaving the relationship

          4) Regain the strength to leave and be independent

     b. See Box 12-4 for reasons victims of violence may have difficulty leaving violent relationships

     c. Leaving a violent relationship is a difficult process that takes specific planning and can take the victim months to years to make it happen

     d. The most dangerous period for the victim is when he or she leaves the violent relationship

5. Assessment

     a. Observe for and document physical and emotional signs of violence; document both subjective and objective information (see Table 12-1)

     b. Observe for jealous, passive, controlling, and/or intrusive behavior in the perpetrator

     c. Determine whether conflict resolution styles in the relationship are authoritative or equal

     d. Do not ask client about whether he or she is being treated violently, since client may not identify the behavior as violence; instead ask more general questions

          1) "Have you ever been pushed or shoved during an argument?"

          2) "Has anyone ever hit, punched, kicked, or slapped you?"

          3) "How are disagreements dealt with in the home?"

     e. Assess beliefs about physical violence and who the victim perceives as responsible for violent acts

     f. Assess social support system (i.e., family, friends, people from church, neighbors)

Box 12-4	
Reasons Victims May Have Difficulty Leaving Violent Relationships	Financial dependency or fear of being financially independent
	Religious/spiritual beliefs about marriage
	Emotional attachment to spouse or partner, traumatic bonding
	Not wanting to view the relationship as pathological
	The cycle of violence contains a period of time where the perpetrator promises to change (i.e., personal counseling, marriage counseling)
	Victim of violence may blame self and feel if he or she only does better the violence will stop
	Fears for safety—perpetrators of violence often threaten to kill partners if they leave; may harm or kill family pets, or abuse children to illustrate this
	Not wanting to disrupt children's lives; perpetrator of violence often threatens to take children away
	Perpetrator of violence may threaten to have victim committed as mentally ill
	Shame involved in admitting involvement in a violent relationship

6. Priority nursing diagnoses
   a. Pain (emotional/psychological or physical) related to the infliction by partner with the intent to cause harm
   b. Ineffective Family Coping related to inadequate support system, poor relationship skills, or unrealistic expectations of either the relationship or the partner
   c. Disturbed Self-Esteem related to unmet dependency needs, repeated abuse, or dysfunctional family system
   d. Hopelessness related to belief in lack of options or inadequate support system
   e. Powerlessness related to lifestyle of helplessness, low self-esteem, or lack of support network of caring others
   f. Ineffective Family Processes related to inadequate caretaking or dysfunctional family relationships
   g. Social Isolation related to inadequate social support or being prevented from interacting with family, friends, or others

7. Planning and implementation
   a. Treat existing wounds and/or other injuries
   b. Assess client's immediate level of danger
      1) Is client planning to leave partner/spouse?
      2) How frequent and severe are attacks? Are they escalating?
      3) Are there weapons in the home?
      4) Is the partner using alcohol and/or drugs? Is the use increasing?
      5) Has the partner ever threatened to kill the client or self?
   c. Client education
      1) Assure client that he or she is not to blame for the violence
      2) Provide information to client about laws, ordinances, and client's rights
      3) Provide referral and phone number of resources such as women's shelters or safe houses (even if the client does not want to use them presently)
      4) Use mutual goal setting—allow the client to decide on goals; this empowers the client and validates his or her strengths
      5) Assist client to mobilize available support systems
      6) Assist with development of a safety plan if client is returning to previous environment (see Box 12-5)

8. Evaluation
   a. Client verbalizes feelings of fears and anxiety
   b. Client acknowledges danger of situation
   c. Client develops a safety plan
   d. Client begins using community resources provided
   e. Client reengages with support systems such as family and friends

9. Violence toward pregnant women
   a. Pregnancy is a time of increased risk of violence

Practice to Pass

You are discharging a client from the emergency department after treatment of injuries from intimate partner violence. The client is returning to the same environment. What would your priorities be for discharge planning? Give five to six examples why persons stay in violent relationships.

Box 12-5	Ask neighbors to phone police if violence begins.
Safety Plan for Continued Violence	Establish code with family and friends to signify violence.
	Plan an escape route to use if the abuser blocks main exit.
	Identify a place to go and how to get there.
	Have an escape bag that has extra clothing for self and children.
	Have children's favorite toys available in a safe place.
	Have extra copies hidden of phone numbers and important documents (i.e., driver's licenses, birth certificates, marriage license, insurance papers, social security numbers, bank account numbers, cash.)

      b. A pregnant woman is most often beaten in the stomach, which can lead to complications of pregnancy such as placentae abruptio, premature labor, miscarriage and fetal loss, or maternal injury such as fractures of the pelvis, rupture of the uterus, and hemorrhage

      c. Etiology: violence can be related to feelings of ambivalence about the pregnancy or partner feeling threatened by attention the woman is receiving due to the pregnancy

      d. Assessment, diagnosis, and interventions are the same as in partner violence with the additional need to assess partner's attitude regarding pregnancy, assessing the fetal health and well-being, and interventions that include prenatal care

C. Elder violence

  1. Elder abuse: physical, emotional/psychological, or sexual injury to an older adult (over age 65); recent findings indicate that 60% of elder injury is inflicted by spouse (overlap with intimate partner violence); is one of the most underreported crimes

  2. Elder violence takes many forms and may be difficult to identify due to elders' reluctance to reveal information out of fear of abandonment or retaliation; can occur in any setting such as the home, extended care facility, nursing home, day-treatment programs

      a. Physical violence: results in bodily harm or injury

      b. Emotional or psychological violence includes the following:

        1) Verbal assaults, threats, or intimidation

        2) Social: restriction of social contacts

        3) Violation of personal rights: forced to act against their will

        4) Unreasonable confinement, forced isolation, or denying privacy

        5) Abandonment or threats of abandonment

      c. Neglect: not providing basic needs (i.e., water, food, shelter)

        1) Deprivation of proper medical care

        2) Providing unsafe environment

        3) Economic: strict control of money, food, clothing, or transportation

  3. There are federal laws to protect elders in most states; nurses need to be familiar with the state statutes governing reporting of elder abuse

  4. Etiology and psychopathology

      a. Perpetrators are usually family members

      b. Perpetrators may have personal problems and a lack of support

      c. Perpetrators may be stressed by caring for elder

      d. There may be a history of family violence

      e. There may be unresolved previous conflicts and power struggles

      f. Violence may be in retaliation for past behavior of elder

      g. Cultural devaluation of elders

  5. Assessment

      a. Physical signs as noted in overview of violence

      b. Assess for symptoms of mental illness in both elder (i.e., delirium, dementia, depression) and perpetrator

      c. Determine if elder is financially dependent on suspected perpetrator or if suspected perpetrator is dependent on elder

      d. Assess interactions within family system for signs of aggression

      e. Establish a therapeutic and trusting relationship, as elder may be hesitant to disclose violence for fear of abandonment or placement in a long-term care facility

      f. Assess for symptoms of neglect

        1) Malnutrition and/or dehydration

        2) Untreated medical conditions (i.e., pressure ulcers, urinary tract infections, and/or poor dental hygiene)

        3) Reports of being locked in a room

    g. Assess for substance abuse in both caregiver and elder

  6. Priority nursing diagnoses

    a. Fear related to the infliction by caretaker of physical, emotional, or financial abuse with the intent to cause harm or abandonment

    b. Anxiety related to fear of revealing the abuser and the consequences

    c. Chronic Pain related to poor health and illness or repeated infliction of physical or emotional pain over an extended period of time

    d. Posttraumatic Stress Response related to having been the recipient of physical, emotional, and/or financial trauma

    e. Ineffective Coping: individual or family related to inadequate support systems, poor follow-up care, or dysfunctional family relationships

    f. Risk for Violence related to being vulnerable, socially isolated, or having inadequate support systems

    g. Low Self-Esteem related to unmet dependency needs, or being physically, emotionally, or financially abused

    h. Hopelessness or Powerlessness related to lifestyle of helplessness, low self-esteem, or lack of support network of caring others

  7. Planning and implementation

    a. Treat client's existing injuries

    b. Assess for untreated medical conditions

    c. Assess imminent danger of client

        1) How frequent and severe are attacks?

        2) Are there weapons in the home, and of what lethality?

        3) Does the elder fear for own life?

    d. Report violence to elders to Adult Protective Services following state laws and guidelines

    e. Provide referral to social services

  8. Evaluation

    a. The client verbalizes fears and feelings

    b. The client's medical condition improves

    c. The client's ability to care for self improves

    d. The client regains dignity and autonomy

    e. The family improves coping style

    f. The elder is placed in alternative living situation

IV. SEXUAL VIOLENCE OR ASSAULT

  A. Description: sexual violence includes sexual harassment, rape, sexual assault, and child sexual assault; it is an intentional act, not of sexuality, but intended to injure and intimidate

  B. Types

    1. Sexual harassment: unwelcome sexual advances or conduct of a sexual nature on the job that creates an intimidating or offensive work environment; is considered a form of discrimination by the Equal Employment Opportunities Commission; two types of sexual harassment:

      a. Quid pro quo: Latin for "this for that" when a person in authority suggests that a job, promotion, or salary will be given or withheld in exchange for sexual favors

      b. Hostile environment: sexually offensive conduct that permeates the workplace, making it difficult or unpleasant for an employee to do his or her job

---

Practice to Pass

An elderly client, with numerous unexplained bruises, is brought to the emergency department by a caregiver. What factors would you assess to determine if the client had been abused or neglected?

!

2. Sexual assault: forceful genital, anal, or oral penetration of the victim by any objects including a penis; includes rape (forced sexual intercourse)
   a. Sexual assault is a crime of violence: 93% of those assaulted are women and 90% of perpetrators are men, but either can be assaulted or a perpetrator
   b. There is no profile for perpetrator; victims can be children through elderly
   c. Types of sexual assault
      1) Date or acquaintance rape: the perpetrator is known to the victim; this form of rape is underreported
      2) Marital rape: occurs within marriage, this is the most prevalent and underreported form of rape, often with concurrent physical violence
      3) Statutory rape: victim under the age of consent; this includes consensual sex between an underage child and an adult
      4) Gang rape: a group of perpetrators often in a ritual manner
   d. Between one-third and one-half of battered women are sexually assaulted by their partners
   e. Men who are sexually assaulted by men are more likely to be beaten and reluctant to report
3. Immediate consequences of sexual assault: in addition to physical injury, pregnancy and sexually transmitted infection can result; victims of sexual assault can experience rape-trauma syndrome (a variant of posttraumatic stress disorder)
   a. Initial response may be deceptively calm, but this usually masks distress, denial, or emotional shock
   b. 25% of clients can have impairment that continues up to one year
   c. There is high level of anxiety and fear related to future attacks
   d. The sexual assault survivor may develop phobic reactions or difficulty with decision making
   e. Flashbacks, violent dreams, and preoccupation with future danger are common
   f. Feelings of guilt, doubts, fear, anger, and hatred of the perpetrator may occur
   g. Subsequent problems with intimate relationships may occur
4. Long-term consequences
   a. Depression (see Chapter 4)
   b. Feelings of helplessness and vulnerability
   c. Posttraumatic stress disorder (see Chapter 5)
   d. Problems with sexuality
5. Cultural specific issues with sexual assault
   a. United States has a higher reported rate of sexual assault than other developed countries
   b. In countries where a young woman's worth is related to her virginity, sexual assault is particularly devastating; to save the family reputation male members of a family may kill the woman or force the woman to marry the perpetrator
6. Etiology and psychopathology
   a. Intrapersonal theory
      1) Perpetrator is emotionally immature, powerless, and unsure of self
      2) Uses sexual assault as a method to exert power, intimidate, or inflict pain
   b. Interpersonal theory
      1) Perpetrators do not have normal interpersonal involvement
      2) Perpetrator is preoccupied with own fantasies
   c. Social learning theory
      1) Society accepts and glamorizes violence
      2) Aggression is learned through family, peers, and culture

      d. Feminist

          1) Sexual assault is the result of deep-rooted socioeconomic tradition of male dominance

          2) Women are devalued by society

7. Assessment

      a. Clients that are brought to the emergency department by police after rape or sexual assault are easily identifiable; other victims who come non-escorted may not be; in addition to current sexual assault, clients should be assessed by past sexual assault

      b. Questions need to be broadly stated: "Has anyone ever forced you to have sex when you did not want to?"

      c. This can be followed with more broad open-ended questions to elicit further history

      d. Explain that this line of questioning is routine and done with every client

      e. Assess for physical injuries and behavioral signs of sexual assault as noted previously

      f. Following sexual assault, subjective and objective evidence needs to be gathered; this may be done by a specialized health care provider

      g. Permission *must* be obtained prior to the taking/gathering of photos of evidence

      h. Provide the client with as much control as possible during the assessment process

8. Priority nursing diagnoses

      a. Rape Trauma Syndrome related to having been the victim of sexual violence executed with the use of force and against one's personal will and consent

      b. Pain related to the infliction of sexual, physical, and/or emotional abuse by a predator

      c. Anxiety related to fear of loss of control, fear of repeated abuse, or fear of revealing the abuser and the consequences

      d. Disturbed Self-Esteem related to unmet dependency needs, questioning of self-efficacy, or unrealistically blaming self

9. Planning and implementation

      a. Initial response must include nonjudgmental listening and psychological support

      b. Identify client's immediate concerns and priorities

      c. Allow client to discuss feelings about assault

      d. Support decision making and active problem solving using mutual goal setting; client's goals may differ from nurse's

      e. If the attack was recent, evidence may need to be gathered; follow facility policies regarding gathering of evidence; obtain permission from client

      f. Test for pregnancy and sexually transmitted diseases

      g. Client education

          1) Reassure client that sexual assault is not his or her fault and survival was the most important outcome

          2) Advise about potential for pregnancy and sexually transmitted disease

          3) Provide information and encourage use of community services, such as survivors groups, shelters for battered women (men), and legal service

          4) If sexual assault is committed by a partner, identify and provide education about options, including staying with client when the perpetrator is present, removing perpetrator through arrest, obtaining protective orders to keep perpetrator away, or leaving perpetrator

      h. Assist with development of a safety plan if client is returning to the environment with the perpetrator

10. Evaluation
   a. Client expresses feelings about the incident, which may include anger, fear, guilt and vulnerability
   b. Client seeks appropriate medical care for problems related to the assault;
   c. Client develops a safety or escape plan
   d. Client identifies support systems and people that are available to assist in dealing with crisis
   e. Client is actively involved in mobilizing support systems

Practice to Pass

You are discharging a client who had been sexually assaulted. What teaching would be most important for this client?

Case Study

You are doing an admission assessment on a child who has multiple bruises on his body. You suspect injuries result from physical violence to the child.

1. What information will you gather from the mother?

2. What physical signs will you look for in the child?

3. What behavioral signs will you look for in the child?

4. What are your priority interventions in caring for this child?

5. What things will you teach the mother?

For suggested responses, see page 301.

POSTTEST

1. An older adult has been admitted to the hospital for dehydration. The client is poorly dressed, has body odor, appears unkempt, and has numerous unexplained bruises. In addition, he states that he has not been receiving his medications from his caregiver. What is the nurse's priority initial action?

   1. Determine if the client is experiencing abuse or neglect.
   2. Contact the appropriate elderly protective services agency.
   3. Explore methods of rehydration attempted at home.
   4. Inquire about medications the client is taking.

2. The nurse is caring for a client who is being treated for migraine headaches. Upon physical exam the nurse assesses old scars on the client's arms and legs. The client confides childhood memories of sexual abuse by the father. What should be the nurse's immediate response?

   1. "Tell me more about your migraines."
   2. "How did you get the scars?"
   3. "How old were you when the abuse stopped?"
   4. "Are you comfortable discussing the abuse?"

3. The nurse is working on a neurological unit. A client with three young children was beaten so severely that she is unconscious and has sustained a traumatic brain injury. Another staff nurse on the unit states, "She was stupid for staying in the relationship; she deserved it." What is the best response by the nurse? Select all that apply.

   1. "Yes, she has a lot of family and friends whom she could have gone to."
   2. "One reason she may have stayed is because of traumatic bonding."
   3. "One reason she may have stayed is the fear of losing her children."
   4. "Women may stay in violent relationships due to fear, helplessness, guilt, or shame."
   5. "Maybe she has come to think violence is acceptable."

4 A mother brings in an eight-month-old infant who is having difficulty breathing. The nurse assesses bleeding in the baby's retinas. The mother states that the child was being cared for by the father while the mother was out of the house. What is the most appropriate initial response of the nurse?

1. Question the mother about the events prior to the respiratory distress.
2. Identify this situation as a medical emergency.
3. Inform the mother that the period of greatest danger has passed.
4. Report the situation to the children's protective services agency.

5 The nurse is conducting a home visit. The nurse observes a five-year-old child wearing a diaper while sucking his thumb, rocking, and banging his head. The child made adequate verbal responses to the nurse's verbal greeting. What would the nurse suspect this behavior to represent?

1. Mental retardation
2. Possible emotional abuse or neglect
3. An indication of autism
4. Pervasive developmental delay

6 An adult survivor of child abuse states, "Why couldn't I make him stop the abuse? If I were a stronger person, I might have been able to make him stop. Maybe it was my fault he abused me." Based on this data, which would be the most appropriate nursing diagnosis?

1. Ineffective Family Coping
2. Social Isolation
3. Chronic Low Self-Esteem
4. Anxiety

7 The mother of a six-year-old client in the emergency department (ED) tells the nurse that the child vomits after every meal. The child has a normal appearance and is in no acute distress. This is the fifth time within three months that the child has been taken to the ED by the mother. The mother states, "This time I won't go away until my child is admitted for a complete and thorough gastrointestinal workup. The doctors say there's nothing wrong, but I know my child is very ill." What should the nurse suspect about what the mother is experiencing?

1. Panic level anxiety
2. Dissociative identity disorder
3. Munchausen's syndrome by proxy
4. Cluster A personality traits

8 The nurse is counseling an extremely distressed female victim immediately after a sexual assault. What is the nurse's most important initial intervention?

1. Reassure the victim that the sexual assault was not her fault.
2. Ask the client to provide a sample of pubic hair for the evidence kit.
3. Collect a serum specimen for pregnancy testing.
4. Teach the client about the risk for sexually transmitted infections.

9 The nurse is evaluating a family in which an 18-month-old son has been abused by both parents. At the initial interview with the nurse, the parents stated that they spank the toddler because he "cries and cries and never tells us what is wrong." The parents are adolescents who are still in high school. The nurse determines that what parental outcome would indicate progress?

1. Less use of spanking for discipline
2. Joint attendance at parenting classes
3. Holding high expectations for their child
4. Recognizing crying as an age-appropriate way to communicate

10 The nurse is conducting an in-service program on risk factors for victims of domestic violence. The nurse would include which items of information about risk factors during the session? Select all that apply.

1. A high school dropout is at higher risk then a high school graduate.
2. Persons of lower income status are at higher risk than those of higher economic status.
3. Gay/lesbian persons are at not risk.
4. Domestic violence cuts across all socioeconomic lines.
5. Domestic violence cuts across all educational levels.

➤ *See pages 251–253 for Answers and Rationales.*

ANSWERS & RATIONALES

Pretest

1 **Answer: 1 Rationale:** The number, extent, and location of the bruises and the mother's vague explanations of the injuries indicate possible child abuse as does the mother's statement that the child was unsupervised while playing. Children of this age should be supervised during play. No information is given about the level of maturity of the mother, but clearly it appears that the parenting is inadequate. While it is true that an 18-month-old is unsteady and will fall often, the nurse would not expect to see numerous large bruises of different stages confined to the back and hips. If tissue fragility was present in this child, it would not be limited to the back and buttocks. **Cognitive Level:** Applying **Client Need:** Safety and Infection Control **Integrated Process:** Nursing Process: Assessment **Content Area:** Mental Health **Strategy:** Notice the extent of bruising and the mother's explanation. Do they seem to "fit" together? **Reference:** Varcarolis, E., & Halter, M. (2010). *Foundations of psychiatric mental health nursing: A clinical approach* (6th ed.). St. Louis, MO: Saunders Elsevier, p. 518.

2 **Answer: 1, 3 Rationale:** Social learning theory states that society's attitude of the use of coercion and force supports levels of violence. Violent behavior is a means to exert power and control over others. Impulse control problems may play a factor in violent behavior. There are many theories for violent behavior, these include intrapersonal theory, interpersonal theory, social learning theory, and gender bias theory. The feminist theory outlines the idea that economic activities perceive the women as powerless and subservient to the male gender. There is no male response theory. **Cognitive Level:** Analyzing **Client Need:** Psychosocial **Integrated Process:** Nursing Process: Assessment **Content Area:** Mental Health **Strategy:** Study and understand the processes of human violence towards others by learning the various theories related to violent behavior. **Reference:** Kneisl, C.R., & Trigaboff, E. (2009). *Contemporary psychiatric–mental health nursing* (2nd ed.). Upper Saddle River, NJ: Pearson Education, pp. 640–642.

3 **Answer: 3 Rationale:** The child's examination shows probable signs of sexual abuse, which must be reported. Nurses are mandated reporters of suspected child abuse. Further data gathering (obtaining a urine sample and assessing the child for other health problems) and teaching the mother about UTI symptoms would be secondary priorities. **Cognitive Level:** Analyzing **Client Need:** Safety and Infection Control **Integrated Process:** Nursing Process: Planning **Content Area:** Mental Health **Strategy:** Apply the "vulnerable person" theory. Meeting the child's safety needs is the first priority for the nurse, who is also legally mandated to report suspected child abuse. **Reference:** Varcarolis, E., & Halter, M. (2010). *Foundations of psychiatric mental health nursing: A clinical approach* (6th ed.). St. Louis, MO: Saunders Elsevier, pp. 519–520.

4 **Answer: 3 Rationale:** The client's safety is of utmost importance. If returning to the violent environment, it is urgent for the client to have a safety plan. Instructing the client to leave the relationship will not help if the client is not ready to do so. Additionally, the nurse should assist the client to make her own decision, rather than trying to impose personal views on the client. Providing information about legal assistance and a list of services that are available are appropriate, but are secondary to assisting the client to plan for personal safety. **Cognitive Level:** Analyzing **Client Need:** Safety and Infection Control **Integrated Process:** Nursing Process: Implementation **Content Area:** Mental Health **Strategy:** Recall that, for varied and complex reasons, the decision to terminate an abusive relationship is very difficult for most victims to reach. Keep the client's needs for safety at the forefront of your thinking. **Reference:** Varcarolis, E., & Halter, M. (2010). *Foundations of psychiatric mental health nursing: A clinical approach* (6th ed.). St. Louis, MO: Saunders Elsevier, p. 521.

5 **Answer: 3 Rationale:** Education and money do not make people immune from violence. It crosses all socioeconomic lines. Violence often begins in dating relationships. It is estimated that 30 to 40% of college students and 10 to 20% of high school students are in abusive relationships. As part of a predictable cycle of violence, abusers typically apologize and promise to stop. However, the reality is that the level of abuse generally intensifies with the passage of time. Abusers are often excessively jealous and possessive. They control the victim's life and isolate the victim from outside family or social contacts. **Cognitive Level:** Analyzing **Client Need:** Safety and Infection Control **Integrated Process:** Nursing Process: Evaluation **Content Area:** Mental Health **Strategy:** Look for an inaccurate statement. The question is asking you to identify a need for continued teaching. **Reference:** Varcarolis, E., Carson, V., & Shoemaker, N. (2006). *Foundations of psychiatric mental health nursing: A clinical approach* (6th ed.). St. Louis, MO: Saunders Elsevier, p. 515.

6 **Answer: 1, 4, 5** **Rationale:** Her pets and children being at risk for abuse and the likelihood of her husband trying to sabotage her career goals are correct. Abuse may include hurting or killing pets, destruction of property, or hurting ones' children. **Cognitive Level:** Analyzing **Client Need:** Psychosocial Integrity **Integrated Process:** Nursing Process: Implementation **Content Area:** Mental Health **Strategy:** Study and understand all aspects of interpersonal violence including emotional abuse and child abuse. **Reference:** Kneisl, C.R., & Trigaboff, E. (2009). *Contemporary psychiatric–mental health nursing* (2nd ed.). Upper Saddle River, NJ: Pearson Education., pp. 640–642.

7 **Answer: 3** **Rationale:** The child will be at risk for depression, both now and in the future. Among other frequent consequences are self-esteem disturbances, feelings of guilt, sexual acting out behaviors, posttraumatic stress disorders (PTSD), and self-mutilation behaviors. There are many long-term consequences of child abuse. Abuse is more devastating if the abuser is a person the child knew and trusted. It is true that many victims of child abuse do themselves become abusers in the future but one cannot predict that this will happen in all cases. Many victims of child abuse are able to have normal, healthy, non-abusive parent–child relationships. **Cognitive Level:** Applying **Client Need:** Health Promotion and Maintenance **Integrated Process:** Teaching and Learning **Content Area:** Mental Health **Strategy:** Consider the fact that sexual abuse is an assault of the entire person: psychological, physical, and spiritual. **Reference:** Varcarolis, E., & Halter, M. (2010). *Foundations of psychiatric mental health nursing: A clinical approach* (6th ed.). St. Louis, MO: Saunders Elsevier, p. 507.

8 **Answer: 4** **Rationale:** The client has been sexually assaulted, and the nurse needs to respond to the client's immediate concerns. Since the student describes occurrences that often lead to a situational crisis response, it is most important for the nurse to allow the student to ventilate feelings at the beginning of the interview. The nurse should listen patiently and supportively, understanding that compulsive retelling helps the victim gradually become desensitized to the sexual assault.

Pregnancy testing and teaching are secondary interventions that can be begun after the client has ventilated feelings about the sexual assault. **Cognitive Level:** Analyzing **Client Need:** Psychosocial Integrity **Integrated Process:** Nursing Process: Planning **Content Area:** Mental Health **Strategy:** Recall that one of the ways of coping with rape is to avoid talking about it. Notice that the client has initiated the topic with the nurse. This indicates readiness and a need to discuss the event and express feelings. **Reference:** Varcarolis, E., & Halter, M. (2010). *Foundations of psychiatric mental health nursing: A clinical approach* (6th ed.). St. Louis, MO: Saunders Elsevier, p. 547.

9 **Answer: 1** **Rationale:** It is vital that the client understand that the pregnancy may be in danger from the abuse. Among possible consequences of abdominal beating of a pregnant woman are miscarriage, placenta abruption, fetal loss, premature labor, and fetal or maternal fracture. The client will need resources, childbirth classes, and assertiveness training in the future, but she must first understand the risk to the baby in order to provide safety for herself and the baby. **Cognitive Level:** Analyzing **Client Need:** Safety and Infection Control **Integrated Process:** Teaching and Learning **Content Area:** Mental Health **Strategy:** Note that this client has sustained trauma to the abdomen. If you were this pregnant client, what would your concerns be? The nurse should have the same concerns and recognize a need to try to provide information that could lead to safety for the victim and her unborn child. **Reference:** Fontaine, K. (2009). *Mental health nursing* (6th ed.). Upper Saddle River, NJ: Prentice Hall, p. 617.

10 **Answer: 1** **Rationale:** A delay in seeking treatment for serious injuries is an indication of abuse. Vague descriptions of the injuries with little detail are more likely to indicate abuse than a detailed description. Anxiety and concern on the parents' part would be expected. Preventing the child from explaining the injuries, not encouraging explanation, would be an indication of abuse. **Cognitive Level:** Analyzing **Client Need:** Safety and Infection Control **Integrated Process:** Nursing Process: Assessment **Content Area:** Mental Health **Strategy:** Look for what appears to be atypical parental behavior. This is the option that is the correct answer. **Reference:** Varcarolis, E., & Halter, M. (2010). *Foundations of psychiatric mental health nursing: A clinical approach* (6th ed.). St. Louis, MO: Saunders Elsevier, p. 514.

Posttest

1 **Answer: 1** **Rationale:** Initial observations of dehydration, unexplained bruises, and poor hygiene indicate possible abuse or neglect, the possibility of which should be assessed immediately. It is premature for the nurse to report the suspected abuse before more data are gathered. Some of the necessary data will come from the history of the present illness and rehydration methods attempted at home and medications the client has been taking at home. **Cognitive Level:** Analyzing **Client Need:** Safety and Infection Control **Integrated Process:** Nursing Process: Assessment **Content Area:** Mental Health **Strategy:** Remember that it is important not to jump to conclusions. Gather data before making a decision. **Reference:** Kneisl, C., Wilson, H., & Trigoboff, E. (2009). *Contemporary psychiatric–mental health nursing* (2nd ed.). Upper Saddle River, NJ: Prentice Hall, p. 553.

2 Answer: 4 Rationale: The migraines may be the presenting problem, but the client is indicating a need to discuss the abuse. A nonjudgmental approach considering the client's comfort level would be best to prevent the client from feeling guilt and shame. The nurse should acknowledge the client's comment and explore what the client would like to share at this time. Asking how the client got the scars and how old he/she was when the abuse stopped is secondary at this point. The client is indicating a readiness to express feelings, not provide data. **Cognitive Level:** Analyzing **Client Need:** Psychosocial Integrity **Integrated Process:** Nursing Process: Implementation **Content Area:** Mental Health **Strategy:** Note that the client has introduced the topic of having been abused as a child. This indicates a readiness and need for further discussion and active support from the nurse. **Reference:** Kneisl, C., Wilson, H., & Trigoboff, E. (2009). *Contemporary psychiatric–mental health nursing* (2nd ed.). Upper Saddle River, NJ: Prentice Hall, p. 563.

3 Answer: 2, 3, 4, 5 Rationale: Four options are correct. There are several reasons for which women stay in abusive relationships. For example, they include traumatic bonding, which is where the client has hope and is looking for meaning in relationships. The abuser may threaten to kill or hurt the children and/or she may have a fear of losing custody. Thinking that violence is acceptable is known as learned helplessness, whereby the victim thinks she has no control, and begins to think of violence as an acceptable way of life. Women may stay in violent relationships due to fear, guilt, shame, hope, and/or financial or emotional dependence. Agreeing and stating that the client has a lot of family and friends she could have gone to is incorrect. The nurse must put all judgments aside and understand the theoretical reasons for why women stay in abusive relationships; in addition, many victims are socially isolated due to being controlled by their spouse. **Cognitive Level:** Analyzing **Client Need:** Psychosocial Integrity **Integrated Process:** Nursing Process: Assessment **Content Area:** Mental Health **Strategy:** Study and understand all aspects of interpersonal violence, including emotional abuse and child abuse. **Reference:** Kneisl, C., & Trigoboff, E. (2009). *Contemporary psychiatric–mental health nursing* (2nd ed.). Upper Saddle River, NJ: Prentice Hall, pp. 640, 650.

4 Answer: 2 Rationale: The respiratory distress and retinal bleeding are symptoms of shaken baby syndrome and represent a medical emergency. The child will continue

to be at grave risk at least until cerebral and ocular bleeding subsides. The events leading up to the distress are relevant but secondary at this time. Informing the mother that the greatest danger period has passed is inaccurate, as the child will continue to be at grave risk at least until cerebral and ocular bleeding subsides. Reporting the incident to the children's protective agency is important, but at this time is secondary to providing emergency care to the child. **Cognitive Level:** Analyzing **Client Need:** Safety and Infection Control **Integrated Process:** Nursing Process: Assessment **Content Area:** Mental Health **Strategy:** Recognize this child's symptoms as a grave consequence of child abuse and a medical emergency of the highest order. **Reference:** Kneisl, C., & Trigoboff, E. (2009). *Contemporary psychiatric–mental health nursing* (2nd ed.). Upper Saddle River, NJ: Prentice Hall, p. 552.

5 Answer: 2 Rationale: The age-inappropriate behaviors combined with capacity to communicate verbally would indicate probable abuse or neglect. If mental retardation, autism, or pervasive developmental delay were present, the child's language skills would be affected. **Cognitive Level:** Analyzing **Client Need:** Safety and Infection Control **Integrated Process:** Nursing Process: Assessment **Content Area:** Mental Health **Strategy:** Notice the incongruity between the physical appearance and the language development of the child. **Reference:** Varcarolis, E., & Halter, M. (2010). *Foundations of psychiatric mental health nursing: A clinical approach* (6th ed.). St. Louis, MO: Saunders Elsevier, pp. 511, 641.

6 Answer: 3 Rationale: Inappropriate self-blame and feelings that a child could have stopped an adult's abuse indicate a low self-esteem. The other three options are possible diagnoses for adult survivors of abuse, but there is no evidence in the situation to support these diagnoses. More data would be needed. **Cognitive Level:** Applying **Client Need:** Psychosocial Integrity **Integrated Process:** Nursing Process: Diagnosis **Content Area:** Mental Health **Strategy:** Note that chronic low self-esteem is just one of many, many possible consequences of childhood sexual abuse. Recognize that this client's statements are very typical of survivors of childhood sexual abuse. **Reference:** Kneisl, C., & Trigoboff, E. (2009). *Contemporary psychiatric–mental health nursing* (2nd ed.). Upper Saddle River, NJ: Prentice Hall, p. 561.

7 Answer: 3 Rationale: Munchausen's syndrome by proxy is characterized by a caregiver, usually a parent, fabricating or causing illness in another person in order to gain sympathy or attention for him- or herself. The mother's statement and the past history of repeated attempts to have the child hospitalized in the absence of diagnosed problems suggest that this rare somatoform disorder might be present. Somatoform disorders are considered anxiety related disorders. While the mother is anxious, she is not in panic level anxiety since she is able to organize and verbalize her thoughts very clearly. There is no indication of more than one personality or alter being present in the mother, which would be the case if a dissociative identity disorder were present. There is no indication of Cluster A personality traits, which present as odd, eccentric, and suspicious behaviors. **Cognitive Level:** Analyzing **Client Need:** Psychosocial Integrity **Integrated Process:** Nursing Process: Assessment **Content Area:** Mental Health **Strategy:** Recognize that these four options are all medical diagnoses. It is useful for the nurse to understand behaviors associated with the diagnoses, but the physician will actually determine these diagnoses. **Reference:** Kneisl, C., & Trigoboff, E. (2009). *Contemporary psychiatric–mental health nursing* (2nd ed.). Upper Saddle River, NJ: Prentice Hall, p. 389.

8 **Answer: 1** **Rationale:** Victims of sexual assault often feel guilty and responsible for the assault. It is essential for the nurse to reassure the client that it was not her fault. Teaching and collecting a specimen for testing are secondary interventions after the client is calmer. Gathering evidence would proceed only after reassuring the client and obtaining permission to gather evidence. **Cognitive Level:** Analyzing **Client Need:** Management of Care **Integrated Process:** Nursing Process: Implementation **Content Area:** Mental Health **Strategy:** Unless the client is suffering grave physical consequences of the assault, attend to the psychological needs of the client first. This is the reverse of the usual priority in caregiving situations. **Reference:** Kneisl, C., & Trigoboff, E. (2009). *Contemporary psychiatric–mental health nursing* (2nd ed.). Upper Saddle River, NJ: Prentice Hall, p. 550.

9 **Answer: 4** **Rationale:** The parents need to learn that 18-month-old children cry as a means of communication. The word "less" in "less use of spanking" makes it

incorrect, since the child should not be spanked for crying. Attendance at parenting classes does not indicate behavior change. Having unreasonably high expectations for children is a continued risk factor for abuse. Understanding normal growth and development will help the parents have more reasonable expectations of the child. **Cognitive Level:** Analyzing **Client Need:** Health Promotion and Maintenance **Integrated Process:** Nursing Process: Evaluation **Content Area:** Mental Health **Strategy:** Note that age of the parents does not point in the direction of any particular option. Older parents could engage in exactly the same kind of behavior as these young parents. **Reference:** Fontaine, K., (2009). *Mental health nursing* (6th ed.). Upper Saddle River, NJ: Prentice Hall, pp. 619–620.

10 **Answer: 4, 5** **Rationale:** Domestic violence occurs in all socioeconomic and educational levels. There is a myth that domestic violence happens only amongst the undereducated and poor. However, due to public education, this myth is changing, whereby society is accepting that domestic violence cuts across all socioeconomic levels. Domestic violence occurs in gay/lesbian couples. **Cognitive Level:** Analyzing **Client Need:** Psychosocial Integrity **Integrated Process:** Nursing Process: Assessment **Content Area:** Mental Health **Strategy:** Discount the choices that represent misconceptions about risk factors for domestic violence. Study and learn that all persons, regardless of socioeconomic and educational status, are at risk. Those with alternative lifestyles are also at risk. **Reference:** Kneisl, C., & Trigoboff, E. (2009). *Contemporary psychiatric–mental health nursing* (2nd ed.). Upper Saddle River, NJ: Prentice Hall, p. 645.

References

Fontaine, K. (2009). *Mental health nursing* (6th ed.). Upper Saddle River, NJ: Pearson Education.

Kniesl, C., Wilson, H., & Trigoboff, E. (2009). *Contemporary psychiatric–mental health nursing* (2nd ed.). Upper Saddle River, NJ: Pearson Education.

North American Nursing Diagnosis Association (2008). *Nursing diagnosis: Definitions and classification 2009–2011.* Indianapolis, IN: Wiley-Blackwell.

Stuart, G. (2009). *Principles and practice of psychiatric nursing* (9th ed.). St. Louis: Elsevier Science.

Townsend, M. (2011). *Essentials of psychiatric–mental health nursing* (5th ed.). Philadelphia, PA: F.A. Davis.

Varcarolis, E., & Halter, M. (2010). *Foundations of psychiatric mental health nursing: A clinical approach* (6th ed.). Philadelphia: Saunders.

ANSWERS & RATIONALES

13 Loss, Grief, and Death

Chapter Outline

Overview of Loss, Grieving, and Death

Assessment of Loss, Grieving, and Death
Nursing Diagnoses/Analysis

Planning and Implementation
Evaluation/Outcomes

NCLEX-RN® Test Prep

Use the accompanying online resource, NursingReviewsandRationales, to test yourself with hundreds of NCLEX®-style practice questions.

Objectives

➤ List at least five physiologic and at least four psychological responses to loss and grief.
➤ Explain the differences between normal and pathologic or dysfunctional grief.
➤ Differentiate between the grief experienced by males and the grief experienced by females.
➤ Identify at least three behaviors associated with uncomplicated, delayed, distorted, and disenfranchised grief.
➤ Describe the purpose of an advance directive.
➤ Explain nursing management of a client experiencing grief, loss, or death.
➤ Identify expected outcomes for the client experiencing grief, loss, or death.

Review at a Glance

abbreviated grief mild anxiety and sorrow experienced for a brief period but genuinely felt

advance directive a general term that refers to a client's written instructions about future medical care, in the event that the client becomes unable to speak or is incapacitated; each state regulates the use of advance directives differently

anticipatory grief anxiety and sorrow experienced prior to an expected loss or death

bereavement status of having lost a family member, friend, colleague, or other significant person through death

closed awareness client and family are unaware of impending loss or death

death cessation of physiologic processes that sustain life; a passing or parting; letting go of this life, or loss of life

delayed grief postponed response in which bereaved person may have a reaction at the time of loss, but it is not sufficient to loss; a later loss may trigger a reaction that is out of proportion to meaning of current loss

disenfranchised grief a response to a loss or death in which individual is not regarded as having right to grieve or is unable to acknowledge loss to other persons

do-not-resuscitate order (DNR) a physician's order of "no code" or "do not resuscitate" for clients who are in a stage of terminal, irreversible illness, or expected death

dying dynamic and individualized process of death

dysfunctional grief unresolved or inhibited grief that does not lead to a successful resolution

euthanasia act of painlessly putting to death persons or animals suffering from incurable or distressing disease

grief a pervasive, individualized, and dynamic process that may result in physical, emotional, or spiritual distress because of loss or death of a loved one or cherished object

health care proxy a document appointing someone else (e.g., a relative or trusted friend) to manage health care treatment decisions when client is unable to do so

inhibited grief suppressed response that may be expressed in other ways, such as somatic complaints (e.g., physically symptomatic on anniversary of a loss or during holidays)

living will provides specific instructions about what medical treatment the client chooses to omit or refuse (e.g., ventilator support) in the event that the client is unable to make those decisions

loss actual or potential situation in which something that is valued is changed, no longer available, or gone

mourning expression of sorrow of loss and grief in a manner understood and approved by culture

mutual pretense a state in which client, family, and health care provider

know that prognosis is terminal but do not talk about it and make an effort not to raise the subject

open awareness a state in which client and individuals involved know about impending loss or death and feel comfortable discussing it, even though it may be difficult

unresolved grief grief that is prolonged or extended in length and severity of response

PRETEST

1 A client underwent a gastric banding surgical procedure as treatment for morbid obesity. Following a 140-pound weight loss, the client's body mass index (BMI) is now 24.8. The client states, "I'm too fat. I always have been." The nurse concludes that this client has a disturbed body image related to which type(s) of psychological loss? Select all that apply.

1. Actual
2. Perceived
3. Anticipatory
4. Permanent
5. Painful

2 Before counseling parents who have recently lost a child to death, it is important for the nurse to have already dealt with personal feelings about death, grief, and loss in children. Having this self-awareness is important for which reason?

1. It assists the nurse to help the parents express their grief fully.
2. It prevents the nurse from being personally affected by the loss.
3. It prevents the nurse from sharing any personal feelings with the parents.
4. It assists the nurse to avoid discussing unpleasant feelings with the parents.

3 A young woman arrives at a routine medical visit, appears depressed, and tells the nurse she is having difficulty dealing with the death of her infant son. The nurse learns the infant died 30 months ago in an automobile accident. The initial nursing diagnosis is Dysfunctional Grieving. Which statement by the client would support this diagnosis?

1. "When children play in playgrounds, it makes me angry that my son will never be able to play like other children."
2. "I sometimes cry in my son's old bedroom because he's not there anymore."
3. "I watch other toddlers in the neighborhood play, and I wish my son were still alive."
4. "I think of my son and I am sad that my new baby will never be able to know his brother."

4 The client whose spouse died four months ago is admitted for inpatient psychiatric care. The client has been unable to work since the spouse's death and has lost 20 pounds. The client cries frequently and says, "No, I won't believe it. It's not true." The client further describes feeling "numb" and "empty." The admitting medical diagnosis is major depression. The nurse identifies which of the following as the priority problem?

1. Dysfunctional grief
2. Disenfranchised grief
3. Distorted grief
4. Normal grief

5 An African-American family who has gathered around their dying grandmother's bed refuses to allow a feeding tube to be removed and to stop feeding her, even after the health care team has stated that nothing else could be done to help her recover. The nurse concludes that the family's resistance to removing the feeding tube is most likely based on which factor?

1. Their refusal to accept the finality of death
2. Their need to try every possible solution
3. Their spiritual and cultural beliefs
4. Their distrust of the health care system

6 A father who recently lost his eldest son to cancer refuses to share his feelings in a support group and has not shown any tears related to the loss. What is the nurse's most appropriate interpretation of this behavior?

1. A common expression of how men grieve loss and death
2. A dysfunctional expression of grief, and the client should be referred to counseling
3. A common expression of denial and refusal to accept death or loss
4. The father's attempt to be strong for the rest of the family

7 A child, aged four, says, "If I can make a big enough wish, my daddy will not be dead anymore." The nurse concludes that the child is doing which of the following?

1. Expressing magical thinking common to much older children
2. Voicing thoughts that are normal for children his age
3. Delusional and should be evaluated by a psychiatrist
4. Making up the story in order to avoid feeling sad and scared

8 A terminally ill 78-year-old female client tells the nurse she does not want her adult children to know she is dying. Later that day when the adult children visit, they tell the nurse that they know their mother is dying but will not talk about this in front of her. The nurse mentions in the inter-shift report that this family's situation is one that can be characterized in which way?

1. Closed awareness
2. Mutual pretense
3. Mutual concern
4. Open awareness

9 A frail 79-year-old female calls the home health nurse and says, "I am a failure, and I can no longer care adequately for my husband who has Alzheimer's disease." She has been his primary caregiver for over five years; now he has become despondent, is unable to ambulate, and is difficult to manage. The nurse determines that which nursing diagnosis is most appropriate?

1. Ineffective Coping related to chronic illness
2. Social Isolation of Family Unit related to altered state of health
3. Dysfunctional Grief related to not accepting personal limitations
4. Caregiver Role Strain related to overwhelming caregiving tasks and expectations

10 The nurse is counseling a client who has lost the spouse through death. Which of the following is an appropriate outcome criterion for the client? Select all that apply.

1. Accept professional assistance if needed.
2. Stop expressing feelings about the spouse's death.
3. Plan a memorial tribute for the spouse.
4. Attend grief support groups.
5. Avoid sharing loss with significant others.

➤ *See pages 269–270 for Answers and Rationales.*

I. OVERVIEW OF LOSS, GRIEVING, AND DEATH

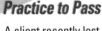

A. Definition of *loss*—the actual or potential situation in which something that is valued is changed, no longer available, or gone

1. Losses are experiences that affect not only the client and the client's family but also the nurse
2. Change in status of significant other
3. Any change that reduces the possibility of achieving implicit or explicit goals
4. Experience of deprivation or complete lack of something that was previously present

B. Types of loss

1. Actual: can be identified by others and can arise in response to or in anticipation of a situation (e.g., death of significant other)
2. Perceived: is experienced by one person but cannot be verified by others (e.g., loss of self-esteem)
3. Anticipatory: is experienced before the loss actually occurs (e.g., terminal illness)

C. Time period of loss

1. Temporary: deprivation and later restoration of something that was previously present (e.g., missing child)
2. Permanent: irreversible deprivation (e.g., paralysis)

D. Circumstances of loss

1. Maturational: results from normal life transitions (e.g., parents feeling sadness when their youngest child leaves for college)
2. Situational: loss occurs in response to a specific event

E. Sources of loss

1. Aspect of self: loss of a valued part of oneself—a body part (e.g., amputation of an extremity), a physiologic function, or a psychological attribute
2. External objects: loss of inanimate objects (e.g., property) or loss of animate object (e.g., family pet)
3. Familiar environment: separation from an environment and people who provide security (e.g., placement in a nursing home)
4. Loved one: loss of a significant person or valued person (or pet) through illness, separation, or death (e.g., death from AIDS)
5. Loss of life: loss of a significant person or loss of one's own life (e.g., terminal illness)

F. Physiological responses related to loss or grief

1. Crying and sobbing
2. Sighing respirations
3. Shortness of breath and palpitations
4. Fatigue, weakness, and exhaustion
5. Insomnia/sleep disturbance
6. Loss of appetite
7. Choking sensation
8. Tightness in chest
9. Gastrointestinal disturbances

G. Psychological responses related to loss or grief

1. Intense loneliness and sadness
2. Depressed mood
3. Anxiety or panic episodes
4. Difficulty concentrating and focusing
5. Anger or rage directed toward self or others
6. Ambivalence and low self-esteem
7. Somatic complaints
8. Guilt

Practice to Pass

A client recently lost a partner of 20 years to acquired immunodeficiency syndrome (AIDS). What physiological and psychological responses by the client would you expect to observe?

H. **Self-assessment and self-awareness**
1. Is critical in order for the nurse to be sensitive and therapeutic with clients who have experienced loss
2. Explore personal attitudes, feelings, and values related to loss and grief

I. **Bereavement, mourning, and grief**
1. **Bereavement**: a subjective response caused by losing a family member, friend, colleague, or other significant person through death
2. **Mourning**: the expression of the sorrow of loss and grief in a manner understood and approved by the culture
3. **Grief**: a pervasive, individualized, and dynamic process that may result in physical, emotional, or spiritual distress because of loss or death of a loved one or cherished object
   a. **Abbreviated grief**: mild anxiety and sorrow experienced for a brief period but genuinely felt
   b. **Anticipatory grief**: anxiety and sorrow experienced prior to an expected loss or death
   c. **Disenfranchised grief**: a response to a loss or death in which the individual is not regarded as having the right to grieve or is unable to acknowledge the loss to other persons (e.g., a gay partner unable to acknowledge the loss of his or her significant other)
   d. **Dysfunctional grief**: unresolved or inhibited grief that does not lead to a successful conclusion
      1) **Unresolved grief**: prolonged or extended in length and severity of response (e.g., after a prolonged period, an individual continues to search for a lost person)
      2) **Inhibited grief**: suppressed response that may be expressed in other ways, such as somatic complaints (e.g., physically symptomatic on the anniversary of a loss or during holidays)
      3) **Delayed grief**: postponed response in which the bereaved person may have a reaction at the time of the loss, but it is not sufficient to the loss; a later loss may trigger a reaction that is out of proportion to the meaning of the current loss (e.g., loss of a pet triggers a suicidal reaction in a woman after not being able to grieve her husband's death three years ago)

J. **Stages of grief**: labels for stages must be used with caution because each individual processes grief in different ways and at different rates
1. Stages should be used as descriptive of the grieving process rather than prescriptive of the grieving process (see Table 13-1)
2. There have been many theories on the stages of grief; the central themes of these theories include the following:
   a. Shock and disbelief (one to three weeks)
      1) Numbness
      2) Denial
      3) Passive
      4) Unaware of others
   b. Searching and protesting (three weeks to four months)
      1) Crying and yearning
      2) Guilt
      3) Intense and conflicting emotions, such as sadness and anger
      4) Empty feeling
      5) Identification and preoccupation with thoughts of loss or death
      6) Dependent
      7) Self-destructive behaviors

Stage	Behavioral Response
Shock and disbelief	Refusal to accept loss
	Stunned feelings
	Intellectual acceptance but emotional denial
Developing awareness	Reality of loss begins to penetrate consciousness
	Anger may be directed at agency, nurses, or others
Restitution	Rituals of mourning (e.g., funeral)
Resolving the loss	Attempts to deal with painful void
	Still unable to accept new love object to replace lost person or object
	May accept more dependent relationship with support person
	Thinks over and talks about memories of the lost object
Idealization	Produces image of lost object that is almost devoid of undesirable features
	Represses all negative and hostile feelings toward lost object
	May feel guilty and remorseful about past inconsiderate or unkind acts to lost person
	Unconsciously internalizes admired qualities of lost object
	Reminders of lost object evoke fewer feelings of sadness
	Reinvests feelings in others
Outcome	Behavior influenced by several factors: importance of lost object as source of support, degree of dependence on relationship, degree of ambivalence toward lost object, number and nature of other relationships, and number of previous grief experiences (which tend to be cumulative)

Table 13-1 Engel's Stages of Grieving

Source: Engel, G. L. (1964). Grief and grieving. *American Journal of Nursing 64* (9), 93–98.

Practice to Pass

A client is expected to die from lung cancer within the next few months. The client's wife tells you, "I can't help with my husband's care right now. He keeps wanting to talk about his dying, and I just can't talk about that right now because it is too hard to lose him." You suspect the wife is experiencing what type of grief? Why?

c. Disorientation (4 to 14 months)
 1) Depression and despair
 2) Apathy and loss of interest
 3) Aimlessness
 4) Disorganization
 5) Insomnia
 6) Inability to maintain work and family responsibilities
 7) Confusion and slowed thinking
 8) Social withdrawal
 d. Reorganization and resolution (14 months throughout rest of life)
 1) Acceptance of loss, letting go
 2) Awareness of having grieved
 3) Ability to talk about deceased or loss without intense pain
 4) New or renewed social relationships
 5) New or renewed interest
 6) Process that may typically last up to one year
3. Kübler-Ross's stages of death and dying were originally intended to be used for individuals dying of terminal illness, but have been used to describe the grieving process of loss
 a. Denial: disbelief or refusal to acknowledge that loss or death is happening
 b. Anger: expression of overt hostility toward loss object, dying person, or others
 c. Bargaining: attempts to negotiate to prolong one's life or to erase the loss

      d. Depression: sense of sadness over loss or death

      e. Acceptance: comes to terms with loss or death

  4. Worden's four tasks of mourning: imply that persons who mourn can be actively involved in helping themselves and can be assisted and influenced by the nurse in resolving their grief

      a. Task I: accept the reality of the loss

      b. Task II: work through the pain of grief

      c. Task III: adjust to the environment in which the deceased or loss person/object is missing

      d. Task IV: emotionally relocate the deceased and move on with life

K. Factors influencing the grief response

  1. Age (see Table 13-2)

      a. Childhood

         1) Preschool children (aged three to five) fear separation from parents and do not understand the finality of death

         2) Children aged five to six see death as reversible

         3) Children aged six to nine begin to accept death as a destructive force and as a final event

         4) Children at age 10 realize that death is inevitable

         5) Adolescents intellectualize awareness of death, but tend to repress feelings about it

Table 13-2   Development of the Concept of Death

Age	Beliefs/Attitudes
Infancy to 5 years	Does not understand concept of death Infant's sense of separation forms basis for later understanding of loss and death Believes death is reversible, a temporary departure, or sleep Emphasizes immobility and inactivity as attributes of death
5 to 9 years	Understands that death is final Believes own death can be avoided Associates death with aggression or violence Believes wishes or unrelated actions can be responsible for death
9 to 12 years	Understands death as the inevitable end of life Begins to understand own mortality, expressed as interest in afterlife or as fear of death
12 to 18 years	Fears a lingering death May fantasize that death can be defied, acting out defiance through reckless behaviors (e.g., dangerous driving, substance abuse) Seldom thinks about death, but views it in religious and philosophic terms May seem to reach "adult" perception of death but is emotionally unable to accept it May still hold concepts from previous developmental stages
18 to 45 years	Has attitude toward death influenced by religious and cultural beliefs
45 to 65 years	Accepts own mortality Encounters death of parents and some peers Experiences peaks of death anxiety Death anxiety diminishes with emotional well-being
65+ years	Fears prolonged illness Encounters death of family members and peers See death as having multiple meanings, (e.g., freedom from pain, reunion with already deceased family members)

Source: Berman, A.J., & Snyder, S. (2012). *Kozier & Erbs' Fundamentals of nursing: Concepts, process, and practice* (9th ed.). Upper Saddle River, NJ: Pearson, p. 107.

      b. Early and middle adult
         1) View loss and death as normal developmental tasks
         2) Potential loss from impaired health or body function
         3) Change in various role functions

      c. Older adult
         1) Loss of health, function, and/or independence
         2) Potential change in living accommodations
         3) Loss of longtime mate or significant other
         4) Multiple losses (i.e., control, competence, and material possessions) and deaths of friends, family, and significant others

2. Significance of the loss
   a. Value placed on the loss person, object, or function
   b. Degree of change required because of loss
   c. The person's belief and values

3. Culture
   a. Dictates customs and rituals used to express grief
      1) In cultures where strong kinship ties are maintained, physical and emotional support and assistance are provided by family members
      2) Spiritual beliefs and practices greatly influence both a person's reaction to loss and subsequent behavior
   b. Describes the nature of life after death
   c. Explains the meaning of death
   d. Defines the relationship between the dead and the living
   e. Designates the processes of bereavement
   f. Delineates the appropriate expression of feelings
      1) Some cultures endure grief internally and privately, favoring a quiet and stoic expression of grief
      2) Some cultures value social support and the outward expression of loss, such as, wailing, crying, and physical prostration
   g. Determines patterns of behavior specific to age and gender

4. Gender
   a. Male or masculine grief
      1) Expression of feelings are limited and toned down
      2) Thinking precedes and often dominates feelings
      3) Focus is on problem solving rather than expression of feelings
      4) Outward expression of feelings often involves anger and/or guilt
      5) Internal adjustments to the loss are usually expressed through activity
      6) Intense feelings may be experienced privately; there is a general reluctance to discuss these with others
      7) Intense grief is usually expressed immediately after the loss, often during post-death rituals
   b. Female or feminine grief
      1) Expression of feelings is more overt
      2) May verbally express for a longer period of time
      3) More communicative about the loss
      4) Usually exhibit a wider range of emotions and openly share feelings with others
      5) More often seek and accept support in one-to-one relationships or as members of support groups
      6) Usually assume supportive roles for other survivors of loss through volunteering or other activities

5. Socioeconomic status
   a. Socioeconomic status often affects the support system available at the time of loss
   b. A loss of function or body part may cause a change in socioeconomic status due to loss of work or vocation
6. Support system
   a. People closest to the grieving individual can often provide emotional, physical, and functional assistance
   b. Because of being uncomfortable with loss or death, support people may withdraw from the grieving individual
   c. Support may be available when the loss is first recognized, but as the support people return to their usual activities, the need for ongoing support is often unmet
7. Cause of loss or death
   a. Views that society places on the cause of the loss or death
   b. Loss or death caused by murder, suicide, or other tragic event may be more difficult to accept and process
   c. A loss or death that is beyond one's control (e.g., cancer) may be more acceptable than one that is preventable (e.g., drunk-driving accident)
   d. Loss of death occurring during respected activities (e.g., police officer in the line of duty) are considered honorable, whereas those occurring during illicit activities (e.g., accidental drug overdose) may be considered the individual's "just rewards"

L. **Definitions and signs of death**
   1. **Death**: cessation of physiologic processes that sustain life; a passing or parting; letting go of this life, or loss of life
      a. Death represents the ultimate loss
      b. Death is part of the continuum of life and as such is a universal and inevitable part of the human experience
      c. Death is often viewed as a mystical event that may generate great fear and anxiety
   2. **Dying**: the dynamic and individualized process of death
   3. Clinical signs of death
      a. Total lack of response to external stimuli
      b. No muscular movement, especially breathing
      c. No reflexes
      d. Flat electroencephalogram
   4. In instances of artificial support, absence of electric currents from the brain (measured by an electroencephalogram) for at least 24 hours is an indication of death
   5. Cerebral death or higher brain death: occurs when the higher brain center, the cerebral cortex, is irreversibly destroyed

M. **Byocak's developmental landmarks and tasks at the end of life**
   1. Sense of completion with worldly affairs: transfer of fiscal, legal, and formal social responsibilities
   2. Sense of completion in relationships with community
      a. Closure of multiple social relationships (employment, commerce, organizational, and congregational)
      b. Components include expressions of regret, expressions of forgiveness, acceptance of gratitude and appreciation
      c. Leave-taking; the saying of goodbye
   3. Sense of meaning about one's individual life
      a. Life review
      b. Telling of "one's stories"
      c. Transmission of knowledge and wisdom

4. Experience love of self
   a. Self-acknowledgment
   b. Self-forgiveness
5. Experience love of others: acceptance of worthiness
6. Sense of completion in relations with family and friends
   a. Reconciliation, fullness of communication and closure in each of one's important relationships
   b. Component tasks include expressions of regret, expressions of forgiveness and acceptance, expressions and acceptance of gratitude and appreciation, expressions of affection
   c. Leave-taking; saying goodbye
7. Acceptance of the finality of life—of one's existence as an individual
   a. Acknowledgment of the totality of personal loss represented by one's dying and experience of personal pain of existential loss
   b. Expression of the depth of personal tragedy that dying represents
   c. Decathexis (emotional withdrawal) from worldly affairs and cathexis (emotional connection) with an enduring construct
   d. Acceptance of dependency
8. Sense of new self (personhood) beyond personal loss: developing self-awareness in the present
9. Sense of meaning about life in general
   a. Achieving a sense of awe
   b. Recognition of a transcendent realm
   c. Developing and achieving a sense of comfort with chaos
10. Surrender to the transcendent, to the unknown—"letting go"; the ego accepts the volition to surrender

N. Legalities related to death and dying

1. **Advance directive** is a general term that refers to a client's written instructions about future medical care in the event that the client becomes unable to speak or incapacitated; each state regulates the use of advance directives differently

   a. **Living will** (durable power of attorney for health care) provides specific instructions about what medical treatment the client chooses to omit or refuse (e.g., ventilator support) in the event that the client is unable to make those decisions

   b. **Health care proxy** is a document appointing someone else (e.g., a relative or trusted friend) to manage health care treatment decisions when the client is unable to do so
2. Organ donation: under the Uniform Anatomical Gift Act and the National Organ Transplant Act, people 18 years or older and of sound mind may make a gift of all or any part of their own body for the following purposes:
   a. Medical or dental education
   b. Research
   c. Advancement of medical or dental science, therapy, or transplantation
3. **Euthanasia** is the act of painlessly putting to death persons or animals suffering from incurable or distressing disease
   a. Voluntary active euthanasia occurs when the person being euthanized has agreed and volunteered for death
      1) Example: a terminally ill client taking a medication to hasten the end of life
      2) Current Oregon law permits voluntary active euthanasia with physician assistance under certain circumstances
   b. Involuntary active euthanasia occurs when the person being euthanized has not agreed or volunteered for death (e.g., the lethal injection of a death row inmate)

  c. Voluntary passive euthanasia occurs when treatment is intentionally withheld by voluntary consent of the individual who is dying (e.g., an individual who has requested through a living will not to be placed on life support for an end-stage condition, such as massive brain trauma)

  d. Involuntary passive euthanasia: occurs when treatment is intentionally withheld without voluntary consent from the person who is dying (e.g., the decision not to treat pneumonia or an opportunistic infection in an immobilized and cognitively impaired long-term clients who have not made their wishes known through an advance directive)

4. **Do-not-resuscitate order (DNR):** a physician's order of "no code" or "do not resuscitate" for clients who are in a stage of terminal, irreversible illness or expected death; the American Nurses Association (ANA) makes the following recommendations related to DNR orders:

  a. The competent client's values and choices should always be given highest priority, even when these wishes conflict with those of the family or health care provider

  b. When the client is incompetent, an advance directive or the surrogate decision makers acting for the client should make health care treatment decisions

  c. A DNR decision should always be the subject of explicit discussion between the client, family, any designated surrogate decision maker acting on the client's behalf, and the health care team

  d. DNR orders must be clearly documented, reviewed, and updated periodically to reflect changes in the client's condition

  e. A DNR order is separate from other aspects of a client's care and does not imply that other types of care should be withdrawn (e.g., nursing care to ensure comfort or medical treatment for chronic but non-life-threatening illnesses)

  f. If it is contrary to the nurse's personal belief to carry out a DNR order, the nurse should consult the nurse manager for a change in assignment

5. Comfort measures only order: a physician's order indicating that the goal of treatment is a comfortable, dignified death and that further life-sustaining measures are not indicated

O. Death-related religious and cultural practices

1. Serve primarily to assist individuals coping with the experiences of loss or death

2. Knowledge of the client's religious and cultural heritage helps the nurse provide individualized care to clients and families, even though they may not participate in the rituals associated with loss or death

3. Dying in solitude is generally unacceptable in most cultures

4. Most cultural heritages support the individual's preference to a peaceful death at home rather than in the hospital

5. Some members of ethnic groups may request that the health professional not reveal the prognosis of a terminal illness or impeding death to a dying client

6. Beliefs and attitudes about death, its cause, and the soul vary among cultures

7. Beliefs about preparation of the body, death-related rituals, autopsy, organ donation, cremation, and prolonging life are closely allied to the person's religious beliefs and cultural heritage

II. ASSESSMENT OF LOSS, GRIEVING, AND DEATH

A. Knowledge: client and family understand the implication of the loss or death

1. **Closed awareness**—the client and family are unaware of impending loss or death

2. **Mutual pretense**—the client, family, and health care provider know that the prognosis is terminal but do not talk about it and make an effort not to raise the subject

Practice to Pass

A client asks you to explain the difference between a living will and choosing a health care proxy. What would you include in client teaching?

3. **Open awareness**—the client and individuals involved know about the impending loss or death and feel comfortable discussing it, even though it may be difficult

B. **Self-care abilities**: client's ability to care for self based on any physical or psychological limitations that may have been altered by the loss

C. **Current coping**: assess how client is coping rather than how he or she should be coping

D. **Previous coping strategies**: use of previous coping skills in dealing with past loss or death

E. **Current manifestations of the grief response**: adaptive or maladaptive signs and symptoms including culturally and spiritually based behaviors

F. **Role expectations**: client and family's perception and expectations of the need to return to work, social, or family roles

G. **Support people's availability and skills**: sensitivity to the client's emotional and physical needs; ability to provide an accepting environment

H. **Advance directive**
1. Does the client have basic information about advance care directives, including living wills and durable power of attorney?
2. Does the client wish to initiate an advance directive?
3. If the client has prepared an advance directive, did the client bring it to the health care agency or can the client locate the advance directive?
4. Has the client discussed end-of-life choices with the family or designated a surrogate, physician, or other health care team worker?

I. **Resources**: availability and familiarity with possible sources of assistance such as grief support groups, religious or spiritual services, counseling services, physical care providers, or hospice programs

III. NURSING DIAGNOSES/ANALYSIS

A. **Bereavement, mourning, and grief**: Grieving; Anticipatory Grieving; Dysfunctional Grieving; Interrupted Family Processes; Ineffective Role Performance; Anxiety; Impaired Adjustment; Compromised Family Coping; Readiness for Enhanced Family Coping; Risk for Loneliness; Social Isolation; Chronic Sorrow

B. **Death or dying client**: Fear; Hopelessness; Powerlessness; Interrupted Family Processes; Death Anxiety; Ineffective Coping; Spiritual Distress

IV. PLANNING AND IMPLEMENTATION

A. **Nursing care goals and interventions for loss and grief**
1. Client goals
    a. Understand personal feelings about and reaction to loss and grief
    b. Able to discuss response and reaction to loss and grief
    c. Resume baseline sleeping and eating patterns
    d. Resume daily activities and roles as the client accepts loss
2. Nursing interventions
    a. Establish rapport and build trust
    b. Support client and family and facilitate grief work (see Box 13-1)
    c. Encourage clients to express feelings and assist them to identify their fears concerning the loss
    d. Accept negative feelings and use of defense mechanisms
    e. Provide client with opportunities to release tension, guilt
    f. Promote an adequate balance of rest, sleep, and activities
    g. Explain grieving and mourning processes and relate to client and family responses
    h. Discuss potentially difficult times such as holiday seasons or anniversary dates

Box 13-1	• Explore and respect the client and family's racial, cultural, religious, and personal values in their expression of grief.

Facilitating Grief Work with Clients and Families

- Explore and respect the client and family's racial, cultural, religious, and personal values in their expression of grief.
- Explain the various common grief responses (e.g., denial, anger, depression, guilt and isolation) and describe ways that the client and family member can identify these.
- Teach the client and family what to expect in the grief process, such as that certain thoughts and feelings are normal (acceptable) and that labile emotions (e.g., feelings of sadness, guilt, anger, fear, and loneliness) will stabilize or lessen over time. Knowing what to expect may lessen the intensity of some reactions.
- Encourage the client to express and share grief with support people. Sharing feelings reinforces relationships and facilitates the grief process.
- Teach family members to encourage the client's expression of grief and not to push the client to move on or enforce their own expectations of appropriate reactions. If the client is a child, encourage family members to be truthful and to allow the child to participate in the grieving activities of others.
- Encourage the client to resume normal activities on a schedule that promotes physical and psychological health. Some clients may try to return to normal activities too quickly. However, a prolonged delay in return may indicate dysfunctional grieving.

    i. Assist grieving person to seek new meanings with both death or other loss, as well as life

    j. Encourage clients to implement religious beliefs and rituals surrounding death or loss

    k. Mobilize the client's support systems

    l. Refer client and family to self-help groups for survivors of loss, families for mentally ill persons, and individuals who are psychiatrically disabled

    m. Validation of client's grief

B. Nursing care goals and interventions for clients and families facing death

  1. Client goals

    a. Client is assisted in achieving his or her potential

    b. Client maintains optimum comfort

    c. Family supports the client and is with client as much as possible

    d. Client and family have the opportunity to discuss what death means and to progress through stages of dying

  2. Nursing interventions

    a. Recognize that client and families have own way of dealing with death and dying

    b. Use silence and personal presence along with techniques of therapeutic communication (see Chapter 1); these techniques enhance exploration of feelings and let clients know that the nurse acknowledges their feelings

    c. Accept and support the client and family's use of coping mechanisms

    d. Accept denial and negative responses from clients and families

    e. Encourage client to participate in decisions

    f. Encourage client and family to discuss feelings related to death and dying

    g. Encourage family to communicate openly with client; acknowledge the family's grief

    h. Support client and family as they work through the dying process

    i. Assist client and family to adapt to changes in roles and lifestyles

    j. Provide appropriate information regarding how to access community resources: clergy, support groups, counseling services

    k. Support staff and seek support for self when dealing with dying client and grieving family

Practice to Pass

A client has just been diagnosed with a life-ending illness. What are your immediate assessments and goals?

V. EVALUATION/OUTCOMES

A. Outcomes of grief and loss—the client and family should be able to do the following:
1. Describe the meaning of loss
2. Progress through grieving and mourning process
3. Share loss with significant others
4. Report decreased preoccupation with loss and resumed involvement in all possible usual activities
5. Report adequate sleep and nutritional intake
6. Verbalize positive expectations for the future
7. Participate in decision making regarding daily activities
8. Recognize events that may result in additional stress on altered function
9. Seek necessary support groups or other resources

B. Outcomes of dying and death
1. Client takes opportunity to discuss feelings about dying and impeding death and eventually acknowledges inevitable outcome
2. Client is comfortable and participates in self-care for as long as possible
3. Client maintains personal control over present situation
4. Client accepts declining health status
5. Family discusses feelings about loss of loved one

Case Study

A seven-year-old male client is expected to die from leukemia. You are the nurse working in the home where the child has gone to prepare for death.

1. Based on the child's age, how would you expect him to view his impending death?

2. What assessment information would you expect to obtain from the child and family?

3. What would be the important nursing diagnoses for this child and family?

4. How would you determine the child and family have obtained goals?

5. Once the child has died, describe the bereavement, grief, and mourning by the family.

For suggested responses, see pages 301–302.

POSTTEST

POSTTEST

1 In a child newly diagnosed with leukemia, which nursing care measure would the nurse identify as a teaching priority for the child and family?

1. Comfort measures
2. Distraction activities
3. Anticipatory grieving
4. Bereavement counseling

2 The nurse is to counsel a mother who recently placed her newborn baby up for adoption. Before beginning the counseling, it is important for the nurse to deal with personal feelings about adoption, grief, and loss. This self-awareness would do which of the following?

1. Prevent the nurse from being personally affected by the client's choice in adoption.
2. Prevent the nurse from sharing any personal feelings with the client.
3. Assist the nurse to avoid discussing unpleasant feelings with the client.
4. Assist the nurse to help the client express grief fully.

3 During a counseling session, a 21-year-old client with schizophrenia verbalizes feelings of sadness and anger about being unable to keep a job or continue attending college. The nurse should formulate which of the following as the most applicable nursing diagnosis?

1. Grief related to perceived inability to achieve developmental milestones
2. Anxiety related to fear of unknown and fear of failure
3. Ineffective Coping related to feelings of hopelessness and anger
4. Dysfunctional Grief related to unrealistic expectations of abilities and lack of achievement

4 The community health nurse arrives at a home for a routine monthly visit. The client, who is crying, invites the nurse in and says, "My mother's funeral was yesterday. I'm so sad." What is the most appropriate action by the nurse at this time?

1. Encourage the client to think about something other than the mother's death.
2. Allow the client to talk about personal memories of the mother.
3. Ask the client to describe what led to the mother's death.
4. Explore the nature of the client's relationship with the mother.

5 A client reports that since her husband's death four years ago, she has experienced migraine headaches and severe nausea each year around the date of the husband's death. The nurse suspects the client is experiencing which of the following?

1. Delayed grief
2. Anniversary grief experience
3. Disenfranchised grief
4. Unresolved grief

6 The nurse works in a crisis clinic. A client arrives in a very agitated state saying, "My life partner of 15 years has died of cancer and the family will not allow me to attend the funeral. They never accepted our relationship." The nurse plans to facilitate the grieving process in this client because circumstances place the client at risk for which type of grief?

1. Delayed
2. Inhibited
3. Disenfranchised
4. Unresolved

7 The nurse informs a 20-year-old client that both parents and two older siblings were killed in an automobile accident. The client screams "No, no!!" while covering the ears and crying. Which of the following types of behavior is the nurse likely to observe next?

1. Denial
2. Depression
3. Bargaining
4. Anger

8 When questioned by a client about what an advance directive or living will is, the nurse should respond that this type of document indicates which of the following?

1. What treatment should be provided or omitted if the client becomes incapacitated
2. Which practitioners should be allowed to provide end-of-life care
3. Details about preferred caregivers for end-of-life care
4. Which family members are to be responsible for making end-of-life decisions

9 The grandfather of a three-year-old client died two days ago. Based on an understanding of normal growth and development, the nurse anticipates hearing the client make which type of comment? Select all that apply.

1. "Grandfather would not have died if I had wished a little harder."
2. "Grandfather will be waiting for me when I die."
3. "Grandfather will be back to take me to the ball game next week."
4. "Grandfather is gone, and now I have to be strong and not cry."
5. "Grandfather and I are going for ice cream tomorrow."

10 The client with lung cancer is expected to die within three months. When working with this client, the nurse assist the client to do which of the following? Select all that apply.

1. Avoid discussing the future or making future plans, as the future is uncertain.
2. Discuss feelings of impending death and acknowledge the inevitable outcome.
3. Verbalize need to avoid taking narcotic analgesics since they can cause clouded thinking.
4. Allow caregivers to provide as much care as possible to reduce stress and to preserve energy.
5. Explore what the person believes about the grieving process.

➤ *See pages 270–272 for Answers and Rationales.*

ANSWERS & RATIONALES

Pretest

1 **Answer: 1, 2** **Rationale:** Actual and perceived are correct. A perceived loss is experienced by one person but cannot be verified by others (e.g., loss of self-esteem or body image). An actual loss can be identified by others and can arise in response to a significant change in a person's appearance, body, or life circumstances, such as weight loss after surgery. An anticipatory loss is experienced before the loss actually occurs (e.g., terminal illness). A permanent loss is an irreversible deprivation (e.g., paralysis). A painful loss is a generalized term that does not have universal meaning. **Cognitive Level:** Applying **Client Need:** Psychosocial Integrity **Integrated Process:** Nursing Process: Assessment **Content Area:** Mental Health **Strategy:** Recognize that this client will experience both positive and negative psychological effects from having had the surgery. Look beyond the obvious and evaluate each option in terms of its relevance to the client in the situation. **Reference:** Varcarolis, E., Carson, V., & Shoemaker, N. (2009). *Foundations of psychiatric mental health nursing: A clinical approach* (6th ed.). St. Louis, MO: Saunders Elsevier, pp. 715–721.

2 **Answer: 1** **Rationale:** Assisting the nurse to help the parents express their grief fully is correct. The capacity for self-awareness allows the nurse to reflect and make choices. Nurses who understand their own feelings and beliefs will be able to be therapeutic when clients need to address issues which are disturbing and difficult. The death of a child will personally affect the nurse, and it is critical for the nurse to share these feelings with others, including the parents. The nurse must be available both physically and emotionally for the parents in discussing unpleasant and difficult feelings. **Cognitive Level:** Understanding **Client Need:** Psychosocial Integrity **Integrated Process:** Caring **Content Area:** Mental Health **Strategy:** Review concepts of grieving. Recognize that the nurse, too, can grieve. **Reference:** Varcarolis, E., Carson, V., & Shoemaker, N. (2009). *Foundations of psychiatric mental health nursing: A clinical approach* (6th ed.). St. Louis, MO: Saunders Elsevier, pp. 163, 569.

3 **Answer: 1** **Rationale:** Feeling anger when watching other children play is correct. Although the loss of a child can be devastating, the ability of a parent to reintegrate involvement in usual activities is important to successfully resolving grief and loss. The client's behavior indicates that she has not moved past the initial stage of grief in which preoccupation with feelings of loss and intense emotional pain are prevalent. The other options are more average responses to the death of a child. **Cognitive Level:** Analyzing **Client Need:** Psychosocial Integrity **Integrated Process:** Nursing Process: Assessment **Content Area:** Mental Health **Strategy:** Review concepts or grief and mourning. Note that the child has been dead for two and a half years. **Reference:** Varcarolis, E., Carson, V., & Shoemaker, N. (2009). *Foundations of psychiatric mental health nursing: A clinical approach* (6th ed.). St. Louis, MO: Saunders Elsevier, p. 718.

4 **Answer: 1** **Rationale:** Dysfunctional grief is correct. The client is showing denial, which is the earliest reaction to loss. This first stage of grieving is normally short-lived, and the grieving person moves on to other grief responses, like anger. The total time for acute grieving is very individualized, but feelings of numbness, emptiness, and active denial of the death four months later indicates that this client's mourning is not progressing normally. Disenfranchised grief is not present because there is nothing in the situation (such as a clandestine relationship) that would prevent the client from expressing grief. The client is grieving the actual loss of the spouse, not another situation, as would occur in distorted grief. This client's reaction is not consistent with the normal pattern of grieving. **Cognitive Level:** Analyzing **Client Need:** Psychosocial Integrity **Integrated Process:** Nursing Process: Diagnosis **Content Area:** Mental Health **Strategy:** Notice the time frame given in the question. Compare this with theories of grief and mourning. **Reference:** Fontaine, K. (2009). *Mental health nursing* (6th ed.). Upper Saddle River, NJ: Prentice Hall, pp. 41–42.

5 **Answer: 3** **Rationale:** Their spiritual and cultural beliefs is correct. Spiritual and cultural beliefs and practices greatly influence both a person's and family's reaction to death and subsequent behavior. The other options may also be correct, but the common organizing underpinnings to each of these options are cultural and spiritual beliefs. **Cognitive Level:** Applying **Client Need:** Health Promotion and Maintenance **Integrated Process:** Nursing Process: Assessment **Content Area:** Mental Health **Strategy:** When one or more options appear to be partially or completely correct, look for an answer that is more comprehensive and can include the other answers. **Reference:** Fontaine, K. (2009). *Mental health nursing* (6th ed.). Upper Saddle River, NJ: Prentice Hall, p. 48.

6 Answer: 1 Rationale: A common expression of how men grieve is correct. Male or masculine expressions of loss or death are commonly limited and less overt. Intense feelings are usually experienced privately with a general reluctance to discuss these with others. Referring the client to counseling would not be indicated at this time because the father is probably not experiencing dysfunctional grief. There are not enough data in the other two options to support them. **Cognitive Level:** Applying **Client Need:** Psychosocial Integrity **Integrated Process:** Caring **Content Area:** Mental Health **Strategy:** Recall information about grief styles of males versus females in U.S. society since there is a lack of other cultural reference in the question. **Reference:** Fontaine, K. (2009). *Mental health nursing* (6th ed.). Upper Saddle River, NJ: Prentice Hall, p. 40.

7 Answer: 2 Rationale: Voicing thoughts that are normal for children his age is correct. Preschool-age children (ages three to five) do not understand the finality of death, but instead may see it as separation. They engage in magical thinking and truly believe in the power of wishes. Magical thinking is most common in preschool-age children. The child is not experiencing delusions or making up a story to avoid negative feelings. **Cognitive Level:** Analyzing **Client Need:** Psychosocial Integrity **Integrated Process:** Caring **Content Area:** Mental Health **Strategy:** Pay attention to the age of the child. Review theories about cognitive development in children. **Reference:** Fontaine, K. (2009). *Mental health nursing* (6th ed.). Upper Saddle River, NJ: Prentice Hall, p. 40.

8 Answer: 2 Rationale: Mutual pretense is correct. With mutual pretense, the client, family, and/or health care providers know that the prognosis is terminal but agree not to talk about it and make an effort not to raise the subject. In closed awareness, the client and family are unaware of impending loss or death. There is no mutual concern. In open awareness, the client and involved individuals know about the impending loss or death and feel comfortable discussing it, even though it may be difficult. **Cognitive Level:** Applying **Client Need:** Health Promotion and Maintenance **Integrated Process:** Caring **Content Area:** Mental Health **Strategy:** Notice that both the client and the family are making a decision independently of each other that they think is in the best

interests of all. Select the option that is comprehensive of all people in the question. **Reference:** Fontaine, K. (2009). *Mental health nursing* (6th ed.). Upper Saddle River, NJ: Prentice Hall, pp. 42–43.

9 Answer: 4 Rationale: Caregiver Role Strain is correct. As the care receiver becomes more chronically ill and the caregiving burden becomes more demanding, a great strain can be placed on the caregiver's emotional and physical health. There is not enough data to suggest ineffective coping, dysfunctional grief, or social isolation. **Cognitive Level:** Analyzing **Client Need:** Psychosocial Integrity **Integrated Process:** Caring **Content Area:** Mental Health **Strategy:** Imagine yourself in this spouse's situation. Can you feel the frustration, fatigue, and strain? **Reference:** Varcarolis, E., Carson, V., & Shoemaker, N. (2009). *Foundations of psychiatric mental health nursing: A clinical approach* (6th ed.). St. Louis, MO: Saunders Elsevier, pp. 760–761.

10 Answer: 1, 4 Rationale: Accepting professional assistance and attending support groups are correct. A major outcome of grief counseling is to assist the client in sharing his or her loss and to accept support from others. It is critical for the spouse to share the feelings of loss and grief with others. A vital part of normal grieving is expressing feelings of loss and grief in a supportive, interpersonal environment, particularly with those who are most significant in the grieving person's life. It is too early to memorialize the spouse; the client must grieve the loss of client first. **Cognitive Level:** Analyzing **Client Need:** Psychosocial Integrity **Integrated Process:** Nursing Process: Planning **Content Area:** Mental Health **Strategy:** Recall basic grief processes. Consider the normal need of the grieving person to talk about personal loss. Recognize the mutuality of loss in supportive personal relationships. **Reference:** Videbeck, Sheila, A. (2011). *Psychiatric–mental health nursing* (5th ed.). Philadelphia: Lippincott, p. 218.

Posttest

1 Answer: 3 Rationale: Anticipatory grieving is correct. The child and family will be overwhelmed with such a life-threatening illness; anticipating the loss of a child would be a priority for the family. The other options suggest pertinent interventions, but during the initial period following learning of the diagnosis, the first need of the family is to react emotionally and begin to adjust to the losses implied by the diagnosis. **Cognitive Level:** Analyzing **Client Need:** Psychosocial Integrity **Integrated Process:** Nursing Process: Planning **Content Area:** Mental Health **Strategy:** Imagine yourself in the situation of this family. Would not your emotional level be very high? **Reference:** Varcarolis, E., Carson, V., & Shoemaker, N. (2009). *Foundations of psychiatric mental health nursing: A clinical approach* (6th ed.). St. Louis, MO: Saunders Elsevier, pp. 711–712.

2 Answer: 4 Rationale: Assisting the nurse to help the client express grief fully is correct. Self-awareness is a key component of any nurse–client experience. The nurse must be able to examine personal feelings, actions, and reactions in order to better assist the client in fully expressing his or her own feelings and thoughts. A firm understanding and acceptance of self allows the nurse to acknowledge a client's differences and uniqueness. In order to be empathetic to the client, the nurse must be aware of his or her own feelings. The other options do not focus on self-awareness. **Cognitive Level:** Applying **Client Need:** Health Promotion and Maintenance **Integrated Process:** Caring **Content Area:** Mental Health **Strategy:** Look at what the question is asking, which is "In what way can self-awareness benefit the nurse?" **Reference:** Kneisl, C., Wilson, H., & Trigoboff, E. (2009). *Contemporary psychiatric–mental health nursing*. Upper Saddle River, NJ: Prentice Hall, pp. 31–35.

3 **Answer: 1** **Rationale:** Grief related to perceived inability to achieve developmental milestones is correct. Schizophrenia most often occurs in young adults who are in the prime of life and attempting to achieve a normal adulthood. The individual experiences many losses, and the nurse should assist the client through the grieving process. The situation does not indicate that the client is experiencing significant anxiety. This situation does not indicate that the client is experiencing impaired coping or that hopelessness is present. Sadness and hopelessness are different emotions. The client's grieving is not dysfunctional, as the client is actively grieving a recent loss. **Cognitive Level:** Applying **Client Need:** Psychosocial Integrity **Integrated Process:** Nursing Process: Assessment **Content Area:** Mental Health **Strategy:** Consider this client's reaction to be normal. **Reference:** Varcarolis, E., Carson, V., & Shoemaker, N. (2009). *Foundations of psychiatric mental health nursing: A clinical approach* (6th ed.). St. Louis, MO: Saunders Elsevier, pp. 715–721.

4 **Answer: 2** **Rationale:** Allowing the client to talk about personal memories is correct. Even though great emotional pain is felt after a loss, it is necessary for the grieving person to talk about memories of the lost person. This process begins early in the grief experience. Encouraging the client to think about something else and asking the client to describe what led to the mother's death would actively prevent the reminiscing that is necessary in early grieving. Additionally, asking the client to describe what led to the death would also change the focus from the grieving person's feelings to a more impersonal and clinical topic. As for exploring the nature of the client's relationship with the mother, while it is true that people with a high level of ambivalence about the lost person may have difficulty resolving grief, this sort of exploration is inappropriate at this time. The client needs to express initial feelings of loss before moving on to other grieving tasks, which include reviewing the relationship. **Cognitive Level:** Applying **Client Need:** Psychosocial Integrity **Integrated Process:** Nursing Process: Implementation **Content Area:** Mental Health

Strategy: Notice that the loss has occurred very recently. **Reference:** Varcarolis, E., Carson, V., & Shoemaker, N. (2009). *Foundations of psychiatric mental health nursing: A clinical approach* (6th ed.). St. Louis, MO: Saunders Elsevier, p. 715.

5 **Answer: 2** **Rationale:** Anniversary grief experience is correct. Somatic complaints may be experienced around the date of a loss. This is called an anniversary grief response and is not a dysfunctional grief experience if the physical symptoms occur only around the specific date of the loss and the individual has otherwise returned to a full life. Individuals who have been together for many years often have these experiences for many years. Delayed grief is a postponed response in which the bereaved person may not grieve sufficiently at the time of the loss but instead has a disproportionate reaction to a later loss, which can be much more minor than the original loss. Disenfranchised grief is a response to a loss, which the individual is not regarded as having the right to grieve, or is unable to acknowledge the loss to other persons. Unresolved grief is a response that is prolonged or extended in length and severity of response. **Cognitive Level:** Applying **Client Need:** Psychosocial Integrity **Integrated Process:** Nursing Process: Assessment **Content Area:** Mental Health **Strategy:** Notice the time period since the spouse's death. **Reference:** Varcarolis, E., Carson, V., & Shoemaker, N. (2009). *Foundations of psychiatric mental health nursing: A clinical approach* (6th ed.). St. Louis, MO: Saunders Elsevier, pp. 715–721.

6 **Answer: 3** **Rationale:** Disenfranchised is correct. Disenfranchised grief is a response to a loss or death in which the individual is not regarded as having the right to grieve or is unable to acknowledge the loss to other persons. Delayed grief is a postponed response in which the bereaved person may have a reaction at the time of the loss, but it is not sufficient to the loss. However, a later loss may trigger a reaction that is out of proportion to the meaning of the current loss. Inhibited grief is a suppressed response to loss that may be expressed by somatic complaints, such as physical symptoms around the anniversary of a loss or during holidays. Unresolved grief is a response that is prolonged or extended in length and severity of response. **Cognitive Level:** Applying **Client Need:** Psychosocial Integrity **Integrated Process:** Nursing Process: Planning **Content Area:** Mental Health **Strategy:** Recognize the extent of this client's aloneness and the absence of a support system. **Reference:** Varcarolis, E., Carson, V., & Shoemaker, N. (2009). *Foundations of psychiatric mental health nursing: A clinical approach* (6th ed.). St. Louis, MO: Saunders Elsevier, p. 718.

7 **Answer: 4** **Rationale:** Anger is correct. Although the stages of grief should be used with caution in labeling expected behaviors and feelings, many clients will experience the five stages of grief as denial or shock, anger, bargaining, depression, and acceptance. Although the stages of grief should be used with caution in labeling expected behaviors and feelings, many clients will experience the five stages of grief as denial or shock, anger, bargaining, depression, and acceptance. **Cognitive Level:** Applying **Client Need:** Psychosocial Integrity **Integrated Process:** Nursing Process: Diagnosis **Content Area:** Mental Health **Strategy:** Recall commonly identified steps in the grief response. Think of grieving persons you have known. **Reference:** Varcarolis, E., Carson, V., & Shoemaker, N. (2009). *Foundations of psychiatric mental health nursing: A clinical approach* (6th ed.). St. Louis, MO: Saunders Elsevier, pp. 708, 716.

8 Answer: 1 Rationale: The type of treatment that should be provided or omitted if the client becomes incapacitated is correct. Advance directive is a general term that refers to a client's written instructions about future medical care in the event that the client becomes unable to speak or is incapacitated. Specific instructions about what medical treatment the client chooses to omit or refuse (e.g., ventilator support) in the event that the client is unable to make those decisions is also included. Advance directives do not specify particular practitioners or family members preferred for providing end-of-life care. When an advance directive document is created, the individual makes the decisions about future treatment to be administered or withheld (which family members are to be responsible). Advance directives are not the same as designating another person to make medical decisions for the individual; this is a specific legal process known as health care proxy or medical power of attorney. **Cognitive Level:** Applying **Client Need:** Management of Care **Integrated Process:** Teaching and Learning **Content Area:** Mental Health **Strategy:** Recall situations in the clinical area in which advance directives have been utilized. **Reference:** Varcarolis, E., Carson, V., & Shoemaker, N. (2009). *Foundations of psychiatric mental health nursing: A clinical approach* (6th ed.). St. Louis, MO: Saunders Elsevier, pp. 663–665.

9 Answer: 3, 5 Rationale: The notions that the grandfather will return to take the child to the ball game and go out for ice cream are correct. Preschool-age children believe death is reversible. They do not have a developed sense of death, and they are unable to understand the permanent impact of death and dying. Children between five and nine years of age believe wishes or unrelated actions can be responsible for death (thinking the grandfather would not have died if the child had wished harder). The other two responses indicate the child is aware the death is permanent. **Cognitive Level:** Applying **Client Need:** Psychosocial Integrity **Integrated Process:** Nursing Process: Diagnosis **Content Area:** Mental Health **Strategy:** Review concepts of major theorists, such as Piaget. **Reference:** Fontaine, K. (2009). *Mental health nursing* (6th ed.). Upper Saddle River, NJ: Prentice Hall, p. 40.

10 Answer: 2, 5 Rationale: Discussing feelings of impending death and exploring what the person believes about grieving are correct. This client needs to be assisted to move through the final developmental landmarks and tasks at the end of life, which include closure and completion in relations with family and friends. This will also assist the family to engage in anticipatory grieving. Avoiding discussing the future would actively prevent the client from moving through the final developmental landmarks and end-of-life tasks. Relief of pain is of highest priority when the client is terminal. The nurse should be aware of the fact that there are means of using narcotic analgesics without causing clouding of consciousness. At end of life, the dying person should be allowed to be as independent as possible in order to preserve self-esteem. **Cognitive Level:** Analyzing **Client Need:** Psychosocial Integrity **Integrated Process:** Nursing Process: Diagnosis **Content Area:** Mental Health **Strategy:** Recognize that providing appropriate end-of-life care is an important nursing role. **Reference:** Vidabeck, Sheila, L. (2011). *Psychiatric–mental health nursing* (5th ed.). Philadelphia, PA: Lippincott Williams & Wilkins, p. 217.

References

American Nurses Association (1991). *Position statement on nursing and the patient self-determination act.* Washington, DC: Author.

American Nurses Association (1992). *Position statement on nursing care and do-not-resuscitate decisions.* Washington, DC: Author.

Berman, A., & Snyder, S. (2012). *Kozier & Erb's fundamentals of nursing: Concepts, process and practice* (9th ed.). Upper Saddle River, NJ: Pearson Education.

Engel, G. L. (1964, September). Grief and grieving. *American Journal of Nursing 64,* 93–98. (Classic.)

Fontaine, K. L. (2009). *Mental health nursing* (6th ed.). Upper Saddle River, NJ: Pearson Education, pp. 40–44.

Kastenbaum, R. J. (2009). *Death, society and human experience* (10th ed.). Upper Saddle River, NJ: Pearson Education.

Kniesl, C., Wilson, H., & Trigoboff, E. (2009). *Contemporary psychiatric–mental health nursing* (2nd ed.). Upper Saddle River, NJ: Pearson Education.

Kübler-Ross, E. (1969). *On death and dying.* New York: Macmillan. (Classic.)

North American Nursing Diagnosis Association (2008). *Nursing diagnosis:*

Definitions and classification 2009–2011. Indianapolis, IN: Wiley-Blackwell.

Stuart, G. (2009). *Principles and practice of psychiatric nursing* (9th ed.). St. Louis: Elsevier Science.

Townsend, M. (2011). *Essentials of psychiatric–mental health nursing* (5th ed.). Philadelphia, PA: F. A. Davis.

Varcarolis, E., & Halter, M. (2010). *Foundations of psychiatric mental health nursing: A clinical approach* (6th ed.). Philadelphia: Saunders.

ANSWERS & RATIONALES

Psychological Adaptation to Medical Illness

14

Chapter Outline

Overview of Psychological Aspects Related to Medical Illness

Associated Common Psychological Symptoms

Medical Conditions Contributing to Psychological Symptoms

Assessment

Nursing Diagnoses/Analysis

Empowering Strategies

Evaluation/Outcomes

Objectives

➤ Identify four *emotional/psychological* responses to acute and/or chronic medical illness.

➤ Identify common clinical symptoms of psychotic disorders due to medical illness.

➤ Differentiate intervention strategies for clients experiencing critical acute illness and chronic illness.

➤ Describe the psychological effects of acquired immunodeficiency syndrome (AIDS) and other life-ending illnesses.

NCLEX-RN® Test Prep

Use the accompanying online resource, NursingReviewsandRationales, to test yourself with hundreds of NCLEX®-style practice questions.

Review at a Glance

adaptive coping an effective or appropriate response to a stressful event

control a feeling that an event can be managed

coping cognitive, physical, and or psychological/emotional attempts to manage stress

crisis an experience of being confronted by a stressful event in which the individual is unable to cope or problem solve

internal locus of control individual believes that his or her behaviors are guided by own choices and efforts

maladaptive coping an ineffective or inappropriate response to a stressful event

precipitating stressors a person's perception of something that results in feelings of anxiety

PRETEST

1 The client was involved in a severe automobile accident and had emergency surgery two days ago. At this time, the nurse should anticipate the need to assist the client to adapt to change or loss in which of the following? Select all that apply.

1. Verbal communication ability
2. Cognitive patterns
3. Body image
4. Personal autonomy
5. Family relationships

2 The nurse is assigned to a client who is hospitalized following a motor vehicle accident. The nurse determines that the client has a strong internal locus of control after hearing the client make which statement?

1. "It was an accident. That other driver cut in front of me and caused us to collide."
2. "Accidents happen, but I'll work hard in physical therapy and get out of here soon."
3. "I've had a lot of accidents before, and the doctors have always made me well again."
4. "When something accidental happens to me, I ask my higher power to take charge."

3 The client has been diagnosed with a cardiovascular disease. When the nurse is teaching the client about disease management techniques, the nurse should emphasize strategies for reducing which of the following?

1. Dependent behaviors with significant others
2. Number of social encounters
3. Urgent approach to non-urgent tasks
4. Amount of time spent in solitary activities

4 The client has the diagnosis of acquired immunodeficiency syndrome (AIDS). The nurse observes that the client is demonstrating changes in behavior that include memory difficulties, declining attention to personal hygiene, and frequent manifestations of angry and hostile behaviors. The nurse assists the client's family and friends to understand this as an indication of which of the following?

1. Rapidly approaching death
2. Reversible symptoms of delirium
3. Chronic impairment of brain functioning
4. Treatable side effects of anti-AIDS medications

5 The client has been diagnosed with a life-changing medical illness. When planning care for this client, the nurse should give priority to assessing for which of the following?

1. Anger
2. Anorexia
3. Apathy
4. Euphoria

6 The client is an adolescent who has gained considerable weight as a side effect of corticosteroid therapy for a chronic medical illness. Considering the client's developmental level, in which area is the client most likely to need support from the nurse?

1. Family relationships
2. Schoolwork
3. Plans for college
4. Sexuality

7 The client has been diagnosed with an acute medical illness. The nurse determines that the client's initial response to the illness will be highly influenced by which of the following? Select all that apply.

1. Ability to use familiar and effective coping techniques
2. Support and availability of friends and/or relatives
3. Socioeconomic and educational level of client
4. Cultural background, beliefs, and practices of client
5. Nature of the physical problem

8 Because the client has frequent episodes of parotitis and lesions of the oral mucous membranes, the school nurse suspects that the client may have bulimia nervosa. As part of the assessment process, it will be most important for the nurse to ask the client about which of the following?

1. Who prepares the food at home
2. How the client is performing at school
3. What part of life the client finds dissatisfying
4. How much weight the client has lost

9 The nurse refers the family of a terminally ill client to a grief support group. The nurse explains that such groups provide members opportunity for which of the following? Select all that apply.

1. Increased social connectivity
2. Elimination of intense emotions
3. Increased opportunity for expression of emotions
4. Decreased feelings of loss
5. Recognition of interpersonal difficulties with the client

10 The client diagnosed with a chronic medical illness arranged for a wheelchair ramp to be built for easier access to the home. The nurse interprets that this client is exhibiting which type of coping?

1. Adaptive
2. Maladaptive
3. Stressful
4. Hopeless

➤ *See pages 283–285 for Answers and Rationales.*

I. OVERVIEW OF PSYCHOLOGICAL ASPECTS RELATED TO MEDICAL ILLNESS

A. Factors influencing response to medical illness: the client's developmental/level, personality type/behaviors, coping mechanisms, precipitating stressors, support systems, resources, and nature of illness

1. Developmental stage: refers to the developmental stage of a client at the time of onset of a medical diagnosis and influences the client's reaction to the illness; the medical illness may impair mastery of the developmental/stage, which further affects how the client copes

a. Medical illnesses that occur when clients are in infancy may interfere with development of trust as per Erikson stages

b. Medical illnesses that occur when clients are in preschool may interfere with development of autonomy as per Erikson stages

c. Medical illnesses that occur when clients are school-age may interfere with development of industry as per Erikson stages

d. Adolescence: medical illnesses that occur when clients are in adolescence; may interfere with development of identity as per Erikson stages, and can isolate adolescent from peers; adolescence when confronted with chronic illness are at high risk for anxiety and/or depression (see Chapters 4 and 5), and possibly suicidal ideation

e. Early/middle adulthood: medical illnesses that occur when clients are in the early/middle adulthood may interfere with intimacy, sexuality, and/or career goals

f. Late adulthood: medical illnesses that occur when clients are in late adulthood may interfere with a sense of integrity, ability to do self-care and other activities of daily living; this lack of autonomy may result in severe emotional stress

Practice to Pass

The parents of an adolescent who was recently diagnosed with a medical illness are concerned with their child's depressed response to the diagnosis. How should the nurse respond?

2. Coping behaviors: a client's response to a medical illness diagnosis is affected by the coping behaviors that the client is able to utilize; **coping** (cognitive, physical, or emotional attempts to manage stress) implies that the client is attempting to lower tension in order to manage the situation effectively; both adaptive and maladaptive coping behaviors are typically manifested

> a. **Adaptive coping** behaviors: utilization of adaptive coping behaviors facilitates the client's ability to mobilize internal/external resources and sustain general homeostasis

> b. **Maladaptive coping** behaviors: utilization of maladaptive coping behaviors, such as severe anxiety and panic, results in cognitive disorganization; this impairs the client's ability to mobilize internal/external resources; ineffective and destructive behaviors may appear, and general homeostasis is not preserved

3. **Precipitating stressors**

a. Are defined as events occurring prior to a medical illness that initiated a stress response of physiological and/or psychological alterations

b. Precipitating stressors can influence a client's response to medical illness because the client may already be in an emotionally compromised state prior to the medical illness diagnosis

4. Support systems: the presence or absence of strong support systems influences a client's response to medical illness; strong family, friend, and community support systems can result in positive responses; a lack of support systems can result in negative responses

5. Nature of illness: a client's response to medical illness may be dependent on whether the illness is of an acute state, chronic state, or terminal state

a. Acute illness: sudden onset, may be caused by trauma from an accident or caused by an illness that is rapid onset in nature such as type 1 diabetes, or a new diagnosis of cancer

1) Acute illness often results in a crisis situation for both client and family

2) **Crisis** refers to an event in which the client's regular coping mechanisms are inadequate to meet needs

3) The client may have severe anxiety and/or panic as manifested by short attention span, inability to concentrate or problem solve, impulsivity, and unproductivity

b. Chronic illness: gradual adaptation to a chronic problem; may be caused by disability from trauma, or caused by an illness that the client must learn to cope with; chronic illness is debilitating in nature; this results in ongoing stress for client and family; the client and caregiver often feel frustrated, hopeless, and fatigued

c. Terminal illness: a terminal illness diagnosis may place the client and family in a crisis mode

1) This type of illness continues to be extremely disruptive to client and family functioning

2) The client often exhibits signs of anger, hopelessness/helplessness, and despair

II. ASSOCIATED COMMON PSYCHOLOGICAL SYMPTOMS

A. **Certain psychological symptoms are common** to clients diagnosed with a medical illness; these include anger, depression, anxiety, helplessness, and hopelessness

B. **Anger**

1. Clients with a medical illness diagnosis may demonstrate behaviors that are indicative of anger

2. These behaviors reflect feelings of helplessness and frustration about the illness, and the effects it has on daily functioning

3. Behaviors likely to be exhibited include demanding types of action, loud verbalization, slamming of items, and/or social withdrawal

C. Depression
1. Clients with a medical illness diagnosis may demonstrate symptoms of depression related to the disruption of daily functioning
2. Signs associated with depression include feelings of helplessness/hopelessness, flat affect, poor eye contact, disrupted eating/sleeping patterns, absence of motivation and compliance, and a decreased energy level (see Chapter 4)

D. Anxiety
1. Clients with a medical illness diagnosis may demonstrate feelings and behaviors of anxiety
2. This reflects feelings of real or imagined threat to body image
3. Anxiety results in autonomic nervous system stimulation; i.e., increased heart rate, increased blood pressure, increased respirations, increased visual acuity, diaphoresis, shortness of breath, and/or restlessness

E. Helplessness/hopelessness
1. Clients with a medical diagnosis may manifest feelings of helplessness/hopelessness
2. Helplessness is defined as feelings of powerlessness associated with the inability to control what is occurring; hopelessness is defined as feelings of despondency, loss of optimism, and an inability to mobilize energy
3. This is reflected in feelings of loss of **control** (feeling that an event can be managed) of the self (individuality) with increased dependence on others

III. MEDICAL CONDITIONS CONTRIBUTING TO PSYCHOLOGICAL SYMPTOMS

A. **Critical/acute illness** may occur without warning and immediately affect a client's daily functioning; clients typically experience feelings of loss of control, anxiety, helplessness, and anger
1. Cardiovascular illnesses
   a. Have been linked to the occurrence of stress
   b. Include myocardial infarction, cerebrovascular accident, and hypertension
   c. Stress levels can influence the course and/or the outcomes of the medical illness
2. Trauma
   a. May be the result of an accident or crime
   b. Behavioral and physiological responses occur and are manifested in client by social isolation, agitation, nightmares, and/or feelings of numbness
   c. The client typically struggles to control episodes of anxiety related to the traumatic event
3. Surgery as the result of a critical or an acute medical condition may be disfiguring or incapacitating; surgical procedures can result in alterations of client daily functioning and changes in the client's perception of self-image
4. Pain can accompany many acute illnesses; the client's response is based on a need to protect oneself from harm

B. **Chronic illness** produces effects that are long term and demand that the client cope with the illness and its effects for a long duration; the onset of these illnesses may be unpredictable and will require ongoing use of adaptive coping mechanisms; lower socioeconomic status increases the likelihood of multiple chronic health problems due to limited health care access and limited financial resources; this may impair adherence to treatment plans
1. Pulmonary diseases
   a. Include exacerbation of chronic obstructive pulmonary disease and asthma
   b. Higher stress levels lead to increased secretions and airway spasms and result in increased episodes of breathing difficulties

Practice to Pass

Family members of a client hospitalized with asthma become upset when the treatment team talks about stress factors and asthma. They feel asthma is "just" a medical illness. How should the nurse respond?

2. Gastrointestinal (GI) diseases
   a. Irritable bowel syndrome, peptic ulcer, and ulcerative colitis are stress-related illnesses
   b. Physiological reaction to stress impacts both the GI tract and the autonomic nervous system
3. Medical illnesses that result in chronic pain can have a profound effect on clients and their adaptive and maladaptive coping behaviors; clients respond to pain in a psychological and physiological manner that requires them to continually attempt to adapt

C. Terminal illness: exemplar HIV

1. Human immunodeficiency virus (HIV) and acquired immunodeficiency syndrome (AIDS) result in an immunodepressed state; persons with these disorders may also have comorbid psychiatric illness that further compromises the primary disease state
   a. Due to severe grief and loss in clients with HIV, assessment of clients with this disorder need to be evaluated for a comorbidity of psychiatric illness
   b. Many stressors: chronic fear of the disease, fear of exposing others to the virus, intimate/sexual disruption, social isolation, stigmas attached to the disorder, impairment in occupational functioning, and problems with insurance place the client at risk for psychiatric problems
   c. Depression and anxiety are often comorbid disorders with HIV
      1) A differential diagnosis of clients with AIDS who may also have anxiety or depression is difficult to differentiate since all three illness can manifest with fatigue, hopelessness, helplessness, weight loss, aching muscles, and diarrhea
      2) Psychiatric symptoms commonly observed in clients with HIV/AIDS include irritability and psychotic symptoms including paranoia, substance abuse, and suicidal ideation
   d. Dementia and delirium are both comorbid cognitive disorders seen with HIV/AIDS
      1) Dementia is a chronic irreversible brain disorder manifested by memory loss, impaired judgment, personality changes, and decline in physical appearance; disturbance in behavior may also occur
      2) Delirium is an acute reversible brain disorder manifested by inattentiveness, cloudy consciousness, apathy, and bizarre behaviors
   e. When applicable, nursing interventions for clients with HIV/AIDS should include those that relate to AIDS:
      1) Dementia and delirium
      2) Changes in body image
      3) Low self-esteem
      4) Preparation for imminent death, referral to hospice
      5) Pain management
      6) Support of family/significant others
2. Other terminal illnesses
   a. The dying client experiences feelings of helplessness and hopelessness
   b. In addition, feelings of depression, anger, and hostility are experienced
   c. The client's response to terminal illness diagnosis is affected by biological factors, cultural implications, locus of control, stages of development, coping mechanisms, coping resources, and support systems
   d. Interventions for clients with a terminal illness should include the following:
      1) Therapeutic communication that encompasses acceptance, empathy, and compassion
      2) Focus on positive aspects of the client's life
      3) Spirituality assessment and reinforcement of spirituality

         4) Support of family and significant others

         5) Allowing the client to have dignity

         6) Allowing the client to have control

         7) Sufficient pain management

IV. ASSESSMENT

A. The nurse uses various resources to collect physical, psychological, and social data

B. The assessment phase includes both subjective and objective data; objective data should include family input, physical assessment, and diagnostic and laboratory findings

C. Psychological assessment

    1. Elicit client's emotional reaction to the medical diagnosis, assess coping mechanisms, resources, locus of control, and support systems

    2. Complete a stress appraisal that includes identification of the source of physical and psychological stressors, number of stressors, duration client endured the stressors, and client's appraisal of the stressors

    3. Assess for symptoms of depression including client appearance, mood, affect, recent weight loss or weight gain, sleep patterns, eating patterns, and/or suicidal ideation

    4. Identify adaptive and maladaptive coping behaviors; identify how these impair or facilitate the client to identify problems, solve problems, and express and analyze feelings

    5. Assess for any substance use, abuse, or dependence; this is crucial during the assessment phase since the substance can be a symptom of or contribute to depression, anxiety, hopelessness, helplessness, unhealthy eating patterns, and problems with sleep

    6. Identify the stage of grief the client is in regarding the medical illness

        a. Clients eventually progress through the five stages of grief; nursing interventions should be planned according to the stage of grief

        b. Five stages of grief occur:

           1) Denial of the medical illness and associated limitations

           2) Anger at loss of control and associated limitations

           3) Bargaining, with a plea for another chance and a seeking of new answers/treatments

           4) Depression, when grieving, occurs due to loss or anticipated loss

           5) Acceptance/adaptation is when the conflicts are resolved and the client begins to participate in care

D. Biological assessment

    1. This type of assessment is done to understand how stress alters a client's internal body functioning

    2. Biological changes can assist the nurse with determining the severity of an illness

    3. Complete an assessment of current and past health conditions that may be contributing to the client's recent level of physical and psychological functioning; both recent illnesses and chronic illnesses alter the client's immune system, thereby raising susceptibility to additional health problems

    4. Conduct a complete physical exam to detect any physical conditions contributing to psychological symptoms; it is important to differentiate manifestations of the medical illness from any manifestations of psychiatric illness so misdiagnosis does not occur

    5. Complete a thorough neurological status exam to reveal current neurological status; current findings provide a baseline level of functioning

    6. Review laboratory results carefully, as these may provide information that is relevant to occurrence of psychological symptoms

    7. Assess the client's current physical functioning such as the abilities to perform activities of daily living and/or exercise; this helps to establish a baseline for a plan of care

8. Assess sleep patterns, note any sleep disruptions (i.e., inability to fall asleep, inability to stay asleep during the night, desire to sleep all of the time); sleep disruptions may be indicative of either physiological or psychological problems

9. Assess nutritional pattern, not problems (i.e., lack of appetite, failure to enjoy previously enjoyable food, and overeating); eating problems can be indicative of either physiological or psychological stress

10. Complete a pharmacological assessment; note pharmacological agents that the client is currently taking that influence their level of physical and psychological functioning

E. **Social assessment**

1. Include a social assessment as part of the total client assessment

2. Complete a social assessment that explores a family history, the client lifestyle, any life-changing events, and presence of social support systems (identify both negative and positive social networks)

3. Explore any recent life-changing events that may have an impact on adaptation to the current illness

4. Discuss the client's lifestyle patterns and any potential impact current lifestyle choices may have on the development and progression of the disease

5. Assess for unique aspects of the client's cultural practices that may influence specific responses to the disease or the need for special nursing interventions

6. Assess family communication patterns, level of cohesion, boundaries, flexibility, overall functioning, and general support

7. Explore community resources and support resources for availability of home health care, respite care, mental health services, and support groups

8. Assess spiritual concerns; note traditional patterns or rituals, and inquire about other forms of spirituality that may be important to the client

9. Complete an occupational assessment: determine if there will be a temporary disruption in work, or if client can realistically continue in current occupation in the future

10. Determine economic status, specifically whether there are finances to support current and future expenses

Practice to Pass

A client was admitted to the hospital with various physical symptoms. The nurse should be sure to assess what major areas of the person's life?

V. NURSING DIAGNOSES/ANALYSIS

A. **Nursing diagnoses** are used to describe health problems and needs so that nursing interventions can be planned

B. **Problems identified may be either actual or potential**

C. **Commonly used nursing diagnoses in the care of clients** requiring psychological adaptation to medical illness include the following:

1. Ineffective Denial related to changes in physical and psychosocial abilities following a chronic or acute medical illness diagnosis

2. Disturbed Body Image related to occurrence of a medical illness

3. Impaired Adjustment related to the client's functional changes following a medical diagnosis

4. Ineffective Coping related to occurrence and effects of a medical illness diagnosis

5. Self-Care Deficit related to client's functional changes associated with a medical diagnosis

6. Risk for Situational Low Self-Esteem related to clients functional changes associated with a medical diagnosis

7. Anxiety related to occurrence of a medical diagnosis

Practice to Pass

A client is feeling depressed about how the right leg appears following a traumatic automobile accident and multiple surgeries to correct problems. What nursing diagnoses should the nurse consider?

VI. EMPOWERING STRATEGIES

    A. Interventions
1. The nurse collaborates with the client and family members to develop a plan of care for the client in which the client's response can be monitored
2. Interventions serve as the foundation for all client care and are subject to change as the condition of the client changes
3. Specific interventions that exemplify empowering strategies include the following:
   a. Increase client control; provide opportunities for client decision making regarding care
   b. Engage in therapeutic interactions: establishing trust, using caring and empathetic listening
   c. Recommend referral to a psychologist, social worker, or psychiatrist when applicable to assist client with adaptation to illness and general support
   d. Assist with stress management—teach relaxation methods, imagery, biofeedback, and necessity for exercise
   e. Reinforce current positive, adaptive coping behaviors and persons' strengths
   f. Implement measures that promote comfort and healing
   g. Utilize spiritual resources—provide opportunities for client to engage in spiritual traditions/rituals; refer to spiritual counselor as needed
   h. Offer educational resources related to complementary medicine if client desires

B. Differential interventions for critical/acute versus chronic illnesses
1. Critical/acute illnesses typically result in abrupt interruption of a client's usual daily activities; this can precipitate a crisis stage if client perceives events as a threat to safety, self-esteem, or self-image
   a. Seek immediate ways to increase client's control
   b. Engage in therapeutic interactions with client and family; encourage verbalization of feelings
   c. Assist with immediate anxiety reduction through use of relaxation techniques
   d. Use firm, direct limit-setting to assist client with staying focused
2. Chronic illnesses typically require ongoing adaptation as long-term effects are unpredictable; chronic illnesses often deplete energy levels, support systems, coping reserves, economic abilities, and may lead to suicidal ideation
   a. Increase self-care responsibilities as appropriate to preserve/facilitate functioning/self-esteem/image
   b. Reward positive adaptive coping behaviors and productive interdependence
   c. Reinforce existing support network linkages and assist client with creating new linkages; identify support groups, self-help groups, and special interest groups
   d. Refer to psychiatric services as necessary
   e. Refer for MSW consult when indicated for short-term counseling or support

VII. EVALUATION/OUTCOMES

A. The client will preserve optimal physiological function
B. Disease process reduction/cessation: the client will learn about the illness and means to manage the disease process (i.e., appropriate diet, exercise, and stress-reduction activities)
C. The client will develop, reinforce, and strengthen adaptive coping behaviors
1. The ability to express feelings related to the medical illness diagnosis and effects of the illness
2. The ability to achieve productive interdependence of client with ongoing support systems, such as family and friends
D. The client will participate in the treatment plan and rehabilitative processes

E. The client will manifest an optimal level of functioning
   1. The client will be as independent in self-care as physically capable
   2. The client will develop or use support systems
   3. The client will manifest decreased anxiety to low to moderate levels
   4. The client will begin to manifest evidence of an **internal locus of control**: clients who believe that they have ability and responsibility to decrease the likelihood of illness or effects of illness have an internal locus of control and are less likely to experience symptoms of distress

Case Study

A 20-year-old female client has been diagnosed with HIV. The client is feeling depressed and hopeless about the future. You are the nurse working with this client.

1. Identify three symptoms indicative of depression.

2. Identify two to three assessments needed in the care of this client.

3. List at least three possible nursing diagnoses.

4. What nursing interventions should you consider in the care and treatment of this client?

5. If the client asks you why she should feel anything but hopeless about the future, how would you respond?

For suggested responses, see page 302.

POSTTEST

1 A client who recently had a leg amputation following a car accident is now ready for discharge. The nurse has been talking with the client about signs and symptoms of depression. The nurse concludes that the client best understands how depression might be exhibited if the client makes which statement?

1. "If I'm not sleeping or eating well or I feel like things do not matter any more, then I should seek help."
2. "If I find myself eating more than usual or having arguments with my family, then I could not be depressed."
3. "I shouldn't worry too much if I have headaches and neck pain. They'd be caused from the accident."
4. "It's OK if I stay in bed a lot. I need to conserve my energy."

2 A client diagnosed with ulcerative colitis is preparing for discharge from the hospital. The nurse concludes that the client understands the relationship between the disease and stress after hearing which statement made by the client?

1. "My symptoms of stress will reduce if I take my medicine."
2. "I am glad I am learning how to manage problem areas in my life."
3. "Now that I have a diagnosis, I don't have to worry about stress any more."
4. "I wouldn't be so stressed if my family treated me better."

3 The client who has acquired immunodeficiency syndrome (AIDS) has a nursing diagnosis of Disturbed Self-Esteem. When caring for this client, which approach will be most important for the nurse to use?

1. Avoid looking directly at the client.
2. Maintain a formal relationship with the client.
3. Keep contact with the client at a minimum.
4. Listen attentively.

4 The nurse is developing a stress management seminar for clients recently discharged from a cardiac care unit. Which concepts should the nurse include in the seminar?

1. Learning to develop a large network of friends
2. Developing additional social activities
3. Personality types and how these influence cardiac illness
4. Use of confrontation as a beneficial way to decrease tension

5 When the client has a chronic medical illness that results in severe disability, it will be most important for the nurse to assess for which of the following?

1. Suicidal ideation
2. Depression
3. Anxiety
4. Helplessness

6 The nurse is aware that a client's pain has both physiological and psychological components. The nurse bases pain management strategies on knowledge that the psychological component of pain comes from the need to do which of the following?

1. Express feelings
2. Protect oneself from harm
3. Feel sorry for self
4. Keep feelings inside

7 The client has a medical illness that is causing a significant loss of independence. Which of the following is the most important intervention by the nurse?

1. Help the client with almost all activities.
2. Avoid focusing on the client during activity time.
3. Try not to give assistance to the client.
4. Include the client as an active member of the treatment team.

8 Before devising an initial plan of care for a client with a chronic medical illness, the nurse should assess which of the following of the client? Select all that apply.

1. Sleep pattern
2. Nutritional intake
3. Anxiety level
4. Financial status
5. Aftercare plans

9 The nurse is conducting family therapy with a family in which one member has a progressively debilitating illness. Which comment by the nurse is most likely to facilitate the family's use of the healthy coping mechanism known as productive interdependence?

1. "No single family member should always be in charge of decisions or caregiving."
2. "All of you should work toward reducing conflict within the family."
3. "All of you should work as a team, both asking for and receiving help from the others."
4. "If the family assumes all responsibility for decision-making, this will reduce the ill person's stress level."

10 A client with a medical illness diagnosis is found to be at a lower socioeconomic level of income. The nurse anticipates that this client is more likely to experience an increase in which of the following?

1. Grief responses
2. Generalized pain
3. Use of defense mechanisms
4. Incidence of other illnesses

➤ *See pages 285–287 for Answers and Rationales.*

ANSWERS & RATIONALES

Pretest

1 **Answer: 3, 4 Rationale:** Since the client has experienced both injury and surgery to the body, changes in body image should be anticipated. Having experienced an accident, this client is now in a situation (acute illness and hospitalization) that is expected to limit the client's personal autonomy. There is inadequate information to suggest that changes in family relationships may occur.

Cognitive Level: Analyzing **Client Need:** Psychosocial Integrity **Integrated Process:** Caring **Content Area:** Mental Health **Strategy:** Look for what is expected to be universally true of clients in this type of situation. **Reference:** Varcarolis, E., & Halter, M. (2010). *Foundations of psychiatric mental health nursing: A clinical approach* (6th ed.). St. Louis, MO: Saunders Elsevier, pp. 592–593.

2 **Answer: 2 Rationale:** The client shows a personal commitment to health and health-seeking behaviors and a willingness to participate actively in the treatment plan. This reflects a strong internal locus of control. The other options suggest an external locus of control. By stating that the other driver cut in front of him or her, the client is blaming others. By stating that doctors have always made him or her well again or asking a higher power to take charge, the client expects that efforts of others will restore wellness. **Cognitive Level:** Analyzing **Client Need:** Psychosocial Integrity **Integrated Process:** Nursing Process: Assessment **Content Area:** Mental Health **Strategy:** Identify the one statement that indicates that the client feels capable of having some control in the outcome of his or her own situation. **Reference:** Fontaine, K. (2009). *Mental health nursing* (6th ed.). Upper Saddle River, NJ: Prentice Hall, p. 31.

3 **Answer: 3** **Rationale:** Many people with cardiovascular disease show Type A personality behaviors, consisting of anger, hostility, a sense of urgency, becoming easily frustrated, and having workaholic-type behaviors. These characteristics may play a significant part in the etiology of cardiovascular problems, and when present, they can complicate treatment and recovery. Dependent behaviors with significant others is incorrect, because it is more common for people with Type A personalities and/or cardiovascular disease to be controlling of others. Number of social encounters is incorrect, because the nature of social encounters, rather than the frequency is more significant in determining the individual's behavior. Amount of time spent in solitary activities is incorrect because feelings of urgency and frustration will not necessarily decline when the person is alone. **Cognitive Level:** Applying **Client Need:** Psychosocial Integrity **Integrated Process:** Nursing Process: Planning **Content Area:** Mental Health **Strategy:** Recall information about the interaction of stress, personality types, and physical illnesses. **Reference:** Kneisl, C., & Trigoboff, E. (2009). *Contemporary psychiatric–mental health nursing* (2nd ed.). Upper Saddle River, NJ: Prentice Hall, pp. 103–106.

4 **Answer: 3** **Rationale:** The behaviors described in this situation are characteristic of clients with dementia, which is a possible late consequence of AIDS. The nurse should understand that the occurrence of symptoms indicates progression of the AIDS illness and that care should be planned accordingly. Rapidly approaching death is incorrect because an individual can live with dementia for some time before death occurs, either from AIDS or another cause. Reversible symptoms of delirium is incorrect because the situation describes behaviors that are characteristic of the chronic progressive decline that is seen in persons with dementia. Treatable side effects of anti-AIDS medications is incorrect because the particular pattern of behaviors that is described are not particularly associated with the side effect profile of drugs used to control AIDS. **Cognitive Level:** Analyzing **Client Need:** Physiological Adaptation **Integrated Process:** Caring **Content Area:** Mental Health **Strategy:** Review usual

progression patterns of AIDS. Recognize that the client and significant others have a right to know what is happening. **Reference:** Kneisl, C., & Trigoboff, E. (2009). *Contemporary psychiatric–mental health nursing.* Upper Saddle River, NJ: Prentice Hall, pp. 577–578.

5 **Answer: 1** **Rationale:** Anger is included in the stages of mourning, as clients grieve for what has been lost. Although clients may experience multiple emotional feelings in response to the diagnosis of a life-changing medical illness, anger is one of the most common ones because of the sudden and often dramatic change in lifestyle. Anorexia and apathy might occur but are not considered stages of grief and mourning. Euphoria is not a common manifestation of grieving, but if it is seen, it is possible that the client has bipolar disorder, and that the loss precipitated a period of elevated affect. **Cognitive Level:** Applying **Client Need:** Psychosocial Integrity **Integrated Process:** Nursing Process: Assessment **Content Area:** Mental Health **Strategy:** Recognize that the client is facing a situation that will require great adaptation to loss. Recall normal steps in grief and mourning. **Reference:** Varcarolis, E., & Halter, M. (2010). *Foundations of psychiatric mental health nursing: A clinical approach* (6th ed.). St. Louis, MO: Saunders Elsevier, pp. 614–615.

6 **Answer: 4** **Rationale:** Since a developmental task of adolescence is dealing with one's emerging social and sexual urges and needs, the appearance of the body assumes great importance. When the body is unattractive to the self and/or others (as in situations of debilitating medical illness or significant changes in body weight), issues surrounding sexuality and identity are common. It is common for adolescents to have relationship difficulties with parents, but this is considered a normal part of adolescence. In this client's situation, present (schoolwork) and future (plans for college) educational plans and activities are not as likely to be directly impacted as is sexuality. **Cognitive Level:** Analyzing **Client Need:** Psychosocial Integrity **Integrated Process:** Caring **Content Area:** Mental Health **Strategy:** Recall theories of adolescent development and your own adolescence. Imagine yourself in this client's situation. **Reference:** Kneisl, C., & Trigoboff, E. (2009). *Contemporary psychiatric–mental health nursing.* Upper Saddle River, NJ: Prentice Hall, pp. 33–35.

7 **Answer: 1, 2, 4** **Rationale:** This client is at risk for developing a crisis response. If balancing factors (social support and using familiar coping techniques) are present, a crisis will not be as likely to occur. If the individual can cope using socially appropriate rituals, a crisis response will not be as likely to occur. Persons of all socioeconomic and educational levels can be overwhelmed with life situations and develop a crisis response. No one is exempt from the possibility of developing a crisis response. The client's response to a situation is not always parallel with the severity of the actual problem. Instead, it is parallel with the client's perception of the problem.

Cognitive Level: Applying Client Need: Psychosocial Integrity Integrated Process: Caring Content Area: Mental Health Strategy: Identify those things that would be useful to any person in a crisis state. Remember that in certain circumstances, all persons are vulnerable to having a crisis response. Reference: Varcarolis, E., & Halter, M. (2010). *Foundations of psychiatric mental health nursing: A clinical approach* (6th ed.). St. Louis, MO: Saunders Elsevier, p. 461.

8 Answer: 3 Rationale: Eating disorders are a manifestation of problems in living and difficulty dealing with emotions and stress. Eating disorders are not about eating per se, but rather about making unhealthy attempts to control emotions and manage stress. The nurse should avoid focusing on food and food-related topics with this client. If this client has bulimia, food is being used to express underlying issues and conflicts. Clients with eating disorders do not typically have declines in academic performance. In fact, many of them are compulsive over-achievers who may be seen as model students. Clients with bulimia may not lose weight and may even be at or near ideal body weight. Cognitive Level: Analyzing Client Need: Psychosocial Integrity Integrated Process: Nursing Process: Assessment Content Area: Mental Health Strategy: Recognize that eating patterns are not necessarily related to biologic anorexia or hunger. Recall that food and eating can convey symbolic messages. Reference: Fontaine, K. (2009). *Mental health nursing* (6th ed.). Upper Saddle River, NJ: Prentice Hall, pp. 319–321.

9 Answer: 1, 3 Rationale: It is likely that increased social connectivity would result in increased social support, since the other persons in the group would also be dealing with grief issues. The work of grieving is best accomplished in a compassionate and supportive emotional environment. Grief support groups are aimed at helping a person to recognize, express, and cope with strong emotions, not eliminate them. It is normal for a grieving person to feel intense emotions. Feelings of loss are normal in grief responses. Grief groups acknowledge this and support healthy expression of these feelings, which must be fully expressed and dealt with so the person can progress healthily through all stages of grieving. Grief counseling does not focus on the deceased, but rather on the survivor and the survivor's coping. Cognitive Level: Applying Client Need: Psychosocial Integrity Integrated Process: Caring Content Area: Mental Health Strategy: Notice that two options indicate positive results, and the remaining ones suggest eliminating or minimizing feelings that are expected and normal in the grieving situation. Reference: Varcarolis, E., & Halter, M. (2010). *Foundations of psychiatric mental health nursing: A clinical approach* (6th ed.). St. Louis, MO: Saunders Elsevier, pp. 616–617.

10 Answer: 1 Rationale: Adaptive indicates that the client is able to mobilize internal/external resources to cope with the chronic illness and its effects. Maladaptive relates to

a response that is negative in nature. This client's response will reduce the stress response, not increase it. This client's response shows realism and adaptation to the stress being experienced, not hopelessness. Cognitive Level: Applying Client Need: Psychosocial Integrity Integrated Process: Caring Content Area: Mental Health Strategy: Notice that three of the responses are negative in character. That should suggest to you that the one that is different is likely to be the correct answer. Reference: Fontaine, K. (2009). *Mental health nursing* (6th ed.). Upper Saddle River, NJ: Prentice Hall, p. 271.

Posttest

1 Answer: 1 Rationale: The client understands the disruption of the accident and that feeling down might be expected, but the client is able to differentiate between mild and more severe depressive symptoms, such as anhedonia and having trouble sleeping and eating. The client does not understand that depression may be experienced somatically (eating more than usual, having arguments with family, or having headaches and neck pain). The client does not recognize that being inactive and remaining in bed could be a symptom of depression, nor does the client recognize that physical inactivity may increase the intensity of depression. Cognitive Level: Analyzing Client Need: Health Promotion and Maintenance Integrated Process: Nursing Process: Evaluation Content Area: Mental Health Strategy: Remember that depression has both psychologic and physiologic components. Reference: Varcarolis, E., & Halter, M. (2010). *Foundations of psychiatric mental health nursing: A clinical approach* (6th ed.). St. Louis, MO: Saunders Elsevier, p. 329.

2 Answer: 2 Rationale: "I am glad I am learning how to manage problem areas in my life" is correct. The client has verbalized that there is a relationship between the disease and stress and is learning how to deal with the stress. "My symptoms of stress will reduce if take my medicine" and "Now that I have a diagnosis, I don't have to worry about stress any more" indicate no understanding of the relationship between stress and gastrointestinal symptoms being experienced. Attributing the stress to the family's behavior indicates blaming, rather than awareness of the relationship between stress and gastrointestinal symptoms. Cognitive Level: Analyzing Client Need: Psychosocial Integrity Integrated Process: Nursing Process: Evaluation Content Area: Mental Health Strategy: Look for an option that indicates a change in the client's attitude. Reference: Kneisl, C., & Trigoboff, E. (2009). *Contemporary psychiatric–mental health nursing* (2nd ed.). Upper Saddle River, NJ: Prentice Hall, p. 103.

3 Answer: 4 Rationale: Listening attentively is correct because it indicates interest and concern about the client and facilitates open communication. The other options indicate that the nurse wants distance from the client. Cognitive Level: Applying Client Need: Health Promotion and Maintenance **Integrated Process:** Nursing Process: Planning **Content Area:** Mental Health **Strategy:** Apply common sense to answer this question. If the client has low self-esteem, could the three "distancing" options be expected to elevate the client's self-esteem? **Reference:** Kneisl, C., & Trigoboff, E. (2009). *Contemporary psychiatric–mental health nursing* (2nd ed.). Upper Saddle River, NJ: Prentice Hall, pp. 153–154.

4 **Answer: 3** **Rationale:** Personality types and how they influence cardiac illness is correct because it indicates knowledge related to how personality types influence cardiac illness. Learning to develop a large network of friends and developing additional social activities do not have anything to do with understanding stress and cardiac disease. Using confrontation is not a beneficial way to decrease tension. **Cognitive Level:** Applying **Client Need:** Health Promotion and Maintenance **Integrated Process:** Teaching and Learning **Content Area:** Mental Health **Strategy:** Notice that one option includes the word *cardiac*. Since the stem of the question does also, this is a clue that suggests that this option is correct. **Reference:** Kneisl, C., & Trigoboff, E. (2009). *Contemporary psychiatric–mental health nursing* (2nd ed.). Upper Saddle River, NJ: Prentice Hall, p. 103.

5 **Answer: 1** **Rationale:** Persons with debilitating illness are at high risk for suicide. When suicidal ideation is present, the nurse should gather other assessment data, including whether there is a specific plan for suicide and a means for carrying out the suicidal act. The areas in the other three options should be assessed, but they do not have priority over determining if a suicide plan has been developed and level of lethality. These last two factors would represent the most severe and dangerous response to physical illness and disability. **Cognitive Level:** Analyzing **Client Need:** Safety and Infection Control **Integrated Process:** Nursing Process: Assessment **Content Area:** Mental Health **Strategy:** Consider that psychological debilitation associated with chronic physical debilitation. Is it not reasonable to think that the two could lead to self-destructiveness? **Reference:** Varcarolis, E., & Halter, M. (2010). *Foundations of psychiatric mental health nursing: A clinical approach* (6th ed.). St. Louis, MO: Saunders Elsevier, p. 637.

6 **Answer: 2** **Rationale:** Protecting oneself from harm describes the normal response that a person engages in when threatened in any way, such as with pain. Feeling sorry for self and keeping feelings inside are inappropriate responses of coping with pain. Expressing feelings is not an option related to psychological nature of pain. **Cognitive Level:** Understanding **Client Need:** Physiological Adaptation **Integrated Process:** Nursing Process: Diagnosis **Content Area:** Mental Health **Strategy:** Notice that two options are stated in judgmental language. Eliminate them without further consideration. **Reference:** Kneisl, C., & Trigoboff, E. (2009). *Contemporary psychiatric–mental health nursing* (2nd ed.). Upper Saddle River, NJ: Prentice Hall, pp. 156–157.

7 **Answer: 4** **Rationale:** Including the client as an active member of the treatment team indicates that the client is a part of his or her own care and supports interdependence. Helping the client with almost all activities does not promote feelings of independence. Avoiding focusing on the client during activity time could lead to client isolation, while trying not to help the client would place undue pressure on the client to feel that he or she should be doing things by him- or herself. **Cognitive Level:** Analyzing **Client Need:** Health Promotion and Maintenance **Integrated Process:** Nursing Process: Implementation **Content Area:** Mental Health **Strategy:** Imagine yourself in this situation. Would you want to give up your independence? **Reference:** Varcarolis, E., & Halter, M. (2010). *Foundations of psychiatric mental health nursing: A clinical approach* (6th ed.). St. Louis, MO: Saunders Elsevier, p. 443.

8 **Answer: 1, 2, 3** **Rationale:** Sleep pattern, nutritional intake, and anxiety level are correct. If the client is not receiving adequate sleep or nutrition, heightened symptoms of illness and psychological distress will occur. Sleep and nutrition are basic physiologic needs. If the client's anxiety level is significantly elevated, the client will not be able to focus on important information about the plan of care. Additionally, heightened anxiety will create physiologic stress responses that can intensify prior existing medical illness and complicate recovery. The nurse does not typically assess financial status of clients, as this is the responsibility of the social worker. Talking about aftercare plans is not appropriate when the nurse is establishing an initial plan of care. This discussion should take place later. **Cognitive Level:** Analyzing **Client Need:** Physiological Adaptation **Integrated Process:** Nursing Process: Assessment **Content Area:** Mental Health **Strategy:** Notice that this is an initial assessment and make it as inclusive as possible. Information from this assessment will form the database from which care is planned. **Reference:** Varcarolis, E., & Halter, M. (2010). *Foundations of psychiatric mental health nuråsing: A clinical approach* (6th ed.). St. Louis, MO: Saunders Elsevier, pp. 336, 588–590.

9 **Answer: 3** **Rationale:** Suggesting that they work as a team to ask for and receive help from the others conveys the information that the ill person and the family all share responsibility for decision-making. It further suggests that each person, including the client, should have an awareness of his or her capacities and limitations and ask for assistance as necessary. Stating that no single family member should always be in charge of caregiving decisions conveys useful information, but the information relates to preventing caregiver role strain, rather than promoting interdependence. Suggesting that all of them work toward reducing conflict within the family conveys useful information and indicates that the family should be a team, but it does not suggest a specific route to productive interdependence for the family. Suggesting that if the family assumes all responsibility for decision-making will reduce the ill person's stress level indicates restricting the client's independence and removing the client from the family team. **Cognitive Level:** Analyzing **Client Need:** Health Promotion and Maintenance **Integrated Process:** Caring **Content Area:** Mental Health **Strategy:** Look for the option that best indicates involvement of all family members as part of a team. **Reference:** Kneisl, C., & Trigoboff, E. (2009). *Contemporary psychiatric–mental health nursing* (2nd ed.). Upper Saddle River, NJ: Prentice Hall, p. 702.

10 **Answer: 4** **Rationale:** The existence of comorbidities is more prevalent in individuals in lower socioeconomic levels.

Research indicates that a lower socioeconomic level does lead to a higher number of illnesses in these clients. No research indicates a specific correlation between socioeconomic level and increased grief, increased pain, or use of defense mechanisms. **Cognitive Level:** Applying **Client Need:** Physiological Adaptation **Integrated Process:** Caring **Content Area:** Mental Health **Strategy:** Remember that extrinsic factors have a significant role in the prevalence of diseases in certain populations. Extrinsic factors include economics and health practices. **Reference:** Vidabeck, S. (2010). *Psychiatric–mental health nursing* (5th ed.). Philadelphia: Lippincott, pp. 145–146.

References

Fontaine, K. (2009). *Mental health nursing* (6th ed.). Upper Saddle River, NJ: Pearson Education.

Kniesl, C., Wilson, H., & Trigoboff, E. (2009). *Contemporary psychiatric–mental health nursing* (2nd ed.). Upper Saddle River, NJ: Pearson Education.

North American Nursing Diagnosis Association (2008). *Nursing diagnosis: Definitions and classification 2009–2011.* Indianapolis, IN: Wiley-Blackwell.

Stuart, G. (2009). *Principles and practice of psychiatric nursing* (9th ed.). St. Louis: Elsevier Science.

Townsend, M. (2011). *Essentials of psychiatric–mental health nursing* (5th ed.). Philadelphia, PA: F.A. Davis.

Varcarolis, E., & Halter, M. (2010). *Foundations of psychiatric mental health nursing: A clinical approach* (6th ed.). Philadelphia: Saunders.

ANSWERS & RATIONALES

Appendix

➤ *Practice to Pass Suggested Answers*

Chapter 1

Page 4: *Suggested Answer*—There are neither universally accepted definitions of "normal" or "abnormal" nor clear parameters of mental health versus mental illness. Mental health and mental illness can be viewed as end points on a continuum, with movement back and forth throughout life. One out of four individuals will suffer from mental illness in his or her lifetime. Everyone is susceptible to mental illness. The continuum could be used to demonstrate to the group how cultural, interpersonal, and individual factors contribute to mental health and illness.

Page 8: *Suggested Answer*—The client is most likely using the defense mechanism of denial. Denial is an unconscious attempt to screen or to ignore unacceptable realities by refusing to acknowledge them. Denial allows individuals to reduce their anxiety and not have to acknowledge unacceptable feelings, thoughts, or behaviors.

Page 8: *Suggested Answer*—Erikson's stage of growth and development experienced by a 72-year-old is "integrity versus despair." Individuals who experience "integrity" accept life as it has been by acknowledging both the good and bad aspects of one's life and maintaining a positive self-concept. This client is not currently achieving Erikson's developmental milestone because he is experiencing "despair." He or she finds life meaningless. He or she has no hope for the future and feels that he or she and others would be better off without him or her. The nurse could assist the client in conducting a life review, which may help this client in finding meaning to his or her life. Life review is a process of systematically evaluating one's successes and failures in life to resolve conflicts and to find meaning.

Page 11: *Suggested Answer*—The brain is the site of all integrative functions that govern our behavior, feelings, and thoughts. Neurotransmission is the electrochemical process in the brain that allows nerve signals to pass from one cell to another at the synapse. The synapse is a microscopic gap between where two neuron cells meet. Neurotransmitters act,

as the word implies, to transmit signals across the synapse from one neuron to another. Serotonin is the neurotransmitter involved with depression. Decreases in serotonin levels can lead to depression. Antidepressant medications are the primary drugs that affect serotonin levels.

Page 14: *Suggested Answer*—

- Risk for Other-Directed Violence related to confusion, memory loss, and intruding into others personal space.
- Chronic Confusion related to memory loss and disorientation to place, time, and situation.
- Risk for Injury related to wandering behaviors and wandering into unfamiliar areas.

Chapter 2

Page 32: *Suggested Answer*—

- Situational crisis is any event that poses a threat or challenge to an individual person.
- Maturational crisis is a stage in a person's life where adjustment and adaptation to new responsibilities and life patterns are necessary.
- Cultural crisis is a situation where a person experiences culture shock in the process of adapting/adjusting to a new culture or returning to one's own culture after being assimilated into another.
- Community crisis is a crisis of a proportion to affect an entire community of people. Natural disasters, armed conflicts, and significant social ills are community crises.

Page 33: *Suggested Answer*—

- The individual's perception of the crisis situation will dictate how the client will react to the situation.
- Past experience or lack of experience in coping with stress will impact how the client will react to the crisis situation.
- Established coping strategies will assist the client in dealing more effectively with the current crisis situation.
- Availability of support persons gives the client the resources needed to deal with the crisis and to return to normal.

Page 34: *Suggested Answer*—

- Marked feelings of tenseness and anxiousness without feelings of fatigue, sadness, and depression
- Elevated motor-sensory behavior
- Elevated systolic blood pressure
- Elevated pulse
- Elevated respiration
- High score for verbal anxiety

Page 38: *Suggested Answer*—

- Depression
- Increased alcohol drinking
- Previous suicide attempts
- Buying a gun
- Stockpiling pills
- Giving away money or possessions
- Loss of interest in favorite activities
- Making or changing a will
- Making funeral plans
- Suspicious behavior
- Recent death of spouse, child, or close friend
- Death of pet
- Major move
- Diagnosis of a terminal illness
- Retirement

Page 39: *Suggested Answer*—

- Removing sharp objects, such as knives, scissors, and mirrors, from the client's possession and access
- Removing toxic substances, such as drugs and alcohol, and ensuring that unit medications are locked
- Removing clothing that could be used for self-harm, such as neckties, belts, shoe strings, stockings, and the like
- Placing the client under close supervision, including one-to-one supervision with a staff member

Chapter 3

Page 52: *Suggested Answer*—In some cases, antidepressants are prescribed for children with ADHD, especially venlafaxine (Effexor) and fluvoxamine (Luvox). More commonly, central nervous system (CNS) stimulants are prescribed. These medications increase the ability to focus attention by blocking out irrelevant thoughts and impulses. CNS stimulants lead to significant improvement in 70 to 75% of cases. The advantage of methylphenidate (Ritalin) and dextroamphetamine (Dexedrine) is that effectiveness is almost immediate, while the same effect with pemoline (Cyclert) may take up to eight weeks.

Page 52: *Suggested Answer*—Common side effects include pallor, a pinched facial expression, dark hollows under the eyes, anorexia, insomnia, headache, and dryness of the mouth. Toxic effects may include overstimulation and sedation.

Page 53: *Suggested Answer*—

- Depressed mood, irritable, aggressive
- Academic difficulties
- Eating and sleeping disturbances
- Severe self-criticism and guilt
- Suicidal ideation and plans

Page 53: *Suggested Answer*—

- Intense mood swings
- Academic difficulties
- Argumentative and/or assaultive
- Risk-taking or antisocial behavior
- Hypersomnia
- Very low self-esteem

Page 56: *Suggested Answer*—Any of the following nursing diagnoses may apply:

- Imbalanced Nutrition: Less than Body Requirements related to reduced intake; purging
- Anxiety related to fears of gaining weight and losing control
- Disturbed Thought Processes related to dichotomous thinking, overgeneralization, personalization, obsessions, and superstitious thinking
- Disturbed Body Image related to delusional perception of body in anorexia
- Powerlessness related to having no control over bulimic patterns

Chapter 4

Page 68: *Suggested Answer*—"You tried to hurt yourself and you are on suicide precautions. That means that someone must be with you at all times, 24 hours per day, until you are no longer a danger to yourself." Communicate to the client the understanding that it may be embarrassing, but the client's safety is the most important concern.

Page 70: *Suggested Answer*—Major depressive disorder is one and a half to three times more common among first-degree biological relatives of persons with this disorder than among the general population. Clients have a right to feel angry about having depression, but it is important to reinforce that parents can't choose the traits they pass on to their offspring. The client can choose how to respond and learn how to make changes to cope with the depression.

Page 71: *Suggested Answer*—Those who are depressed do not have the energy to talk or participate in an assessment for any longer than 15- to 20-minute segments. The client may be slow to respond as well, so the nurse needs to be patient with the client and allow sufficient time for client responses. The client who is diagnosed with a bipolar disorder is not able to concentrate for any longer than this, nor may the client be able to focus long enough to sit still for even this amount of time. The nurse also needs to know that this client may not always give accurate information.

Page 77: *Suggested Answer*—Five short-term goals for this client could include any of the following:

- Be free from self-inflicted harm.
- Engage in reality-based interactions.
- Demonstrate appropriate use of boundary setting with staff and other clients.
- Be oriented to person, place, and time.
- Express feelings directly with congruent verbal and nonverbal messages.
- Express anger or hostility outwardly in a safe manner.
- Participate in formulation of discharge plan.

Five long-term goals for this client could include any of the following:

- Be free of psychotic symptoms.
- Demonstrate functional levels of psychomotor activity.
- Demonstrate compliance and congruence with medication knowledge and regime (if prescribed).
- Demonstrate an increased level of coping with anxiety, stress, and/or frustration.
- Demonstrate appropriate coping if a loss or change occurs.
- Identify discharge plan and components.
- Verbally contract and begin to demonstrate compliance with plan of care components.

Page 85: *Suggested Answer*—The plan should include the following points:

- There is no clear evidence as to why the therapy works. There are indications that early morning light causes circadian rhythm shifts.
- Therapy involves a large time commitment.
- Usually clients spend 30 minutes to several hours each day in the light source depending on the light strength (2500 lux is usually administered).
- Antidepressant effects can be full, partial, or not at all.
- If effective, results will usually be seen after two to four days and therapy is complete after two weeks.
- Maintenance consists of sitting in front of the lights for approximately 30 minutes each day.
- The therapy is usually necessary during the fall and winter months when the client is affected by the disorder.

Chapter 5

Page 103: *Suggested Answer*—It would be useful to explain to the client that while there is some evidence of a genetic predisposition to anxiety, many theorists believe anxiety is learned or acquired. It would also be helpful to explain to the client that new ways of coping with anxiety, regardless of its cause, can be learned.

Page 103: *Suggested Answer*—You should explain to the client that anxiety can occur in anybody at any time, and it is important to consider anxiety when designing a nursing care plan for the client. You might also explain that physical illness can increase anxiety, and anxiety can lead to physical illness. In addition, there is some evidence that admission to a hospital may increase a client's level of stress. Nurses need to be aware of how the admission process is affecting the client.

Page 107: *Suggested Answer*—Not all over-the-counter medications are safe for everyone. Benadryl can interact with other prescribed and non-prescribed medications, as well as alcohol. Benadryl can suppress the central nervous system and can be habit-forming. Because Benadryl interferes with REM sleep, the quality of the client's sleep may decrease over time, leading the client to periodically increase the dosage to maintain the desired effect. Conveying information related to actions that facilitate sleep would also be helpful.

Page 109: *Suggested Answer*—Because agoraphobic clients frequently are fearful of leaving their homes and being trapped in situations they cannot escape, the first action would be to assess the client's motivation and ability to participate in this group. It may be necessary for a helping person to accompany the client to the first few meetings to provide reassurance to the client and to promote safety. Teaching a relaxation exercise the client can use before and during the meeting might also be helpful. Assisting the client to contact the group leader before attending the first meeting might reduce some anticipatory anxiety.

Page 110: *Suggested Answer*—It is important to allow the client to discuss this fear openly and honestly and to take this concern seriously. Neglecting this important issue will increase the client's level of anxiety. The client should be reassured that this fear will be taken into consideration when planning nursing care. Whenever possible, medications should be given orally. During procedures where blood is involved, allow the client to avert his or her eyes. Do not ridicule this behavior. Teaching relaxation techniques might be useful. If the fear seriously limits the client's ability to obtain healthcare, some consideration might be given to involving the client in developing a systematic desensitization program.

Chapter 6

Page 122: *Suggested Answer*—In somatoform disorders, anxiety is manifested by physical/bodily symptoms. The physical symptoms facilitate the individual's dependency needs for nurturance, attention, and assistance and allows for the individual to avoid acknowledgement of the psychological conflict.

Page 123: *Suggested Answer*— Primary gain is the symbolic resolution of unconscious conflict that decreases anxiety and wards off the psychological conflict from conscious awareness. A secondary gain is the advantage a person gains from being ill. This gain may be in the form of sympathy, empathy, disability benefits and/or attention; persons with somatization disorders do not consciously/intentionally seek secondary gain.

Page 127: *Suggested Answer*—Anxiolytics are used to treat anxiety in clients with somatoform disorders. Depression is treated with antidepressants such as the SSRIs and SNRIs.

Page 127: *Suggested Answer*—A gradual resumption of responsibilities will help to prevent the client's anxiety from escalating, and will likely be more successful than an attempt to rapidly resume normal roles and responsibilities.

Page 127: *Suggested Answer*—One could teach family members to reinforce verbal expressions rather than symptoms using examples of situations that are reflective of the family's experience, or through attempting to role play such situations.

Chapter 7

Page 142: *Suggested Answer*—Explain to the client that stress or conflicts can cause anxiety. When that anxiety becomes too great, the mind can do many things, automatically, to protect the client. One of those things is dissociation. Dissociation is like being split off from reality or "spacing out." Although it is protective, dissociation can also impair how the client lives because she can lose full awareness of what is occurring.

Page 142: *Suggested Answer*—

- "As a child or as an adult, have you ever been physically hurt or abused by anyone?"
- "As a child or as an adult, have you ever been emotionally hurt or abused by anyone?"
- "As a child or as an adult, have you ever been sexually touched by anyone against your will? Abused sexually by anyone?"

Page 143: *Suggested Answer*—Because visual imagery is created by internal stimuli, when you try to reduce stress, there is a tendency to dissociate, or "space out," especially if you already have a pattern of dissociating. If you feel dissociative, focus on external stimuli—what you can see, hear, and feel physically—which will "ground" you to reality, to the present by distracting you and interfering with the dissociative process. If you want to use stress-management techniques when you are not feeling dissociative, you could try progressive muscle relaxation or deep-breathing accompanied by counting inside your head. Stress-management techniques that are physical in nature are more grounding than those that are more mental or internal.

Page 143: *Suggested Answer*—Anti-anxiety agents are extremely effective in reducing anxiety but are physiologically addictive, with the client developing tolerance (and

withdrawal symptoms when the drug is removed). The agents are also psychologically addictive, and clients can come to believe they cannot cope without medication. Thus, anti-anxiety agents are best used to decrease anxiety to a lower level where the client can learn non-pharmacological techniques to control anxiety.

Page 143: *Suggested Answer*—Clients often dissociate or split off their affect off from an experience so that even horrific events are recounted with minimal emotional expression. This ability to dissociate affect from the traumatic event serves to numb. When a survivor of trauma remembers those events with appropriate affect, the nurse can expect anger, great fear, or sadness to be expressed freely.

Chapter 8

Page 156: *Suggested Answer*—Personality disorders are diagnosed when personality patterns or traits are inflexible, enduring, pervasive, maladaptive, and cause significant functional impairment or subjective distress.

Page 160: *Suggested Answer*—The personality disorders that may manifest with brief psychotic episodes are the cluster A personality disorders: paranoid, schizotypal, and schizoid personality disorders. Low dose atypical and typical antipsychotic agents may be prescribed on a short-term basis to alleviate brief psychotic symptoms in clients with these disorders.

Page 160: *Suggested Answer*—Individuals diagnosed with antisocial personality disorder frequently use manipulation to control others and their environment. Intervening in this behavior pattern by setting limits that deter the client from manipulating others is a small step toward effecting behavioral change. In addition, clients diagnosed with antisocial personality disorder frequently display diminished impulse control. Setting limits helps clients maintain impulse control in order to protect themselves and others from injury.

Page 161: *Suggested Answer*—Individuals diagnosed with borderline personality disorder tend to engage in dichotomous thinking or splitting—they tend to see themselves and others as all good or all bad. This tendency to idealize or devalue the self and others results in unstable interpersonal relationships. It is frequently reflected in rage directed at the self (self-mutilation) or at others (injury to others). Providing cognitive therapies assist clients to see that there is good and bad in all of us; this step helps decrease dichotomous thinking and protects client safety, decreases subjective distress, and improves functioning.

Page 162: *Suggested Answer*—It is designed to support client safety by decreasing the risk of suicide or self-mutilation through the use of anti-harm contracts, close monitoring by both staff and client, identifying triggers and patterns related to self-destructive behavior, and identifying alternative coping strategies.

Chapter 9

Page 177: *Suggested Answer*—Having knowledge about a genetic predisposition to schizophrenia can be helpful to family members and clients. The power of this knowledge can assist individuals in identifying early signs and symptoms of the illness for early intervention and prevention of acute, crisis states of schizophrenia. This knowledge may also be helpful for reproductive counseling services. Research indicates, however, that genetic factors alone do not cause the development of schizophrenia. Other factors, such as the environment and psychological effects from maladaptive relationships, seem to play an important role in the development of schizophrenia.

Page 178: *Suggested Answer*—When clients are experiencing psychosis, they are not in touch with reality. They are disoriented and their safety is in jeopardy. The safety of the client, others around them, and yourself is priority. The environment must be secure and free of potentially dangerous elements. There should be low levels of stimuli and increased vigilance of the client. The client will most likely need to be medicated to treat the psychosis and decrease agitation. Only after safety issues are addressed could other interventions be carried forth. Reality orientation techniques are important interventions to bring the client back in touch with the real world. Providing emotional support to the client and the families may help decrease anxieties and fears. There may also be a need to assist the client with activities of daily living (ADLs) during the period of active psychosis.

Page 178: *Suggested Answer*—Clients with medication non-adherence problems may be appropriate candidates for antipsychotic depot injections. These depot injections only need to be administered every four to six weeks depending on the clients' therapeutic reactions to the medication. Before the depot injection is given, an oral form of the medication must be administered to the client to assess for any adverse reactions to that medication. If an adverse reaction to the oral medication does occur, then the depot form of that medication should not be administered.

Page 180: *Suggested Answer*—A simple tool used to screen for tardive dyskinesia (TD) is the Abnormal and Involuntary Movement Scale (AIMS). This scale assesses for abnormal, involuntary movements of the tongue, face, trunk, and extremities of the body. The client is observed in several body positions. Severity of the symptoms of abnormal, involuntary movements is rated on a scale of zero to four. Zero is the score given for no signs of abnormal, involuntary movements. A score of one to four is given for increasingly severe signs of abnormal, involuntary movements. A client that receives any score other than zero needs to be referred for further evaluation of possible TD. The AIMS should be administered to the client every three to six months while receiving antipsychotic medications.

Page 181: *Suggested Answer*—One of the most important interventions that may prevent relapse is education. Educating family members or significant others about early signs of behaviors indicating relapse is a priority. Early intervention will help decrease the number and severity of relapses. Client and family education regarding the need for medication adherence, management of side effects, need to report any adverse reactions, and possible drug interactions are imperative. Other important interventions include referrals to appropriate community support systems, improved housing conditions, financial assistance programs, and access to medical and psychiatric clinics for follow-up care.

Chapter 10

Page 193: *Suggested Answer*—Possible causes of confusion in clients with a fractured hip (or other trauma) include the following:

- Substance-induced delirium from ingestion of alcohol or pain medications such as narcotics, muscle relaxants, or benzodiazepines
- Psychosocial stress related to pain or the unfamiliar acute hospital setting
- Poor cerebral blood flow caused by complications from the fracture, such as fat emboli, pulmonary emboli, blood loss, shock, and tachycardia
- General medical conditions occurring concomitantly in older adults such as atherosclerosis, arrythmias, vitamin deficiency, diabetes mellitus, COPD, and liver and kidney disease
- Diseases that predispose clients to falls and fractures, such as dementia of the Alzheimer's type, Parkinson's disease, chronic alcoholism, and vascular dementia

Page 194: *Suggested Answer*—

- Most important to obtain would be the client's vital signs, especially temperature (indication of infection) and blood pressure (indication of cerebral blood flow).
- Questions regarding the onset of confusion, illicit drug use, allergies, medication history, medical history, and previous episodes of confusion should then be asked to determine possible underlying causes.

Page 196: *Suggested Answer*—

- Medications to treat mood (particularly depression) include the selective serotonin reuptake inhibitors such as fluoxetine (Prozac), paroxetine (Paxil), sertraline (Zoloft), and nefazodone (Serzone).
- Medications to treat anxiety could include lorazepam (Ativan), trazodone (Desyrel) and buspirone (Buspar).

- Medications to treat psychotic features include atypical antipsychotics such as olanzapine (Zyprexa), quetiapine (Seroquel), and risperidone (Risperdal), and possibly haloperidol (Haldol) if needed.

Page 200: *Suggested Answer*—

- Stage 1 (typically lasts one to three years): client has difficulty performing complex tasks related to a decline in recent memory; forgetfulness, missed appointments; clients has insight into and are frightened by their confusion; declines occur in personal appearance, orientation, concentration, and judgment
- Stage 2 (lasting approximately 2 to 10 years): client has poor impulse control with frequent outbursts and tantrums; labile emotions; wandering or aggressive behavior, psychotic episodes such as hallucinations and/or delusions, progressive aphasia, hyperorality, and perseveration occur, as well as aphasia, agraphia, and a variety of agnosias
- Stage 3 (lasting 8 to 10 years before death occurs): continuation of hyperorality, binge eating, hyperetamorphosis, the need to compulsively examine and touch every object in the environment, progressive deterioration in motor ability, response to environmental stimuli, and cognitive function

Page 201: *Suggested Answer*—

- Respond to her concerns in a nonjudgmental, open manner. Use therapeutic techniques to encourage the wife to explore her feelings. (e.g., "This must be very hard for you. What other feelings do you have?")
- Make arrangements for her to meet with a counselor (e.g., nurse clinician, social worker) to identify feelings and define a plan to regain a sense of control and facilitate grief work.
- Encourage her input and maintain her involvement in her husband's care to help reduce feelings of guilt. Suggest she assist routinely in feeding her husband or other tasks without overwhelming or creating a sense of obligation.
- Provide information regarding appropriate support groups in the community.
- Encourage the wife to stay with the client and help arrange outings or home visits for holidays and special occasions.

Chapter 11

Page 215: *Suggested Answer*—Ask your client what he or she is specifically concerned about. Based on his response, you can encourage him or her to call the local substance dependence treatment facility and discuss his concerns with a trained professional. If the son has alcohol-dependence issues, you could refer your client to Al-Anon to learn more about how alcohol has affected the family dynamics and how to begin healing.

Page 219: *Suggested Answer*—You need assessment data that focuses on the use of mood-altering substances. This includes a physical assessment/systems review, personal family assessment, chemical use assessment, medication assessment, OTC or nutritional supplement assessment, social history assessment, and laboratory value assessment.

Page 219: *Suggested Answer*—You are concerned the client may be experiencing tolerance. Tolerance is identified by a need for markedly increased amounts of a substance to achieve intoxication or desired effect, or markedly diminished effect with continued use of the same amount of the substance. This could mean that the client would need a higher dose of pain medication for pain relief and that the client might have an addiction problem. You may need to discuss your concern with the physician that the client may need an increased medication dose and also educate the client about signs and symptoms of substance abuse.

Page 223: *Suggested Answer*—The concern is that the client may be drinking or experiencing a reaction to an ingredient in the cleaning solution. You ask her to come to the office and bring the cleaning solution in its original container. If the intoxilyzer reading is negative, but you still have reason to believe the client was drinking, the physician may order a urine or blood drug abuse survey. If there is no indication that the client has been drinking, then exposure to alcohol occurred from contact with the cleaning solution or another product. In that case, preventing exposure to the product will minimize the likelihood of a reaction.

Page 224: *Suggested Answer*—The client needs education on the dynamics of substance dependence including signs, symptoms, and defense mechanisms. You recognize that she is in the precontemplation or contemplation stage of change. You will take a laid-back approach using reflective listening and validation. You will help her discuss both the positive and negative aspects of alcohol use.

Chapter 12

Page 240: *Suggested Answer*—Child: physical signs of sexual assault include frequent urination or dysuria; venereal disease or gonorrhea of throat; pain or difficulty walking or sitting; foreign matter in bladder, rectum, urethra, or vagina; sleep problems such as insomnia or nightmares; bruises in genital or rectal area; rashes or itching in genital area, rectum, or vagina; scars in labia or rectal fissures.

Behavioral signs include overly sexualized behavior, seductive or advanced sexual knowledge, fear of a particular person or place, promiscuity or prostitution, compulsive masturbation or precocious sexual play, sexually assaulting another child, unexplained gifts or money from questionable sources, drop in school performance, sudden onset of enuresis or encopresis, excess anxiety, compulsive bathing, running away from home, suicide attempts, and self-destructive behaviors such as head banging.

Parents: relationship with child, stressful situations in life, history of childhood sexual assault in either parent, social isolation, unrealistic expectations of child, maladaptive coping mechanisms, problems with impulse control or low self-esteem, substance abuse in either parent. Traits of the family: father—domineering, impulsive, or physically abusive; mother—passive and submissive, battered. Structure of the family system: closed with rigid rules and rigid external boundaries. Enmeshment: internal boundaries poorly defined and characterized by excessive dependence on family members for physical and psychological needs, role reversal.

Page 241: *Suggested Answer*—Child: provide for protection of the child by reporting violence against child following facility's policies; treat child's injuries; reassure child that violence was not his or her fault and that the child will be protected.

Parents: approach with non-punitive manner. Do teaching on reporting process, normal growth and development, anger management, stress management, parenting skills, communication skills. Teach appropriate disciplinary methods, the availability of and need for treatment for substance abuse if indicated. Provide resources available to them such as Parents Anonymous, support groups, parenting classes, or employment counseling if indicated.

Page 243: *Suggested Answer*—Assess for imminent danger of situation: escalation in violence with increase in severity or frequency of attacks, weapons in the home, increase in use of substances, threats of homicide, or suicide by perpetrator.

Develop a safety plan: ask neighbors to phone police if violence begins. Establish a code with family and friends to signify violence. Plan an escape route if the abuser blocks main exit. Determine a place to go and how to get there. Keep an escape bag available in a safe place with extra clothing for victim and children, children's favorite toys, and cash. Keep hidden and available extra copies of important papers such as driver's licenses, birth certificates, marriage license, insurance papers, social security numbers, bank account numbers, and important phone numbers.

Provide information about resources available: community resources, crisis line numbers, women's shelters or safe houses, legal assistance.

Page 245: *Suggested Answer*—Client: has the client experienced verbal assaults, threats or intimidation, restriction of social contacts, violation of personal rights, unreasonable confinement, forced isolation or denial of privacy, abandonment, or threats of abandonment? Is there evidence of denial of needed food, clothing, or medical care, or misuse or misappropriation of client's funds? Is the client financially dependent on the caregiver? Is client mentally ill or abusing substances?

Client's physical status: malnutrition and/or dehydration, untreated medical conditions, poor hygiene, lack of dental care, bruises, broken bones, healing fractures, unusual pattern of bruises or lacerations such as rope burns on ankles or wrists.

Caregiver: relationship with the client, personal problems, a lack of support systems, increased level of stress in caring for elder, a history of family violence, unresolved previous conflicts and power struggles, evidence the behavior may be in retaliation for past behavior of elder, attitude toward the client, evidence of mental illness or substance abuse. Are there signs of aggression within the relationship?

Page 248: *Suggested Answer*—

Reassure clients that sexual assault is not their fault and survival was the most important outcome.

- Advise about potential for pregnancy and sexually transmitted disease.
- Provide information about community services such as survivors' groups, shelters for battered women, and legal service.
- If sexual assault is by a partner, provide options: staying with perpetrator, removing perpetrator through arrest, obtaining protective orders to keep perpetrator away, or leaving.
- Assist with development of a safety plan if the client is returning to the environment with the perpetrator.

Chapter 13

Page 257: *Suggested Answer*—Clients dealing with loss and the families of these clients often experience many physiological and psychological responses. Physiological responses may include crying and sobbing, fatigue, weakness and exhaustion, insomnia, and loss of appetite. Psychological responses may include intense loneliness and sadness, depressed mood, anxiety or panic episodes, difficulty concentrating and focusing, anger or rage directed toward self or others, ambivalence, and low self-esteem, as well as somatic complaints.

Page 259: *Suggested Answer*—You suspect the wife is experiencing anticipatory grief. Anticipatory grief is the process of disengaging or "letting go" that occurs before the actual loss or death has occurred. Significant others and family members may withdraw emotionally from the dying client in order to disengage or begin the "letting go" process for themselves. They may find it too difficult to provide physical as well as emotional support because they will be confronted with the reality of death.

Page 263: *Suggested Answer*—Males and females often express grief differently. Traditional approaches to bereavement counseling are designed to facilitate feminine grief.

Most counselors emphasize showing empathy; some encourage, even insist, that the griever reminisce about the loss, experiencing and then expressing painful feelings. Masculine grievers find the focus on feelings unhelpful and may resent being urged to express them. Male or masculine grief is usually limited and toned down; thinking precedes and often dominates feelings; focus is on problem solving rather than expression of feelings; outward expression of feelings often involve anger and/or guilt; and intense feelings may be experienced privately.

Page 264: *Suggested Answer*—An advance directive is a general term that refers to a client's written instructions about future medical care, in the event that the client becomes unable to speak or incapacitated. The client can choose between developing a living will or identifying a health care proxy or both. A living will or durable power of attorney for healthcare is a set of specifically written instructions about what medical treatment the client chooses to omit or refuse (e.g., ventilator support) in the event that the client is unable to make those decisions. A health care proxy is a document appointing someone else (e.g., a relative or trusted friend) to manage health care treatment decisions when the client is unable to do so.

Page 226: *Suggested Answer*—The nurse would assess the client's and family's current knowledge and understanding of the implication of the illness and impeding death, the client's ability to provide self-care, the client's and family's current and past coping strategies, current manifestations of grief, role expectations and role changes, availability of support people, client's knowledge and documentation of advance directives, as well as need for community resources. At the end of life, the nurse intervenes in ways that bring comfort to clients and families, even when hope for cure is gone. Promoting an environment that supports and fosters the completion of the essential tasks of bringing closure to life and relationships is the primary goal of nursing.

Chapter 14

Page 275: *Suggested Answer*—"It sounds like you are very concerned. However, it is typical that people feel somewhat depressed about a diagnosis that may disrupt one's usual level of functioning. Adolescents often feel upset as they are also struggling with issues related to self-image and self-esteem."

Page 278: *Suggested Answer*—"The occurrence of medical illnesses can be influenced by stress. Higher stress levels can result in an increased number of asthmatic episodes."

Page 280: *Suggested Answer*—Important assessments include psychological, biological, social, subjective/objective symptoms, family/significant other reports, and diagnostic reports.

Page 280: *Suggested Answer*—Priority nursing diagnoses include Disturbed Body Image and Risk for Situational Low

Self-Esteem related to functional changes associated with medical illness diagnosis.

➤ *Case Study Suggested Answers*

Chapter 1

1. The nurse demonstrated two attentive skills toward the client that communicate respect for individuals. First, the nurse approached the client and asked permission to sit with her. She used a broad opening to ask the client how she was doing. Second, the nurse offered herself by sharing with the client that she had an hour that she could use to spend with the client.

2. When the nurse approached the client and asked her how she was doing, the client leaned away, maintained a rigid posture, avoided eye contact, and only nodded her head in response. The nurse reacted by leaning back and crossing her arms over her chest to create what she thought would be a less threatening posture. However, leaning away from the client and crossing her arms over her chest communicated distance and unavailability to the client. In addition, the nurse communicated to the client that she would spend an hour with her; however, when the client would not respond, the nurse assumed the client did not want to talk and left after only 25 minutes. This was inconsistent communication. This would foster mistrust and lack of confidence in the client's feelings toward the nurse.

3. A depressed client often is quiet and non-communicative. Clients experiencing depression often have difficulty identifying their own feelings and thoughts. The client could have been using the time to collect her own thoughts in order to communicate her feelings and thoughts more clearly to the nurse. The client may have been testing the nurse's trustworthiness by seeing if the nurse would do what she said she would do by spending the hour with the client, whether the client spoke or not.

4. Instead of initially reacting to the client by leaning back and crossing her arms over her chest, the nurse could have better communicated by leaning forward and having an open posture. Leaning forward and having an open posture communicates willingness to be present with the client. Once the nurse offered an hour of her time for the client, she should have stayed the entire hour even though the client did not want to share. This would have promoted trustworthiness. The nurse could have communicated that it was okay for the client to be silent and that the nurse would sit with her in silence for the hour or until the client was ready to share. Silence is an effective therapeutic technique.

5. The nurse assumed the client did not want to share. Instead of confirming with the client her assumption, she acted incorrectly on the client's silence. The nurse may have been uncomfortable with silence and felt the need to leave the situation. Nurses must understand the importance of silence as a therapeutic technique and respect a client's need to not share while remaining in the presence of the client.

Chapter 2

1. Risk factors for this client include the following:
   - Age of 15 years
   - Males are higher risk than females
   - Declining school performance (grades and dropping football)
   - Recent losses: parents undergoing divorce
   - Drug use
2. Priority nursing diagnoses include the following:
   - Risk for Self-Directed Violence related to feelings of loss and hopelessness
   - Ineffective Individual Coping related to situational crisis (suicide attempt) and relocation
   - Hopelessness related to perception of worthlessness
3. Nursing interventions include the following:
   - Establish a therapeutic relationship.
   - Ensure the safety of the client by communicating the potential for suicide.
   - Stay with the client.
   - Listen to the client's concerns.
   - Give the client a message of hope.
4. This client will do the following:
   - Experience no physical harm to self.
   - Set realistic goals for self and future.
   - Express some optimism and hope for the future.
5. The nurse should take the following precautions:
   - Initiate suicide precautions.
   - Begin to establish trust.
   - Establish in each 24-hour period a verbal contract to not harm self.
   - Offer positive encouragement for the client remaining free of injury.
   - Ensure a safe environment: remove sharp objects, toxic substances, and clothing that could be used for self-harm, and place client on close supervision.

Chapter 3

1. Information about the behaviors that the boy displayed as an infant and as a small child would help make an accurate assessment. For instance, consider his ability to concentrate, ease of distractibility, overt acts of hostility, the manner in which he deals with frustration, and specific learning problems.

2. Ask the mother questions about behaviors such as physical aggression and cruelty to people and animals, anger, and no indication of guilt or remorse for actions.
3. The boy has the ability to communicate with others and is not severely socially impaired. He exhibits no ritualistic behaviors or unusual motor behaviors that are associated with autistic disorders.
4. CNS stimulants increase the child's ability to focus attention by blocking out irrelevant thoughts and impulses. Some stimulants are effective immediately (Ritalin and Dexedrine) and they lead to significant improvement in 70 to 75% of ADHD cases.
5. There are several interventions that could be helpful for this client. Socialization enhancement will increase his or her ability to negotiate stressful interpersonal situations with his siblings, parents, and classmates. It will also help him or her develop a more positive self-perception. Self-esteem enhancement allows a shift in focus from negative behaviors to positive behaviors, making the client feel better about him- or herself.

Chapter 4

1. Initial questions should include topics related to suicidality, reason for being brought/coming to the unit, and recent significant stressors (within the last few months) that may have contributed to this manic state/relapse. It is also important for the nurse to assess the presence of hallucinations, flight of ideas, or delusions. The following are examples of appropriate questions:
   - "How did you get to the hospital today?"
   - "Have you ever been hospitalized before? Where? When? For how long?"
   - "Do you feel you want to hurt yourself right now?" If yes, inquire about a plan.
   - "Has anything happened in the last few months that you think could be significant to your being here today?"
   - "Are you hearing voices or seeing things that are unusual?"
   - Can you tell me what you usually do on a typical Tuesday from the time you get up in the morning until you go to bed at night?"
2. Based on the intake assessment data, this client will need to have a physical examination, safe environment, and frequent checks by health care workers until the staff is sure the client is no longer a safety risk to self or others.
3. This client will probably be prescribed lithium carbonate (lithium) PO. If the assessment data indicates, she may also be given a benzodiazepine or an antipsychotic if necessary until the effects of the lithium can be seen (two to four weeks). Then these medications can be slowly withdrawn.

4. The nurse will recognize the cues indicating fatigue/need for sleep and will do the following:
   • Decrease environmental stimuli in room and common areas.
   • Restrict intake of caffeine (coffee, tea, cocoa, cola, etc.).
   • Offer small snack/warm milk at bedtime or when awake during the night.
5. Nursing interventions to assist with nutrition would include the following:
   • Record intake and output.
   • Offer small amounts of food frequently, preferably finger foods.
   • Offer client beverages frequently.
   • Monitor weight and laboratory studies as indicators of effectiveness.

Chapter 5

1. Based on what is known about this client, either Social Isolation or Impaired Social Interactions would probably be the most appropriate nursing diagnosis.
2. Additional information related to the client's level of self-esteem, quality and quantity of social support, and effective coping strategies used for similar problems would be essential. Specific examples of the client's perceptions of stressors in social situations that lead to anxiety, and examples of interactions with other people that have been both positive and negative, would also enhance understanding of the client.
3. Several steps may prove useful to achieve this outcome. Such steps might include the following:
   • Establishing a trusting one-to-one therapeutic relationship with the client
   • Encouraging the client to verbalize feelings about interactions with others
   • Teaching and role-playing interpersonal skills
   • Introducing the client to other people on the unit
   • Assisting the client to identify people on the unit with whom she might like to interact
   • Involving the client in an activity she enjoys, and ask one other person to join in the activity
   • Gradually including more people in the activity
   • If the client's anxiety increases beyond the moderate level while engaged in an activity with others, allowing the client to leave the activity and discussing the incident with her
   • Providing positive reinforcement when the client interacts with others
4. Because the client complains of muscle tension, the best relaxation technique would be some form of progressive muscle relaxation.
5. The first step would be to ask the client to clarify what feeling "more comfortable" means by asking for specific examples of what the client would like to accomplish. Changes in behaviors and feeling could then be compared to baseline data. The staff could keep a record of the frequency and duration of the client's interactions with others and compare findings over time. Direct observation and evaluation of the quality of interactions with others would provide useful information. Asking the client to use a diary to record relevant information could provide a useful self-assessment tool. Using a standardized assessment tool to measure the client's level of anxiety before and after interactions could provide more objective data for the evaluation process.

Chapter 6

1. Pain symptoms are "real" and the nurse should not dismiss them as "only in the client's head." In order to not reinforce the pain symptoms, however, the nurse must assess the pain before and after the client receives analgesics with a concerned but matter-of-fact attitude. Because the client's pain symptoms may be his predominant way of expressing him- or herself and because he or she is unlikely to be aware of the relationship between mind and body, the nurse should also encourage him or her to talk, to express verbally his concerns or difficulties in his or her life. If the pain is significant, talk *after* the medication has taken effect. If easily distracted during the assessment, the nurse may encourage verbalization at that time.
2. Chronic pain often results in hopelessness, helplessness, irritability, and other symptoms of depression.
3. The nurse should acknowledge the client's pain and the use of medications, but help him or her to understand the role of other therapies such as group therapy that may help him or her decrease his or her stress (hence, muscle tension and pain): "When you are hurting, it's hard to think about going to group or thinking that talking will help. Talking about what is going on in your life can help reduce stress, because pain is worsened when stress causes an increase in muscle tension."
4. Somatoform disorders, of which pain disorder is a part, often originate when clients are unable to verbally express problems, conflicts, or dependency needs. Pain disorder is not caused by consciously wanting to avoid work, nor is it "pretending" to have pain. Rather, the pain symptoms "speak" for the client.
5. The nurse could teach the client about the stress-tension-pain cycle, thus setting up the groundwork for relaxation training techniques. Autogenic training, progressive muscle relaxation, and visualization are all effective relaxation training techniques. In addition, the teaching plan could include the effective use of medication (noting the effect of alcohol on pain medications), distraction, and physical activity.

Chapter 7

1. Given the diagnoses of both depression and dissociative identity disorder, several safety issues should be anticipated. First, physical safety may be an issue if the client is suicidal; hence, initial and continued assessment for suicidal ideation is indicated. Physical safety may also be jeopardized by self-mutilation. Although rarely lethal, self-mutilation can be serious with deep burns or cuts that require extensive treatment if severe. Different alters (personalities) may also be more self-destructive than others, and talking about difficult memories in therapy may produce sufficient affective instability and pain that the client feels self-destructive. The emotional safety of the client is also an issue. Having experienced a childhood of abuse, the client does not readily trust or feel safe.

2. Dissociative disorders are rare and fascinating, but they are painful in origin and painful to endure. Talking with the nursing assistants about dissociative identity disorder and its origins, including the dehumanization of the child, may help them see the client not as a curiosity, but as a human being struggling to cope. In addition, introducing the nursing assistants (individually) to the client will reduce the exotic nature of the disorder and create an opportunity for a therapeutic relationship with all staff members.

3. "Mapping" (sketching) the personality system, noting age, gender, and other characteristics, including which alters share consciousness and memories, can decrease confusion. The client's alter personalities may be helpful in creating the map, depending upon the level of acceptance of the diagnosis and the cooperation of various personalities. The host personality is initially unaware of the alters. Additionally, when unsure with whom you are speaking, the nurse can ask, "With whom am I speaking?" or "Who is here now?" when the client is nonverbal.

4. All family members are affected by the behavior and mood of the client with dissociative identity disorder. Family therapy can be helpful in a number of ways. First, teaching the family about the disorder names and identifies the phenomenon so that imagination and fears do not fill the information gap. Second, children are keen observers and are quite aware of the client's affective and behavioral "switches," and they need to learn to deal with, and not manipulate child alters, in particular. Third, family members can learn how to help the client avoid dissociating and how to handle hostile personalities. Finally, the family therapist can work with the family's own interactional patterns so that the family is a healthy place for all members as healing takes place.

5. It is not uncommon for even professional staff to doubt the validity of the disorder itself, or to make the error in logic that an effect (getting "attention" during hospitalization and therapy) is the intention. The possession of material resources or even good family support will not prevent the pain of dissociative identity disorder, nor will it prevent *any* mental disorder. Both family and material resources can make the healing process less difficult, but not easy. The nurse may be uneducated, manifesting countertransference, or have issues regarding power in relationships (seeing and concerned with client manipulation).

Chapter 8

1. Priority nursing diagnoses include the following:
   - Risk for Violence, Self-Directed (Self-Mutilation) related to intense emotional pain including rage and a sense of emptiness coupled with poor impulse control
   - Impaired Social Interaction related to overidealization and devaluation of the self and others
   - Disturbed Personal Identity related to feelings of emptiness

2. The priority goal is maintenance of client safety—client will not harm herself. Secondary goals include to begin to recognize the tendency to dichotomous thinking—idealizing and devaluing others in response to a fear of abandonment, and to begin to recognize the effect of a feeling of emptiness on functioning and mood.

3. Nursing interventions include the following:
   - To maintain client safety, the implementation of an anti-harm contract, staff and client self-monitoring, and identifying behavioral triggers and alternative coping strategies are all important.
   - As a step in diminishing the tendency toward dichotomous thinking, the nurse can assist the client to recognize thoughts and behaviors that indicate it is occurring.
   - As a step in enhancing the client's sense of self, facilitating methods for her to identify her own strengths is important.

4. It is especially important to promote client collaboration in the maintenance of her own safety. Her collaboration in the development of the other goals will depend in part on her level of insight into the effect of her behavior on her functional impairment and subjective distress.

5. The nursing interventions should be evaluated in relationship to the goals—the most important goal being maintenance of client safety.

Chapter 9

1. Clients with a diagnosis of schizophrenia, paranoid type, typically present with auditory hallucinations and delusional thought processes. Delusions are usually of

a persecutory type. This client may appear hostile and angry. Disorganized speech patterns, disorganized behaviors, and flat or inappropriate affect are not present to any significant degree.

2. This client's priority of care is safety of self and others. During an acute phase, safety is a critical issue. As a result of this client's paranoid delusional system, potential for violence is high. Environmental safety factors should include a milieu free of potential harmful objects/sharps and special client observation protocols/vigilance.

3. Several nursing diagnoses may be appropriate for this client's plan of care. The nursing diagnoses that are *most likely* to be included consist of the following:
   • Risk for Violence Directed at Self or Others
   • Disturbed Thought Processes
   • Social Isolation
   • Disturbed Sensory Perception
   • Defensive Coping

4. Paranoid schizophrenic clients have difficulty establishing trust as a result of their suspicious delusions. Several interventions may be helpful to begin fostering trust with this client. The nurse must be consistent and honest with the client. Communication must be clear and concise. Promises should never be made to the client. The nurse should avoid challenging the content of the client's delusions. Objectivity must be maintained, and the nurse should listen actively to the client's verbalizations. Maintaining the client's personal space and using touch carefully is important. The nurse may offer the client food and beverages in closed, sealed containers. The client's care should be provided by staff members consistently assigned to him or her.

5. This client has had multiple hospital admissions because of a history of poor medication adherence with antipsychotic medications. To prevent this problem from repeatedly occurring in the future, the nurse may explore several interventions. First of all, the reason for the poor medication adherence must be determined. It may be that the client is having adverse reactions or side effects from psychotropic medications. If this is the reason, an option may be to change to another antipsychotic medication with a different mechanism of action. Anticholinergic medications may be helpful. Other reasons for poor medication adherence may be a lack of support systems at home. Support systems are very important for prevention of exacerbation in chronic illnesses such as schizophrenia. Community resources must be explored before this client is discharged from the hospital. Administration of antipsychotic medications in the form of depot injections should be explored for overcoming non adherence issues.

Chapter 10

1. The initial assessments to make include the following:
   • Baseline vital signs, which are necessary to ascertain signs of infection, cardiac arrythmia, or vascular problems
   • Mini-Mental State Examination, which is important to determine an objective measure of cognitive impairment for future comparison
   • Head-to-toe physical assessment, concentrating on abnormal findings to determine a possible physiological cause for the confusion
   • Further pertinent information; if any family members are present, ask them to provide further information regarding preferred routines, food likes and dislikes, and family information that would be helpful when communicating with the client

2. The three nursing diagnoses that are appropriate in the care of the client consist of the following:
   • Risk for Injury or Trauma related to episodes of confusion
   • Disturbed Sleep Pattern related to sundown syndrome
   • Anxiety related to fear of cognitive deficits and unfamiliar surroundings

3. The outcome/evaluation criteria that might be appropriate for the client include the following:
   • The client will be free of injury as evidenced by absence of falls, burns, or bruises.
   • The client will sleep five to seven hours per night and remain calm and quiet in the evening.
   • The client will verbalize decreased anxiety and intact orientation to person, place, and time, especially in late afternoon and early evening hours.
   • The client will return to predelirium functioning.

4. Four nursing interventions aimed at promoting safety and security for the client and her family could include the following:
   • Eliminate distracting background noise or shadows. Leave light on in bathroom.
   • Place bed in low position; lower one side rail to prevent client from crawling over the foot of the bed to get up.
   • Provide a simple, structured environment with consistent personnel to minimize confusion and provide a sense of security and stability in the client's environment.
   • Allow client to have familiar objects around her to maintain reality orientation and enhance self-worth and dignity.

5. Your response to the client's daughter might include the following:
   • Encouraging the daughter to reflect the underlying feeling of concern (e.g., "You miss Daddy. It must be lonely here without him.")

- Encouraging the daughter to discuss topics that are meaningful to her mother, such as past events occurring in the family; bring and discuss photos of her children and grandchildren
- Explaining that reality orientation and validation therapy that is geared toward the person and place rather than to the time is more effective in decreasing confusion

Chapter 11

1. Important additional information includes the following:
   - Blackout or lost consciousness: blacking out or passing out can be related to one's use of alcohol or other substances.
   - Changes in bowel movement: persons using alcohol and/or drugs frequently can experience changes in bowel movement. Changes range from diarrhea related to drinking to constipation related to using pain medications frequently. Withdrawal from narcotics can cause diarrhea.
   - Weight loss or weight gain: persons using alcohol or drugs regularly may experience weight loss/gain and/or poor nutritional balance.
   - Experiencing stressful situations: stress can precipitate an increase in drinking; stress can also result from drinking or using drugs regularly.
   - Sleep problems: persons using alcohol and/or other drugs experience all sorts of sleep problems. One may start using alcohol to promote sleep, but once someone develops tolerance, sleep is more difficult.
   - Chronic pain: persons experiencing chronic pain may use drugs and/or alcohol to self-medicate.
   - Concern over substance use: if friends and relatives worry about substance use, it is generally because there is something to be concerned about.
   - Cutting down on alcohol consumption (or drug use, prescription medications, gambling, or addictive behavior): if a person feels that he or she must cut down, it is usually because there are problems.
   - Infections—systemic, viral, sepsis, or localized infection: IV drug abuse and alcohol abuse can cause these medical problems: hepatitis, HIV, TB, endocarditis, kidney abscesses, unexplained urosepsis, syphilis, and infection/abscess at local injection sites.
   - Anorexia, nausea, vomiting, hematemesis: cirrhosis can be caused by alcohol abuse or narcotic abuse.
   - Cardiac rhythm disturbances: persons who regularly abuse cocaine suffer from electrocardiographic abnormalities.
   - Dyspnea, wheezing, tachypnea, wheezing cyanosis: cocaine abusers suffer from abnormal pulmonary function tests.

- Flank pain radiating to groin, hematuria, urinary frequency: alcohol abuse can cause pathologic renal conditions.

2. The nursing assessment should focus on the following body systems:
   - Gastrointestinal
   - Liver
   - Cardiac
   - Respiratory
   - Neurologic
   - Endocrine
   - Reproductive
   - Nutritional status

3. The following lab values would be helpful:
   - Gamma glutamyl transferase (GGT)
   - Aspartate aminotranferase (AST)
   - Alkaline phosphatase (AK)
   - Lactate dehydrogenase (LDH)
   - Mean corpuscular volume (MCV)
   - Urine toxicology and blood screen for drugs of abuse is also an essential component of the substance use evaluation.

4. Obtain the following information:
   - Type of substance used
   - Type of compulsive behavior
   - Pattern/frequency
   - Amount
   - Age at onset
   - Age of regular use
   - Changes in use patterns
   - Periods of abstinence in history
   - Previous withdrawal symptoms
   - Date of last substance use/compulsive behavior
   - Ask about each substance or behavior separately.

5. Focus is on client safety by including the following:
   - Maintain safe environment.
   - Orient client to time, place, and person.
   - Maintain adequate nutrition and fluid balance.
   - Monitor for beginning of withdrawal signs and symptoms.
   - Create a low-stimulation environment.
   - Monitor vital signs and withdrawal symptoms: nausea/vomiting, tremor, paroxysmal sweats, anxiety, agitation, tactile disturbances, auditory disturbances, visual disturbances, headache or fullness in head, disorientation, and sensorium.
   - While female clients may have been initially screened for pregnancy, they should be screened later in the episode of care to be sure that any medication use potentially harmful to the fetus is minimized. Alcohol is the most harmful drug of all to the fetus.
   - Monitor for delirium tremens, psychotic symptoms, and suicide/seizure risk.

- Administer the withdrawal medication: anticonvulsants; benzodiazepines, sedative vitamins, or other medications as ordered thiamine help to prevent confusion and other mental status changes.
- Maintain adequate nutrition and fluid intake.
- Maintain normal comfort measures.
- Monitor for covert substance use during detox period.
- Provide emotional support and reassurance to client and family.
- Provide reality orientations and address hallucinations in a therapeutic manner.
- Advise client of the depressive uneasy feelings and the fatigue that is usually experienced during withdrawal.
- Begin to educate the client about the disease of addiction and the initial treatment goal of abstinence.

Chapter 12

1. Important information to gather includes the following:
   - Do the details about the cause of injuries match the actual injuries?
   - When did the injury take place; was there a delay in seeking treatment?
   - Relationship to the child; family structure; patterns and methods of discipline; unreasonable expectations of the child; problems with pregnancy, labor, or delivery with this child; substance abuse in the family; history of family violence; mother being battered.
   - Availability and use of support systems; social isolation.
2. Current injuries: unusual pattern such as bite marks, burns in shape of objects, or glovelike burns from immersion in hot liquids; bruises in various stages of healing, especially on head and neck; bald spots that would indicate hair pulled out; old fractures, scars, welts, lacerations, or internal injuries.
3. Behavioral extremes such as rage, aggression, or passivity; fear of parents or caregiver; apprehension when other children cry; verbal reports of abuse; hyperactivity; distractibility or hypervigilance; disorganized thinking; self-injurious or suicidal behavior; running away from home or illegal behaviors; school performance; poor relationships with peers; inappropriately dressed for weather; regressed behaviors such as enuresis, encopresis, and thumb-sucking.
4. The child's safety and well-being would be the priority. Report the suspected abuse following facility policies and procedures; reassure the child that he or she is not to blame; treat the child's immediate injuries.
5. Mother needs to be approached nonjudgmentally and taught normal child growth and development to reduce unrealistic expectations of the child that are often present with child abuse. If the mother is not the abuser, she should be taught how to keep the child safe. Teach parenting skills, anger management, stress management, communication skills, and what resources are available to the family.

Chapter 13

1. Adults often believe—or want to believe—that children do not understand death and should be protected from all death-related situations or discussions. The facts are quite different. Children are naturally curious about loss, dying, and death. Furthermore, no child is too young to experience the anxiety associated with separation experiences. Children between the ages of five and nine years understand that death is final; however, they believe their own deaths can be avoided. Many of these children will fear the dying and death process because they may associate death with aggression or violence. They may view death as a person who comes and takes them away from their family. In addition, these children may experience guilt or shame because they believe past wishes or unrelated actions are responsible for their death.
2. Assessment of children and family members in the grieving or mourning process includes an accurate perception of the loss from their viewpoint. The nurse begins by identifying the loss and the family's perception of the impact of their loss. The nurse should use the opportunity for the child to express his concerns through conversation, play, drawing, and writing. The nurse should seek to understand the nature of the family's attachment to the lost child, assess past experience with loss, and determine the impact those have on the family's present experience. It is important for the nurse to assess cultural rituals and rules about mourning to understand the unique experience of grieving individuals.
3. Important nursing diagnoses for the child and family who are experiencing impeding death include Fear, Hopelessness, Powerlessness, Risk for Caregiver Role Strain, Interrupted Family Processes, Impaired Adjustment, Ineffective Coping, and Spiritual Distress. Possible nursing diagnoses for survivors of a family member who has died include Anticipatory Grieving; Dysfunctional Grieving; Social Isolation; Ineffective Role Performance; Risk for Altered Parenting; Compromised Family Coping; and Readiness for Enhanced Family Coping.
4. Living with loss is a normal but very stressful part of life. When coping with loss through grieving or mourning, people may respond in adaptive or maladaptive ways. Some never lose their sense of despair. The loss of a child is one of life's most difficult losses. When evaluating the family's movement toward goals, the nurse should evaluate the family's personal understanding of their feelings about and reaction to loss and grief, the family's ability

to discuss their response and reaction to loss and grief, whether family members have resumed baseline sleeping and eating patterns, and have resumed daily activities and roles as they accept their loss.

5. Once the child has died, the family will experience bereavement. Bereavement is a change in status caused by losing a family member, friend, colleague, or other significant person through death. The family will experience a shifting mix of feelings, including disbelief, anxiety, anger, sadness, and confusion. This condition is known as grief. The family will express their bereavement and loss to others in ways that are culturally patterned. This is known as mourning.

Chapter 14

1. Symptoms of depression include feelings of hopelessness/helplessness, flat affect, poor eye contact, disrupted patterns of eating or sleeping, absence of motivation/compliance, and decreased energy level.

2. Important assessments include spirituality, cultural, biological, psychosocial assessments; also assess developmental level and coping skills.

3. Nursing diagnoses include Ineffective Individual Coping related to occurrence and effect of medical illness; Situational Low Self-Esteem related to function changes associated with medical illness diagnosis.

4. Nursing interventions include empathy, compassion, spirituality reinforcement, support, dignity, control, and pain management.

5. "It sounds like it is difficult to find meaning in your life."

Index

Page numbers followed by b indicate box; those followed by f indicate figure; those followed by t indicate table.